FATE

THE TRINITIES

A NOVEL BY CHRISTOPHER SOCHA

House of Muralann

Canadian Cataloguing in Publication Data

Socha, Christopher
Fate : the trinities : a novel

ISBN 1-894498-16-X

I. Title.

PS8587.O38F38 2002 C813'.6 C2002-900288-5
PR9199.4.S693F38 2002

House of Muralann
192 Spadina Avenue, Suite 308
Toronto, Ontario, Canada M5T 2C2

To all those who find themselves
under the moon and the stars.

Acknowledgements

Thanks to all those who have supported me in all that I do: Mum, Tata who now knows peace, my clan, my Calgary clan, NF, AQ, DH, JK, JSR, DS, FK, RF, JB, SS, EP, JR, KH, MG, ND, MK, KR, LP, TM, AS, XVI (enough said!), Atomic (much missed), the Well, Surface, party people, all those who bring life to the night, all you coat, cover, door, bar people, Star Trek, the Bilderbergers, the blessed Boheme family, Maria Bartiromo, all those who know who they are, and of course 'Lina!

PLUR

Table of Contents

Prologue

Many people say that eyes are the windows into the soul but only a few believe that what one sees out of their eyes is in fact a representation of their inner spirit. Our sight is our doorway to the soul. If one could cut through all the complex layers of reality one would only see their own reflection. It is no wonder then that all people seek to see is a place of belonging, or more specifically, a place to call home.

To reach completion in life, one has to find their way to the home of their soul within reality. Here is the tale of how a trinity of souls found their way home.

1
The Explorer Fate

Her name is Fate. She is many millions of systems away from her home. She has been exploring the universe and existence for years. The journey has brought her to where she now finds herself on the path, on another dead world. Fate has found herself in an environment of miserable decay built by an expansion of the plaque of Cronos layering itself in age surrendered sloth that had been growing since the beginning of time. Where life once thrived there now stood only rusted monuments of extinct despair.

Fate flew to a nearby structure to survey this wretched world she had descended upon. It was like staring into the ocean and seeing beneath its depths that it had held some civilized structure that had become assimilated by the life forms that came to cover a once pristine sea that had lived as in a lifeless decline. There was only one difference: on this world, the sea had not given life a chance to renew itself, and the march of the dead was all that remained. On this world there was only rust, and this made Fate shudder. She realized extinction on this world meant only a decay into nothingness.

The sun began to set on this once great city, and wherever there was a mirrored surface, the city was alight as if it was burning itself out, only to be reborn in its glorious, yet decrepit, form, ready for the next dreary shine of the day ahead.

Fate decided it was time to leave, and as she flew away from this world, she shed a tear of pity for this once great world not realising this tear contained enough altered genetics to seed this world with life once again.

As she flew into the glory of flight in space, something whispered to her. She had heard this voice before. The voice was one she thought she would never hear again. It was as if the sorrows of this world reminded her of her own, and had brought the voice to her. She wondered if this would be a return to paradise. This calling reached into her, and without hesitation, she went off to meet her destiny.

Φ

She could hear the voices calling her from some strange place in the universe. It was a siren's call, and Fate had heard as much as she could take. Fate flew faster and faster through the heavens towards a strange destination where a voice still called to her. It was a voice heard when Fortuna looks to one, and for the Fate it was something more.

Lately, she had become bored of exploring the universe. The only thing that kept her going was the novelty of seeing as many curiosities of existence as possible. Yet the quantity of curiosities, like the flames of Sarasvati, had begun to wane.

Though on this journey to what will be the current path, the joy of traveling the universe had returned to her once again. The stars, galaxies, and other unique traits of space carved a path for her to follow; a waking path of Morpheus to walk upon. Perception leaves one to never know if this is an example of altered reality, or of our own imaginations. Fate looked to find the clarity of what was Delphi. The Fate is certainly tricky in that respect, a blind seer of what is and is not existence.

She flew like lace blowing in the wind. She was elegant, yet still unsure of herself. If this was her final destiny, was she ready for it? Well, she had to be! This would become her final destiny. Then her eyes came upon something she had never seen in all her travels. It was a curious thing indeed. Dark violet luminescent smoke strands grew ahead of her across space; seemingly just another nebula, and seemingly normal enough. The one novelty of this phenomenon was a genuine dirt road that lay out of it. This was the path that the Fate would follow.

2
The Aristocrat

On the path of destiny strolled a very aristocratic, dapper chap, a very tall man with a figure that always seemed to be in the action. He is the Aristocrat. He is wealthy man with a subtle, diplomatic and grandiloquent way. A sense of power earned through both evolution and enlightenment. His only weakness was his inability to decide upon a role for his path to glory. At times, his soul cried out in a vain hope to win over a path towards glory.

It seemed only a moment ago that he was home. So there he stood on his porch, on his plantation, on his tropical island, playing a game of chess against his own strategies, and gambits never before chosen but gambits now taken alone. Then something called to him to leave his game. He somehow knew that this was his chance. The Aristocrat's sense of curiosity led him towards the path going to the beach. There was a flash of light as the Aristocrat was like a George VI stride that disappeared into the sky.

In one moment, the Aristocrat found himself in another place, on a path, on a scene one might see in a dawn over a silent Wessex where sound had yet to flow into its cityscape. Realizing that it might take a while before anything meaningful might happen on this quiet landscape, the Aristocrat lit up a finely tailored cigarette for the lurid stroll.

He realized that he was glad to be here on this path. He believed that boredom is the greatest burden upon any aristocrat. This was going to be an exciting time, and this would be a splendid reason to live.

Then the Aristocrat came upon something that intrigued only his perverse sense of wonder. The path became dark. To the left and the right of the path stood rows of tombstones and ivory memorials.

A lone figure struck his attention. There was a slender, gentle girl there but with the black garb of one returned to an evolved crusade long forgotten. She was a strange sight indeed: a youthful looking girl, a lean monastic sculpture adorned by light mauve eyes, and a dynamically placed swirl of wander swept hair with a visage of tearful serenity. The Aristocrat thought that anyone bold enough to pull off mauve hair deserved his attention. However, he was too distracted by other matters to even ask her name. If not for the matter of the dismal hue of the environment, the Aristocrat would have found something familiar about her. So the Aristocrat put forward a query, "Whose graves are these?" in a tone that was diplomatic, yet directly adversarial. He lightly tapped his timeless gentleman's cane, a cane of obsidian, onyx, and polished ivory tusk, into the finely cut flatness of an ancient cobblestone ground. His tap was a friendly nod that he was a powerful soul.

She spoke softly with a touch of angelic sympathy as if she had walked for far too long a path that darkness had followed, and longed to escape from it. The response certainly put a bizarre anxious quirk in the Zone 14 inspired battle plan of the Aristocrat. The words came simply, yet truthfully.

"They are ours."

3
The Tale of Existence

The monuments of death were most definitely that of their kinsmen. Of that there could be no doubt, for the two were on the path of souls. Before the two were monuments without names but they were in the style known to the pair. The feeling of what it was was enough to know. But these were not monuments to death but rather monuments to lives once lived.

The Fate showed the Aristocrat the truth of this reality. She waved her tender hands, and all became clear. Finding clarity in the middle of this reality showed one that these tombstones were simply part of a place where memories of past lives are kept. The Fate had exposed a pattern to these lives. Truly, these were their own.

Their souls were born out of lives once lived and as if each followed the path where a basic multi-dimensional puzzle was being put together. The path was its own enigma. Reality was a muddled version of itself and the last piece was being put together here.

The Fate and the Aristocrat both knew that this was the final step towards a higher consciousness, towards the evolution of the path of their souls towards liberation. This was the final piece of the puzzle. The Fate and the Aristocrat gave each other a look of acknowledgement that it was time to strike up an alliance; an alliance that would work hand in hand with solving this enigma.

They both walked the path together each about a body width apart from the other. There was a feeling that came upon the Aristocrat. These two beings had been together before in other times, yet both were still slowly becoming unaware of this. A far different sense now came over them. A feeling grew that they were being watched by fierce eyes. Something strong was lurking in the distance.

4
The First Test

The Fate and the Aristocrat walked further down the path. They came upon a sunny field of evenly spaced out lilac bushes; luscious violet fields lathered by an almost white sun that stretched across their vision. This was the view of a silent utopia, and a trap, a place where the pair would be hunted by what was out there. The Aristocrat seemed quite intrigued. All this was hitting the Fate like a psionic boom as she surveyed this field of illuminated vibrancy. The Fate thought it ironic that this was the ideal place to be attacked in the garden of her favourite colour and the colour of her soul. She concentrated, and brought forth weapons to her hands.

Fate was an arsenal, and these rifle-like, high order telekinetic creations were not just simple musings; they were lethal. The Fate tossed one of the rifles, each roughly the size and similar in shape as that of an MP5, to the Aristocrat, and motioned for him to cover the other side of the field. He understood, and quietly, swiftly moved in that direction. He was like Fowler stepping up to the pitch. The Fate made herself alone in the vivid fields in an attempt to draw out of those sweet smelling pastures whatever was out there.

If she had time for pause, the action seemed far too habitual. She flirted with her hair, and checked the charge of her psionically-created rifle. Still, she took this opportunity to embrace the nature of this place. The vibrancy of the colours of this place was almost enough to put her mind at ease but it also heightened her senses enough to hear the first sounds of the impending attack. She enjoyed the silence for a moment.

Then the attack came from above. Something strong descended from the heavens like a tearing across Apollo's cheek. This tear was vicious. The Fate was able to escape the falling bomb by side stepping through folded space to return to this reality on a nearby vantage point.

When the dust settled to the ground after the thunderous impact, in the debris field, one could see that at its centre was something powerful. Though the Fate did not know why, she knew she stood before the great Hunter. There stood a powerfully built man about ten feet in height adorned in black and ruby hued garb. She asked him whether he came as a friend or as a foe. The Hunter did not reply. Fate looked to the broken and burnt flowers beneath her feet before her impatience got the better of her. That is when the second wave came.

The attack came from both the Fate and the Hunter. Both expected the other to attack, and in fact they did so at the same time. Faster than thought they charged at one another, and both crackled open the air around them to surge with energy. Their eyes surged, and pulsed with an intensity that was only further enraged by both of these powerful beings missing their opening offensives. Their techniques may have been different but they were both devout to their disciplines.

Blow after blow was exchanged in all manners of forms, booms, and thunder. The conflict began to take the course of the combatants trying to overpower one another in tests of strength. Most fights usually end up in grappling, and this one was no exception. The Hunter was far superior physically but the Fate was privy to certain thought techniques.

Her thoughts flowed into advanced psionic ribbon flows and sliced through the mind of the Hunter. A powerful thought forced the ether around the combatants to split them apart. There was only one flaw to this technique: some part of it would return to each of them. So both of them stood there feeling the effects of having their minds wounded but still ready to attack one another in spite of their bloodied noses from where the dogs of war had nipped them.

There stood a man, of blond and silver streaked hair, a giant of war with the eyes of a great lion, and a young looking girl with mauve hair, and with ethereal violet eyes that seemed powerful enough to tear open reality. Then suddenly both the Fate and the Hunter started to laugh deeply and uncontrollably because both knew that each was a warrior of honour just by their styles of engagement. Each had a role in waging war on the forces of darkness that infested their paths, and that was enough to make them friends along with being allies in this walk down the path. These soul paths linked in some way from a time long ago.

At the furthest corner of the laughter, handshakes, and arm holding was a long buried sadness that it ever had to come this at all. There was an even deeper sadness that both the Fate and the Hunter could not quite remember, yet it lurked somewhere beyond them.

In this world, such sacrifices had to be made in the search for purity. It was a shame, but it was also an affirmation of the souls possessed by these individuals and how far each was willing to go. The Aristocrat glided through folded space to where Fate and the Hunter were situated. The Aristocrat had taken the diplomatic sense to observe this one out. Since things had gone the way of allegiances, the Aristocrat felt it was time to make an entrance and surprised those on the path as if he were Radzinski. He gracefully bowed before the pair, and gently took a hand from both the Fate and the Hunter. Now that the ruckus was over, the Aristocrat felt it time to lead the trio back onto the path.

5
The Dark Dream

The Trinity of souls walked further down the path to a place of darkening skies, when something happened to the Fate. It happened to the others as well but it took her away before she could have time for concern for her comrades. She felt as if she were flashed into a *transual* place, or a place that was filled with both trance and sensuality. But this path had an eeriness about it. The pace of this hinterland was very slow, and most dreadful. This was a place of darkness.

It was a surreal dreamscape of coal black skies, and the place was filled with death. Fate was blinded by the darkness. She could not see but she could feel. Things moved beneath Fate. Things snapped, slipped, and hissed beneath her. These things scurried around and about her. The Fate sighed into the air with a subtle fury. Her actions were instinctual but her motions were silenced, slowly and panicked. This place was a step away from limbo.

Slowly and surely she moved above the menace. Fate knew that the scourges below needed to be purged from this place, or she would not survive. She acted. She created a high intensity photonic pulse within her womb. The light of one like Hebe's purity burst out of her in all directions. It overwhelmed this place of the dark. She expelled every ounce of power within her. Fate then fell quietly to the ground.

As Fate lay on the ground in a fetal position but with her head held up, she found clarity in the darkness. She had a dazed, drained feeling. But it was not over. She found another strength within herself. She quickly picked herself up, and started to run. A few small fires were dotted across this landscape and now she could see the evil that was exposed from its shadows. It was a wasteland of black, scaly sinister *naga* and *habu*.

Decaying rats littered every other space of soil. What lay before Fate was a desolate Earth, a dark waste-land. The hellish creatures though significantly reduced in number still retained the complete violent intensity of their dead ilk. The Fate ran though a darkening field, avoiding the snapping and lunging vermin that surrounded her, and kept moving.

She avoided the creatures of cold blood as if they were armies of the greatest brutality. She even managed to crush a few of the vile things with her tender feet that swiftly moved through the prison of darkness running for freedom. But as sick as this environment was, something was just as wrong within her. By having made such an attacking move to kill such evil, the Fate left herself open to being without defenses at the wrong time. The Fate started to decay internally from the disease of this place.

Fate continued to run as hard as she could though she was far too groggy to know why anymore. She choked back her tears. She had run to the point where her lungs were almost bursting out of her chest, and if not for the pain, she would have forgotten her humanity. She had never needed her lungs before but they were failing her now. She thought she was without direction but the Fate soon realized why she ran aimless as if hoping for a precipice: it was to make a final stand.

As her skin dried itself into coarse leather, her hair and her teeth fell out. A morning plaque had built the desire for thirst that seemed never likely to be assuaged. She had lost her immunity against this place but Fate was still hopeful that she would make it out alive. Fate needed a miracle. She felt within herself a strength she still clung to in spite of her collapsed immunity. She still possessed the strength to bring into this reality her sword, and her auto-rifle.

The tsunami of evil gathered to be empowered in its fullest extent once again. The vermin and the snakes oozed quickly towards her knowing of the weakness of her current state. The Fate started to shoot wildly in all directions. Blue light flashes filled the air along with the stench of her attackers' charred filth. Fate even had enough force of will to slice a few of these critters down with her sword, opening their vile flood gates and she was made to be covered in the rancid, odious blood, and the sour venom from the darkly fierce creatures she had slain.

The Fate began to falter in this conflict and she fell once again to the ground only this time to become covered in the cloak of Death, and the Death of all. She became separated from her weapons. She was utterly alone.

The serpents bit into her and their venom began to fill her veins. She was poisoned. The vermin gnawed on her and scampered all across the Fate's now wilted body. The evil enveloped her and she began to drown within it. The Fate was washed away to the edge of a deep dark abyss like crude oil sliding down the side of a barrel. The Fate began to loudly scream into the muted darkness. The end was near.

"NO! NEVER! I WILL NOT SUBMIT! I WILL ONLY DIE IN THE ARMS OF PEACE AND FREEDOM!"

Her thoughts became her only means of liberation. The Fate still had a spark within her and it was a similar transcendent thought: burn everything. The only darkness that should be left in this place is the darkness of its ashes after burning in the fires of purity.

All at once this reality began to explode with fire. The mind-fires were more ferocious than anything in this realm. As she fell deeper into the abyss the fires came to burn so brightly and so fiercely that the Fate herself was reduced to ashes along with all the evil that existed in this place. The fire burned so aggressively that it consumed this place into nothingness. This place was left a void. It was left a memory.

A swirling whirlwind of red and white flame fell onto the path from the heavens until all that one could see, after the smoke blew away, was a very crisp crater left as the aftermath in the middle of the path. Like a Phoenix, the Fate pulled herself out of the hole that was left in the ground. She was alive but scarred. Fate still carried the dread and the fear within herself. When the Aristocrat and the Hunter found her, she was still screaming.

6

The Other Divergence, The Other Nightmares

Apparently, the Hunter and the Aristocrat fell to darknesses that the Fate had experienced but ones sorrowfully suited to their perspectives. For the Hunter, the nightmare was especially severe.

The Hunter faced a battle with demonic thieves of purity. He faced a scaly labyrinth full of scrawny weasel-like demons that dug their claws into his back. They attacked him from all angles, and he could not defend himself fully from the onslaught. The demons tore at him with lightning speed in piranha like attacks, giving him barely enough time to turn his head to see his tormentors.

He fell into this realm so easily, and secretly he loved this as if they were one. This was the Hunter though, he scoffed at anything that considered him to be prey. The Hunter then set about an efficient ruse to kill these gangly creatures while continuing to work towards the exit of this tomb like maze. This prison would not become his tomb. Pretending not to see the pursuing quarry, the Hunter then twisted around one hundred and eighty degrees, and one by one snapped the necks of these horrific beings that had a penchant for attacking from behind.

The labyrinth became clogged with the dirty corpses of hell spawns, and the ground had become flooded with the mucous, viscous sludge that these demons considered their blood. Though the Hunter's back was shredded, his ears bitten away at, his body slashed and stained with his warrior's blood from the initial demonic attack, he continued to make progress while all the time relishing in exterminating the things that infested this place of constant war.

It was a feeling of victory for the Hunter, yet it also cost him a sweet white rose from the garden of his soul. For one should know that for every world this man has conquered, and for everything evil that this man has hunted to extinction, a supreme capture of a lost Robinson in the harmattan, has been taken away from him. A price paid for his path. For to fight dragons, one must become them.

But the Hunter is, and will always be, a man of many fragrant virtues from the music of serenity that played in his thoughts to his words of passionate clarity his mind created. He seemed sculpted in the sound of Van Dyk. It was a shame that every time he thrust his sword into darkness, a part of him would die as the price for becoming a more superior beast. At his core, the Hunter was beyond destruction but this nightmare world seemed to leave him mortally naked. But the sand blown winds of time could never hope to reduce him. No one would miss a sonnet if it meant victory. But the Hunter always did, and that is why he always would remain true.

He made his way to the final passage. His zealous exuberance caused him to not just snap the necks of the demons of the infestation that constantly attacked him but to rip their carcasses clean in half as well. He did so with his strong, mammoth bare hands snapping demons with back breakers that one like Adams would flinch at the sight of. Taking life from the legion of sinfulness was such a rush for the Hunter that he actually started to laugh uncontrollably in a hysterically naughty manner whenever he heard the sound of shattered neck bones. In this labyrinth, the Hunter was able to laugh with great regularity as he was so efficient with his craft.

The Hunter gave up the formality of technique simply to let the demons attack him in larger groups than they already had. He found it quite glorious to see how many he could kill at once. One can suppose that is why the Hunter was struck by such a thunderous bolt of stern irony. The Hunter was so drunk with zeal in pursuing extermination that he somehow had travelled through the entire maze without ever actually going towards the direction of freedom. He had gone through the entire structure to end up at the centre of the demonic enigma. All the while he had killed all that had darkly opposed him along the way. The ground, the dirty earth, had grown inches thick with skeletal sludge, and from the air, a rain fell of soiled blood.

The scene around the Hunter had transformed before him. For he was now standing in the garden of his soul. It was no longer a place of utopian delights but a place of dried out and wilted possibilities. Where once aromas of majestic dreams filled the air, it now only stank of rot and decay. For there were no longer the vibrant colours of life to illuminate his being, and there were only the black thorny coils of poetic fossils left to remain.

The Hunter did not scream as the Fate had when released from this debacle but he did feel like someone had blown a cold wind on his soul, and felt it was time to re-evaluate his methods. He stood on the path upon his return and thought of the pyrrhic nature of his absolute victory.

Φ

For the Aristocrat, this experience beneath the dark waters of limbo was a frightful time of leaving control behind as if he were a keeper faced with a Inzaghi strike. Reality became a putrid soup for the Aristocrat. His heart oozed out of his chest and beat alongside his body, floating along in a starkly tantalising way. The Aristocrat's eyes wiggled out of their sockets and spiralled wildly in a vain search for something to focus sight upon. His body was left to become a puddle of flesh. The Aristocrat's mind was being invaded by beings without souls that could only be considered slaves.

Beings without souls, or slaves, are beings submissive to existence and exert no control over it other than by the proportions of their herded infestations. Slaves are dealt their roles in the area of life, and never move beyond their programmed state. They are beings that do not learn to transcend their surroundings. Hence, these beings are never granted absolution. Their existence until they become ready for liberation is one of purgatory. Slaves forever lost. A slave alone can be easily be ordered about and ordered to die but these were a mass, a tumour of the purest vile.

This invasion was an exception. This was a mindless revolt of slaves. Slaves could never bring order to any civilisation but they can bring about a downfall of any civilisation when left to ignorantly try to emancipate themselves. The demonic stubby and sand dwelling beings of constrained decay with the teeth of rodents were left to wander aimlessly through the mind of the Aristocrat. These creatures marched about the mind of the Aristocrat, and where these slaves went, plague beyond bubonic and the misery of final despair followed.

The Aristocrat had to act with promptness, or else this revolt of slaves would collapse his mind. He felt a sudden enlightenment of thought. There was only one solution to this predicament. The Aristocrat swiftly went about duplicating his essence within his mind. Within his mind where reckless slaves now stood, an Aristocrat, or rather a sliver of his being now stood above each debauchery of the parasitic infection. His mind became a hallway of doors.

With one hand to hold a door open and another to adjust grappling leverage, the Aristocrat began to grab them by the scruffs of their necks. The Aristocrat became a being of infinity, briskly pulling upon the necks of the members of the slave revolt and majestically gave each one of the insects a hard booting and a proper thrashing. The strongest foot became the strongest kick, and like Redknapp, he knew what to do. Each of the slaves flew through the voids beyond the doors, and back into the chains of reality. Only Aristocrats and the Aristocracy remained but the halls of the Aristocrat's mind in their restored serenity were left to silence. There was nothing to share his peace with.

He became unsure of his direction. All that he was, came to be was his once again but with its meaning still lost. There was far more that lay beyond in other doors but these doors were locked. The Aristocrat could not open them even with all his might. To have his meaning locked away made the Aristocrat wonder if that was the purgatory he faced. He felt that this realisation gave him far more distress than the experience of having his mind, his soul invaded by the minions of inferiority.

Φ

In a mere moment, the Aristocrat was transfigured away from the inverted bliss of the realm of nightmares and the sullen internal battle. He returned to the path so that the Trinity, those who were now the Trinity of the great path, walked again as if re-forged and without trauma. There was an unusual air amongst the Trinity as they walked the path. The answers he sought, like those sought by those who joined him, came in trinities. These incidents seemed to prepare the Three for what they expected to be the second wave ahead of them.

The wave did not come but something else caught their attention. An object came to appear upon the path. Where the path once stretched out beyond forever for the eye to see, it now became difficult to see beyond the object as the realm now became shrouded in thick rolling mists. This obscurity was of no concern for those on the Triad's path as the object was what captivated the Trinity's attention. It seemed to hold great significance over them.

The Hunter stretched out his hand to use touch to remember what the device was. Before almost becoming frustrated, the Hunter remembered. Fate remained silent but the knowledge was also within her. The Aristocrat who was also a connoisseur of technology, was fascinated to see that it was a transport pad, and his expertise that was never lost to him, noted to his comrades that there were pre-set co-ordinates to transport three life-forms to the lower surface of the moon of Earth. Both the Aristocrat and the Hunter looked at each other, and wondered aloud to the Fate as to what might be there. It was still a muddled a prospect for the Hunter and the Aristocrat.

It seemed to represent a choice without logic but it held all that is logic to the Fate. It distressed her. She moved away from her comrades, and turned to speak to them. Her comrades wanted answers to their gathering and again the Hunter and the Aristocrat asked Fate as to what was there. So sorrowful were her words that the Fate could barely bring them out. But her simple, painful explanation halted the others in their tracks. Her answer was simply,

"My Home."

7
At'Lann

The Trinity found themselves in an ice filled passage on the moon of 'Earth' after being whisked from the path by the transport. And now they had come to a familiar location. Though far away from the Human settlements, the air was breathable, and the gravity hardly felt artificial. The walls of immense ice glowed with a brilliant gleam. The place had frozen many things and the arctic like cold air was enough to preserve the exhalations of the trinity to remain as if for eternity in the air around them.

The Fate walked ahead of the Aristocrat and the Hunter towards a sheer wall of ice. She pointed with a lamented heaviness at the wall spread out before her. The Fate then gave the Aristocrat an expression of understanding and then the Aristocrat gracefully knelt on the ground with his hands spread out before him. He had an expression of serene, quiet concentration on his face that Shiva might admire.

The molecules in this cavern of ice had begun to shift at a quantum level. The wall of ice began to melt. A thick skin of water formed over the ice and then rolled towards the ground. The ice beneath it gradually began to shrink. It was too much for the frozen air of the cavern as it became drowned in steam. When the steam reduced itself to flowing below their knees it became a simpler mist and ice as thick as light bulb glass that fell quietly in a crinkling to the ground. Where a wall of ice once stood, now a very tall door was now before the trinity. A door made of a substance that combined the look of urethane with the rigidity of steel. This very large, very massive onyx door had to the left of it a bright, pastel coloured control panel protruding from a barely visible onyx wall that was still partially obscured by tons of ice.

Fate moved in a sad, yet proud way towards the control panel and keyed in a very long series of decryption sequences. As she pressed the final key, clicking sounds began to echo across the entire ice chasm. Then the sound, of what could only be described as a turbine kick starting itself, rattled across the stillness. The sound thundered heavily throughout the air.

The massive door whooshed itself up into its hiding place high inside the thick onyx wall, and the trinity could finally see what lay before them. The Fate felt bittersweet by unlocking this door but this would complete the circle. For she knew this would unlock so many other forgotten doors. What the Trinity gazed upon was a tunnel of squarely chiselled moon rock illuminated gibbously by smooth blue light strings running along the base of the walls.

A large, gracious white light poured from the end of the passage within the moon. As the Fate, the Aristocrat, and the Hunter passed through the door, a wind of change blew through each of them. Only the Fate knew of what it truly meant. The circle was indeed drawing to a close. She could feel the breeze left by the wind. It was at last coming together.

At the end of the passage, the light that shined upon the Trinity became even more powerful. The light burst out towards them, and the Trinity began to walk towards it with the Fate ahead of the others. What the Trinity saw before them at the end of the passage could only be described as the wonderful joyous sadness of seeing what once was thought of as forever lost.

It was like finding what once was Piast, lain to rest, and waiting to awaken. This feeling struck the Fate as well but her complete knowledge of this place of home was far more comprehensive than either the Aristocrat or the Hunter. For this was her home, and the Aristocrat now seemed to remember more of Fate's once lush place of origin. Though something was still amiss.

As the three walked, they felt what lay at the end of the passage was temporally frozen. Time in this place had a dust covered feel to it. Time literally had been stuck in one spot within this place for so many forgotten ages it was difficult to say for how many ages could have passed over it.

One could feel that this place, Fate's home, had been this way for so long that even Fate herself had almost forgotten the way it was left. Fate did have the ability to return the balance of time to this place. She did not even have to use her own powers to do so as it was a good thing that there was another bright pastel coloured control panel that caught their attention. It was at the last opening to this place that gigantic could not describe that the three gazed upon a world within a world. This underground place bordered on continental grandeur.

The Fate again keyed a sequence into this second terminal, and things began to change. Time once again began to move in the Trinity's here and now as Cronos's way became liberated. The Trinity was then greeted by the sound of water finding freedom to flow once again. The waters began to flow everywhere. Sorrowfully, the sweet sounds of flowing waters were followed by nothingness. If not for the soothing waters this place would be ruled by silence but the waters did surround something greatly magnificent.

Stretching out for as far as the trinity of souls could see was water and light as great as the sun all within the sole satellite of the blue planet. In the centre of this vivid place of forever was a strikingly intricate island off the shore of an even more spectacular long stretch of land surrounded by immense waters. The water jostled luxuriously around these gems that rose above the light blue sea at its central point deep in the underground.

On these islands was something that could only be thought as remembered, yet almost forgotten. On these islands rose gigantic, pristine cities composed of onyx pyramids, garnet ziggurats, emerald domes, various oceanic pastel coloured spires, and towering monuments that brought out feelings of arousing contentment by any who would chance to truly view such wonders.

On the smaller island, at its centre rose three grand pyramids, each in a row with two of equal height with the central pyramid ascending to be by far the largest and the tallest. This unique pyramid was so disproportionate in its close proximity to the other two pyramids that it left these pyramids to probably feel rather dwarfed. But the larger pyramid did overshadow the other two, it was merely far too immense.

This pyramid was far more eye catching than any other on the smaller island. On its angled walls grew countless rows of lilac trees fully in bloom grown with the real beauty of what once was the home firth of their path. The scent from their fragrant flowers surprisingly filled this entire place throughout all its enormity now that time in the lunar underground had begun to flow back into continuance.

Here was the place Fate knew of as home and so much more. Here was At'Lann. And part of At'Lann, residing on the smaller island was what once was and still was the city-state of 'Mura. Whenever the Fate was not out exploring existence, she lived in 'Mura, and her residence was in fact this very lilac pyramid. She pointed to it with a humble smile, and as acknowledgement to the others that this was their destination.

The Hunter and the Aristocrat surveyed this wondrous place with deep curiosity. They had been here before, yet this was not their home, and yet part of it was. To be certain, it was Fate's but their homes were somewhere else, ones they could feel were close by. Though a home shared is still a home. Something else besides that particular revelation struck both the Aristocrat and Hunter as odd. For here stood great cities but cities without any life in them at all.

There was only the sound of silence, and a silence that could never be enjoyed. Not even birds flew in the sky and nothing was swept across the pristine waters, the still fields, and empty streets. No fish swam in the waters, and no songbirds flew in the air. Most terribly, no people bustled through the grand boulevards. It was as if, at the height of this civilisation, all life from it was stripped away. What was left behind was a perfect place, a utopia, robbed of its perfection.

The Trinity floated solemnly over the passionately depressed waters flying like silk in a summer's breeze to the lilac pyramid that Fate called her home. They returned to the ground on a high balcony situated on the far side of the pyramid. The structure was so large that on its balcony one could put an entire phalanx of soldiers. The fact was not lost on this Trinity, and this fact was especially felt by the Fate. For this place, for all its peace, seemed another fallen ruin from a long ago path of war.

They walked through the opening of what seemed like an aerie of the lilac pyramid and into a very expansive imperial state-room. At its left side were a cornered row of black cherry coloured couches made of a union of leather and silk rounded in an Atomic sort of way. Besides the furnishings, it was for the most part a mauve draped room, with lower than expected lighting, a cathedral high ceiling. Its most striking feature was its platinum and black double helixes adorning the mauve background walls that made for a minor colossal square of simplicity atop the pyramid.

Each of the three took a seat on the pneumatically molecular conforming couches, and had a moment to relax before the Fate came out with revelations and realizations. This place was indeed a tomb. It represented the last remnant of a once grand imperium that had somehow been made to suffer with the finality of extinction. In spite of the warm environment, it was full of frigid lamentations. The air had no one to warm but the three who came in from the punishing cold outside. It was merely a comfortable memorial. Each part of the path of the three as one felt this. It could not be escaped; it permeated them. Only the plants seemed oblivious.

This place felt like neatly abandoned palace for what was once a great throne. A place where royalty once paraded, and now its barren halls strode the highest knight left alone by all the dead. Fate was all that remained. Her home was a tomb but it did not always used to be. For they could feel its remnants in the sweet, tranquil air. One could feel a great purpose emerging in this gathering of souls. A gathering to take a stand to complete the path that always had been there, and the path that always would remain.

Fate then stood and faced the Hunter and the Aristocrat. Her stance was of one that would tell the greatest of revelations. She more than had their attention. With an inspiring voice to both the Hunter and the Aristocrat, the Fate asked them if they remembered this place and of the life that once flowed through it. She could see the answer on the tips of their tongues as their long ago memories were stirred. Fate decided to refresh their memories somewhat. She told them of the demise of the At'Lann Imperium, and began to speak of all they had lost.

Though the Hunter did not recall ever being here before this day, he did remember knowing of this place, of the people who once lived here, and he remembered the Imperium. Though this was not the true home of the Aristocrat, he did remember once calling this place to be like one before *upanayana* path, and one far beyond it. He remembered existing here in the days before. And for quite a long stretch of time he happily recalled. And like the Fate and the Hunter, the Imperium of long ago had once been his home.

The pieces of this cosmic puzzle were quickly falling into place. The Fate walked toward the Aristocrat with a slow and delicate pace, and knelt down before him. She looked deeply into his eyes; the eyes of one shaped by what seemed a clerisy's blade like her own and saw that he wields it just as well. Seeing the memory within him, she asked him confidently if he remembered her name.

Time seemed to cloud over the horizon of remembrance for a few moments. They now walked the path atop a frozen descent. And then a burst of light brought forth revelation.

'Lîna.'

The words of the Aristocrat brought a wind of life back to At'Lann and sunshine once again shined on 'Lîna's soul. His remembrance was enough to fill 'Lîna with pride once again of she who became the path of Fate. The utterance of her name, after being lost so long to being locked in the ages past, drew the circle together. The Trinity started to uncover the earth that had been buried like mountains over their memories. They were once of the same path long before they began this final odyssey.

Now was the time when their paths merged again after so many ages away from each other, forcing themselves to forget the cataclysm of their future's past. So long ago that even time came very close to eroding meaning and the purpose they had left behind. Time had put their souls into a listless sleep but now the Trinity truly awakened. Their eyes became wide open to their reality once again. The Trinity brought together almost felt truly alive with purpose and regained meaning. A measure of freedom returned to them.

The Fate grasped the Aristocrat's lower arms before she embraced him with heart-felt contentment, and in her thoughts she could feel him call her by her name of fondness. She rose from the couch where the Aristocrat had been sitting, continuing to hold him as she brought herself up. She only let go to bring herself to the Hunter to embrace him as old veteran warriors would when reunited but also in the way of comrades of idealism. She released him to let him unite with the Aristocrat. The pieces were once again almost whole.

8
'Lîna

When the Trinity first met on the ethereal path, there was a hidden familiarity. Now their circle of truth was almost complete. 'Lîna 'Mura was the catalyst for this trinity in a manner of ways.

Many ages before the dawn of this universe, there existed another reality. Different beings inhabited the universe. Not so different from what remains from the age of that which this trinity of souls called home, yet different nonetheless. On the moon of the blue planet now called 'Earth', there existed an extraordinary civilization. This first civilization and one of the first civilizations of the universe, existed amongst the lush green forests of the moon left to them by those on the path ahead.

Once the lifeless moon flourished with life, with beings, and with balance. All at a level greater than that of what this Fate called E'de, and at levels the once azure, emerald gem and spherical planet had never truly known yet shared for eternity. On this place existed the gifts of achievement left by the gods that came before. This place was once a flourishing civilization. Even the universe itself felt bestowed with this culture that existed in union with nature, and with a people that lived to explore existence though few left At'Lann. They were the children of the first great peace. A peace so great that war itself could not shatter it but all good things did come to an end.

Their bond with life gave these people the ability to create life on the moon and to let the life already there thrive. The building materials were already there, life simply had to be reconstituted to have it emerge. Theirs became the first path onto what is above civilization and what remains its very essence. This covenant was what made what was once a colony into an empire, and the people who were once of At'Lann always remembered this. They lived with eternal gratitude to what they had been bestowed by reality.

It was a place where an infinite array of plants, trees, flowers, and animals once covered the surface above that which now blew around the Trinity in the tomb. All but a zephyr in death throes was left to freeze and burn a parched silver soil. The sweet, aqua hued air that was once an ocean of delights for the lungs was now only rendered to be nearly fully breathable yet somehow still remained stale. But they each remembered a time when At'Lann was a far different place.

On the far side of the moon, above what now rests under rock, the civilization that once radiated with a beauty that once walked to be unbound by the sun and delight of her rays of light upon the waters of L'unn, now seemed only a faraway empty place. This was once a place where the waves lay silently asleep when the wind nestled down with them to dream under a sky of stars that still burned with life. Surrounded by the great oceans, the city-states of At'Lann and 'Mura stood out as golden treasures on what was once the emerald moon of E'de. Fate remembered the peace of home. And she remembered the place that once was a peace torn away, and she remembered their path.

At'Lann ruled 'Mura, and 'Mura ruled At'Lann. She remembered a time before the Imperiatrix of the Imperium came to embody the very nature of the At'Lann. The royal heads of state lived in the centre of At'Lann while their children governed 'Mura. In the last 'Mura line, there were three daughters of At'Lann with the eldest being 'Lîna 'Mura, the heir to an empire and an existence. Her sisters were Za'szu 'Mura and 'Zaya 'Mura. These sisters of 'Lîna's were much younger than her but had taken a more active role in the state affairs of 'Mura. 'Lîna the heir apparent had no desire to lead her people. Her heart was with her people but her heart was elsewhere as well.

Though the King and Queen disapproved of their heir's path, they knew that she would never be complete if she did not heed the logic of her true calling. Daily governance was not in many parts of 'Lîna's nature. She was something more. With great frequency, 'Lîna would leave At'Lann and 'Mura to explore as much of the universe as she could. Even from her early days, 'Lîna was always an explorer.

The galaxies themselves were her early playground, and she became sometimes their only explorer. She could swim the universe for millions of light years at a time. Though most of space was known then, she sometimes made it to remote sections never seen by the At'Lann before. Exploration was what made 'Lîna into herself; it completed many parts of her soul.

When the Fate did return home, one of her greatest pleasures was to share philosophies with the ambassador for the Lon'tus Commonwealth. The Lon'tus and the At'Lann cultures had been friends since their first moment of contact and shared a common origin.

Like 'Lîna, the Ambassador was of great lineage as well. Ambassador Nul'lus and 'Lîna shared a commonality that their friendship easily found a path for them to share and walk. Both were to become masters of their domains, and in youth Nul'lus's soul grew beside 'Lîna's. Their shared path of youth moulded them into becoming what they now were. As 'Lîna lived to become the Fate, so too did Nul'lus live to become the Aristocrat. Their roots were formed in At'Lann. It was so long ago, but they both remembered all they had lost from their golden age in the darkest of days.

For something terrible had happened to this existence. It was also a time when 'Lîna would go on to create the At'Lann Imperium and become its Imperiatrix. It all came to a close with the most damning and taxing of prices. At'Lann was left an empty shell, an eternal ascetic tomb. The Trinity came to remember the Lon'tus and the world of the Hunter, H'Raka, which was also left to languish as relics of another time. As the trinity of souls would discover, they were drawn together to amend the eternal sorrow. With the final circle drawing closer together, the die was cast.

As the Fate would explain, when life was given to the At'Lann Imperium, so too was life given indirectly to the path of this trinity. In understanding Imperiatrix 'Lîna 'Mura 'Lann, one must understand the events that brought her into being. As the Fate would remember and recall the events of the past, the purpose of the path of souls would begin to emerge.

Their future remained in the past. The past, once lost to them, was the true objective of the Trinity. With their union that began again on the path, a hidden opportunity was at last unburied. After the fall of the great Imperia in the ages past, Fate came to possess a technology that, when powered by this trinity, could bring them back to undo the eternal sorrow.

Altering reality was a relatively easy task for any member of this gathering of three but all of reality would require a complete, co-operative symbiosis of their power. Each possessed a quality that the other required. Their ship was ready to sail as if towards a Balearic sunset sky; a sky that blessed those like Tiësto.

The trinities of Fate and Fates were drawn together for one final stand. A stand that could be considered the first step towards mending the shattered dream. Memories were becoming clear, and each of them knew what to do. Their very being was their very cause after all. Their final answer to their equation of life lay in the past where they once shared a path. Perhaps this was for the last time this trinity would enter the gateway they had made in time.

They did not want to return to psionic cemetries. The Trinity would leave this behind them to bring about a future that would not leave them abandoned to what they had become. Their very souls did not want to be tombs themselves any longer. This was the crucible.

9
The Locusts and The Siege

Before time, and many ages beyond that, existed a reality that was far different than all others of its day. The universe was luxurious, so very lavished with life. Space was not dark but was aglow with the various colours of life. In this universe existed an explorer, and heir to the throne of one of its great civilizations.

She was so young, and oh so innocent. So full of life in her ways that wherever she roamed, beautiful life would spread to grow around her. She might have seemed the greatest of nymphs but she was much more. She was the potential of all those who knew her. She brought something wondrous to existence. For she was the child of destiny.

She flew from galaxy to galaxy, from space to space, and from system to system, from the very moment she could pilot her own ship. Her parents initially were quite disappointed by her choice in vocations before her duties would take her to the throne but there could be no other way. They had wanted her to be a proper ruler, and leader, a model for their people. Though she was a very capable leader, 'Lîna 'Mura chose to devote her life to the exploration of existence.

Her younger sister, Za'szu grudgingly respected her choice. She used to fight constantly with her sister Za'szu in their days as children, and usually as to who would lead At'Lann. 'Lîna always wanted to be an explorer so she merely used to posture and play along, to assuage her sister Za'szu's overly competitive antics. Eventually, an arrangement was made. When her time came she would rule, and when she explored, Za'szu would lead. Since 'Lîna postulated that she would return home for only brief periods of time, it was more than a fitting arrangement for the two siblings.

'Lîna even transferred the principality of 'Mura to her worthy hands. This was one of the things that made each of the sisters appreciate the personalities of the other. Though each sister did not have any lusts for mere political power, each made this point, their shared path of agreeable disagreement, to compete over. Even though the power of rule for its own sake matters very little to them, life was made far more fascinating by this friendly tug of war.

Things were not always this way; they evolved to become better. Once they stopped competing with one another, they were able to enjoy being sisters. That led them to love one another as sisters should. When she left home on her ship to explore the universe, 'Lîna's sister was the last one in fact to give her a warm hug good-bye.

'Lîna's youngest sister 'Zaya, had a different, yet just as special a bond with her eldest sister. Since she was offered fewer pursuits in the Monarchy, she had chosen the sciences as her path. 'Zaya, like 'Lîna, had chosen an unorthodox path in life. Her being had just as much joie de vivre as 'Lîna felt with every step on her path in life. They looked out for one another on the same path. 'Zaya was the future to 'Lîna just as much as 'Zaya was to 'Lîna. Their innocent enlightened souls gave each of them a special bond to share and covet. They would always protect one another and would do the same for 'Za'szu. They would do the same for their parents, and for all those who share their path. They would always be family of blood and souls.

That was four years ago but she was still 'Lîna 'Mura, the explorer, the sometime ruler of 'Mura, and heir to all of At'Lann. It all seemed blink of time, a lifetime ago. She found herself many millions of galaxies away from home. 'Lîna was feeling content, and happy on the world of the Lit'vaa.

As her ship orbited the grassy, green world, she found herself sitting and laughing with some cute looking creatures on a rock. 'Lîna was amidst a knoll of long-stemmed, reed like plants. Her glittering mauve hair flew like silk in the wind. She smiled and swayed on her rocky seat, all the while being entertained by the furry, friendly ursine Lit'vaa. The sounds of Chicane seemed to fill the air with sonic bliss.

The Lit'vaa, quite cub like in design, having white fur and with fangs both serrated and hyperbolic, did not possess a spoken language, yet they were quite intelligent as they could communicate with 'Lîna telepathically. Nearly all days for the Lit'vaa were spent munching on Zuku (the simple plant life that covered this world), lying around in the sun, or playfully biting one another. When off-worlders came to visit, they went of their way to hear their stories, tales, and in return the Lit'vaa would entertain their guests. Pleasantness almost existed as a pheromone from these creatures. They knew only of a love of life and they kept their ways simple; to love land and be loved by it.

As the smaller Lit'vaa scampered about the small feet of 'Lîna. The larger ones, the size of Polar bears, sat in circles around the seat of 'Lîna. She told them of her home of At'Lann, of a society that lives in union with their genetics and theology of consciousness. She told them of the great oceans and lush forests. She told them of a peaceful people that gained contentment by their place as thinkers in the universe.

'Lîna also told them of the forest planet of L'unn (the lunar satellite and home to the At'Lann) orbits, E'de. E'de was the At'Lann term meaning world of oceans and island jungles, it seemed only fitting. She told them of E'de, the colonial planet and of the large, warm-blooded creatures native to that world. Creatures with large sharp teeth, and large sharp claws that the Lit'vaa were excitedly amused to hear of.

Using her basic psionic techniques, she created a holographic display above and between her raised hands and thoughts. The Lit'vaa were quite amazed by the snapping motions and power of their teeth, and perplexed by the curious behaviour shown in 'Lîna's animated psionic holograms. Though she could have shown them telepathically, she opted to entertain them with a visual bit of glamour as well. The Lit'vaa more than appreciated her efforts.

The Lit'vaa later asked her if any At'Lann existed on E'de, and she told them of the Hy'Bor colonies. She had not been to these colonies personally as they were a separate political entity. The Hy'Bor had taken a path separate from the At'Lann. There were no diplomatic relations between Hy'Bor and At'Lann, so Hy'Bor was one of the few places in the universe that was restricted for 'Lîna to travel to.

She did know the Hy'Bor were a small but profiting colony by their location on a larger planetary body that allowed them a larger surface area to expand across. Their way was the path towards planetary industrial expansion while the At'Lann ways were sometimes followed the ways of an anchorite. Her species indeed had ways that one might call those of an anchorite: isolationis and reclusivity. 'Lîna made it a point for the Lit'vaa to know that her people were the more evolved species.

'Lîna respected what she had heard of the Hy'Bor and the colony they built using the many interesting natural resources of E'de. Still, 'Lîna was taught from a young age to be a nationalist so her opinions were quite biased. The Lit'vaa seeing such a pretty girl before them took it all with stride. For they could see she never cared to concern herself with the genetic politics of her state she told the Lit'vaa of. She only thought the best of all life in the universe.

Since the Lit'vaa could not get enough of 'Lîna's stories about her home, she continued with more. She even told them of her sisters, and how the warm-hearted Lit'vaa reminded 'Lîna of one of her sisters who, like the Lit'vaa, liked to playfully nip her. 'Lîna was having fun telling these stories of home, simply by watching the equally content seated Lit'vaa chewing on Zuku.

After the tales were told and the entertainment was over with for the day, 'Lîna walked alone to the top of a large green rolled and rolling field. She stared out to the stars and milky glitter of the galaxy in the Lit'vaa horizon. She then looked into the sun that lit the Lit'vaa home world. Her psionically smoothed silver trident edged tiara sweetly reflected the rays of sunshine.

'Lîna thought of this place and all like it as her home. Reality was a very large place but all of it was hers to enjoy as something to feel at home in. Life was beautiful for 'Lîna, all of it. Nothing could fill one with wonder like feeling the happiness of existence. She knew her role. She had purpose of her own designs. This was bliss. And then in another moment, that belief was almost shattered.

Even the Lit'vaa could feel it. It was like a storm cloud of darkness and dread had suddenly spread across the entire universe. Space itself seemed to darken all at once before 'Lîna's very eyes. Abruptly, 'Lîna felt the urge to leave the lovely world of the Lit'vaa without so much as a farewell. She knew they would understand. She was needed in At'Lann. 'Lîna had her ship bend reality, and she folded aboard. 'Lîna compulsively keyed the sequence into the navigational controls to fold space and return home.

Home. She could feel the dark omen already there. She knew something dreadful had happened to her world. It was a feeling of complete violation. 'Lîna wondered what evil could possibly have caused this. She never saw the near future before her. This hit her like a bolt of blue.

Her ship, a construct that looked like two large metallic and grizzled triangles intersecting one another at a right angle, and had three circular purple coloured points of propulsion lay at the end of each thick triangle. 'Lîna's ship, a At'Lann scout class vessel, the Kalu'ko, started to vent an exhaust, a light mauve mist into space. The Kalu'ko, named after the founder of At'Lann, was powered by 'Lîna herself. Since mauve was her colour in life, the mist effect was a reflection of her abilities.

These mists reacted with space to create a rumbling, churning water like passage through it. In an instant, her ship was gone from its orbit of the Lit'vaa planet, and in another instant would emerge in 'Lîna's home system of Tr'Lann. Then before her eyes, was a siege of locusts.

Thousands of dark invading ships swarmed the entire system. The heavens seemed to burn. This was a pillaging force of evil, the ultimate darkness, had stretched its tentacles out to cover any planet or place where life existed. It tore through her empathic soul, the horde's effects could be even felt within 'Lîna as the darkness seemed to eat its way into the white veil of her innocence. It was almost too much to bear.

After she emerged from folded space, 'Lîna wisely activated a cloak field over her ship. She needed to assess the damage done, and would need a moment of time to formulate a counter-attack. So quickly was she thrust onto the path of war that even 'Lîna was unaware. This was the destiny of her basic instincts had taken over. She had a duty to protect her people. She always knew of this possibility even though it seemed so remote to her.

Though the Kalu'ko was designed by 'Lîna as a deep exploratory vessel, the ship still maintained ten decks, ample, luscious living quarters, and with 'Lîna's tolerated permission, the most advanced weapons systems of the At'Lann. The navigational control area, however, was a rather tight fit. The heat of the situation as well as the lack of space may have caused 'Lîna to break into a humid sweat. Her body had never perspired before this day as she had that affliction removed from her genetic structure before she was even conceived. 'Lîna chose to have her emotions fuel her sweat as the crisis made for a rare exception.

Status reports, emergency messages, warnings, and cries for help flashed out to her from the Kalu'ko's interface to her worried position in her command chair. When she finally finished her hidden trek to At'Lann, she found L'unn and At'Lann in flames. Apparently, these dark ships were engaged in intentional acts of twisted *seppuku,* and were flying their demonically aggressive ships at full speed into the surface of L'unn.

Before 'Lîna could feel the true horror of it all, her ship was struck. She attempted to engage the weapons system of her ship but it was to no avail. Even her vaunted technology was taken off-line. The ship was being hit with some strangely configured energy fire. She was discovered. She had become a captive pursuit.

Without hesitation, 'Lîna reached up to grab a very large gravimetric photonic pulse-rifle that was held by fasteners on the third wall of the navigational control area. 'Lîna was not sure how to approach war but she did know how to handle a weapon. It was after all, a royal duty. Though preferably a pacifist, 'Lîna had been trained in the arts of defence. Even with her power, she was taught to think of a rifle as one of your best friends in battle. Just because she was a person of peace did not mean she was not prepared to fight.

The ship was tearing itself apart. The sound of burning, bending metal almost sounded like a dying banshee. The first private ship she ever had was about to be destroyed. She could feel it. It was time to set the balance right. She had no time to think of the coming demise of her long time companion. Her thoughts barely had time to wave goodbye to the Kalu'ko. She only had to ready herself to face the enemy. 'Lîna knew it was time to make a move.

10
The Most Bitter Retreat

The ship was going to explode. There was no question of that any longer for 'Lîna as she watched the interface holo-panels go into a data flow cardiac arrest. She changed reality and jumped, while phased, through the hull of the Kalu'ko and out into space. 'Lîna then changed her molecular structure once again to become solid in the vacuum. With a gentle farewell stroke of her hand, she watched as her last moment of her bond with her ship, the Kalu'ko. Her ship began to drift into the orbital current.

As she has always known, breathing in space is quite simple and it had taken her lungs only a short moment to adapt to the wide open and consuming vacuum of space thanks to her At'Lann genetics. That gave her some time to get past the white flame explosions that consumed her ship. She had a moment for a solitary dirge for her ship that once was her home but was now only flames. She had to leave her old days of peace behind her as 'Lîna found herself entering the gates of Hell.

As she tightly gripped the large poly-metallic rifle that she had brought with her, 'Lîna no longer had time to look back. Her silver and emerald hued metallic rifle was shaped like a rectangular and cubist shaved smooth ghetto blaster, which made for one big gun. 'Lîna saw the ensuing cataclysm before her eyes. This was a tragedy of truth, her home was being raped by a path of destruction. Her sense of peace had been deflowered. It was bleeding. Her home was burning. She had come home to horror. The locust like ships of the dark fleet bombarded L'unn and E'de with energy pulses of Chernobyl concentrated hurls of destruction.

At that moment, one of their largest vessels intentionally drove itself to colliding with E'de. The resulting blast was probably was severe enough to wipe out an E'de continent as the mantle crumbled. With her augmented sight, a gift of her being, 'Lîna could see the very crust being debauched by those that marked her world for Death. Though the heat of the inner E'de reduced the once gigantic monstrosity of evil to simple molten metals, the wave of onslaught, spread quickly across E'de. 'Lîna had never watched an extinction before. It paralyzed her psyche for an instant.

As the shock-wave finished its destructive path, the E'de became an opaque sphere of burning dust, of burning earth. Such evil, 'Lîna thought as she could feel the terrible shock of it all. 'Lîna felt as if something truly vile had shredded the veil of order that lay across reality. A reality now that seemed to suffer with stigmatic tortures and kidnappings by neo-Ravanas. 'Lîna felt as if she were swimming in the fermented remains of the dead. 'Lîna's emotional state would have to wait for another day as she now had to stand as she never had before as she now became targeted by the guns of the vile invasion force.

These crafts of utter evil began to shoot at 'Lîna with photonic rotted orange hued, rodent claw girandole like pulses as if she were a clay pigeon. 'Lîna had anticipated this and she reflected their tainted photonic energy back at the enemy. Back at the ships of the dark invaders with twice the fury as the insipid energy had been flung at her. The enemy vessels, like hyper-obese dung beetles, exploded in gluttonous burning bile flames.

As 'Lîna flew towards At'Lann, those who wanted to destroy 'Lîna and her world, burned behind her with a now dark red flame. Telepathically, 'Lîna could begin to feel the fear, the despair of her people. She could even smell the stench of rotted brimstone that was left in reality by the attackers of her world. She could not probe beyond the burned shells of the dark minds of the invaders. She could not locate any member of her family. 'Lîna tried to hope for the best. But she did find the mind, the soul, of a friend on At'Lann who would aid the cause of her people.

As she neared the At'Lann city-state, she used her own abilities to bolster the protective ethereal shields, and to strengthen the shield enough to keep the dark invaders from inflicting any further damage. At the very least this effort may save most of the ecclesiastically lined city from being completely toppled. Her thoughts became those of protecting the ships of At'Lann's fleet that were stationed on her world. She could not make contact with the At'Lann fleet that was thinly positioned across the galaxy. She hoped her fleet would survive. She would need them if they did.

She could see in her mind her friend's physicality and she flew to his location. The enemy was engaging him and her people on her home-soil. Her friend offered a solution. There was one option to this chaos. 'Lîna knew there was no other choice, and so 'Lîna instructed her friend to meet her outside of the At'Lann House of the Monarchy. He would more than comply. As she neared her domestic defence objective, she then hovered over the mass cities of At'Lann. 'Lîna's home had gone through the very inferno of what the ancient Greeks called Hades.

The city was a splintered fracture of itself. Smoke billowed from the great fires that randomly lined the streets of 'Lîna's home. Fire is usually a pure element but that day it burned like a tainted oil fire. As 'Lîna flew above the great roads that led to the heart of At'Lann, she began to hear the screams of lost innocence. The people of At'Lann were being murdered, being slaughtered, before her very eyes. The shadow filled invading entities were culling her race. Extermination seemed to be their only creed.

This truly was an army one would see sent to herald the death of Death. For At'Lann, it seemed like the beginning of Ragnarok. The future itself seemed to no longer have a path into a continuance of forever. Pandora's box had been flung open with utter viciousness of a Stalin unbound. But the At'Lann were a power to be reckoned with and would not be conquered into eternal submission so easily. At the bottom of Pandora's box lay the hope At'Lann would need. Resistance could now be seen.

One against one, legion against legion, and army against army; there would be no surrender of their home. To prevail, to keep goodness alive, the At'Lann were fighting back. Even with cannons to their left and to their right that thundered and volleyed, the At'Lann refused to die. Weapons fire filled the air, and the sound of struggle filled the sky. Fire fights raged across the city. 'Lîna could hear the sounds that only At'Lann defence technologies could emanate like the most enhanced cathedral organ. She even had to swerve while soaring to avoid an errant blast. It was then that 'Lîna set sight upon her trusted friend Nul'lus, the ambassador on L'unn for the Lon'tus Commonwealth.

He stood beside the third corner of the greatest of all At'Lann pyramids; the pyramid of the Regency. He was not alone. Nor was he resting. Soldiers from both At'Lann and those of the diplomatic house of the Lon'tus stood with him. They stood beside each other to defend a large circle of short stone. They were in battle and they fired rifle shot after rifle shot at the dark invaders who were beginning to creep up on their position.

These were valiant men with the courage of defiance in the face of death like those who slew the Me-109 beasts over Calais. 'Lîna lightly descended from the air to the centre of the flat, slightly raised, vanilla grey stone circle. Nul'lus tapped the ribs of a mauve, peach, thickly trimmed black At'Lann soutane clad male soldier of L'unn that was to his left. He did the same to a sierra ash clad Lon'tus soldier to his right with the same aristocratic motion to enclose the circle and continue firing. Nul'lus then turned around and entered the circle where 'Lîna awaited him.

The enemy that came at them were necro-catalysed warriors and the walking dead surrounded their position. He moved with a whispering quick glide to embrace 'Lîna in a sweet and serious kind of way. Though they faced the siege 'Lîna felt almost safe that she faced it with her best mate from Lon'tus. And she wondered what had become of Lon'tus in the path of the dark storm. Terror had seized the day.

It had been so many years since 'Lîna had last laid eyes upon Nul'lus, who was now the Lon'tus Commonwealth Ambassador to At'Lann. His family, once part of the Lon'tus delegation, had made 'Mura home until Nul'lus came of age to properly assume the post. He had been her friend since the time 'Lîna and Nul'lus both shared in lessons from their wise Royal Tutor, B'Dak, who taught the pair the ways of the universe and of paths like Doshin So. There was no time, however, to reminisce.

'Lîna and Nul'lus both knew what was at stake. They could feel it. Swift action must be taken to save the cities, and defeat the enemy on the ground. The citizenry must be protected. Nul'lus was more than willing to lend a hand for a people and a friend close to his heart. He could feel that this onslaught was everywhere. Something had let slip the tides of Armageddon.

Elsewhere, the fleet was on its way. 'Lîna could see them surging ahead to

At'Lann. It gave small comfort to her heart. What gave 'Lîna the most heaven felt contentment in a time of crisis was that Nul'lus was so selfless as to aid her. She did not have to even ask anything of him. It was, after all, his idea as much as it was hers. 'Lîna and Nul'lus looked at each other with a sense of sense of serene, dedicated confidence. The time was at hand to do what must be done. 'Lîna then knelt on one knee and slid her slender index finger along the stone surface in an elongated triangular diamond type pattern.

In the circle, a large square slab of peach coloured marble stone materialised into reality beneath where 'Lîna and Nul'lus stood transforming the stonework into a gateway. The square that they stood upon within the circle began to seamlessly descend into the underground. As the slab of stone descended to another place beneath the surface of L'unn, 'Lîna had a brief moment of time to turn her thoughts inward.

She knew the only way she was going to go through this was to honour her people. It was her ultimate duty to protect them. She was home to see to the defence of the state. Even though the thought to carry out this protocol that was not her own, it would become her own. Somehow the inherent knowledge of the crafts of war came to her while she was still in space returning home from Lit'vaa. She had never been in battle before but she was bestowed with grace under pressure. The thought to seek out Nul'lus when she could not find her noble kinsmen had been a wise one.

'Where are my sisters? Did they survive?' 'Lîna wondered as she did her best to conquer her anxiety. Then she came to feel not even the most minor psionic (an enhanced high order flow of telepathy that exists in a form beyond energy) trace of her parents. There was a great urgency in Nul'lus's eyes to turn the evil tide but he also withheld something painful.

The two were acting in the absence of power for the sake of At'Lann. 'Lîna peered into Nul'lus's secret truth for this act of urgency. She had already felt the truth, the validation of it hit her with a passive strength. For there was no one else who could fill the void left. This had become her fate for no other reason than by the emotional void that 'Lîna felt in her soul. Her Mother, her Father were both dead. Nul'lus was not able to keep it from her. What was their directive, their protocols in times of crisis had become thrust unto 'Lîna like the devastated beauty of Europa nearly destroyed by far too many wars. Hers became the burden and the joy of protecting At'Lann. She did find solace in this truth by the support of Nul'lus. The full impact of this emotional blow would have to wait.

'Lîna swallowed hard to bury the pain. She had to keep her focus on the task at hand. The only thing that would be on her mind would be the drastic measures about to be undertaken to protect At'Lann, and the lives of those around her. Mourning would be for the time after, for the moment was at hand. 'Lîna knew what to do to carry through the saving grace, and it was within her as much as the pain she hastily buried.

As the stone slab came to rest on a glittering silver ground, Nul'lus had become just as prepared as 'Lîna. He had also used this time to hone his mind to the mission, and laying the concerns of his people aside, was ready to take the final steps to fulfil what would be the first mission of the new war.

There was a silent acknowledgement between Nul'lus and 'Lîna as they walked through a small heptagonal mechanised tunnel lit by the darkest of garnet. They walked toward a bright light at its end. They strolled a pace apart but 'Lîna and Nul'lus had found a new rapport for each other arising from this critical mission. Their bond that began with playful days of study became something more with each passing step. It was like taking first steps with your brother, and Nul'lus had always been the brother that 'Lîna never had.

'Lîna had always respected Nul'lus for the grace of his being and his noble dreams. He had the most worthy of characters with the one of the strongest of minds. If she were going to go through this with anyone, 'Lîna felt quite blessedly thankful that the fates had chosen Nul'lus to be the one at her side for this particular action.

At the end of the passage lay a large black lit spherical chamber. A chamber that was about a storey high and overgrown with a near white lattice layering of ultra conducting technology imposed over an aquamarine background. 'Lîna and Nul'lus moved to the middle of the chamber. Piously, they stood straight and touched each other through the palms of their hands in a vertical way. The two stared into each other with the expression of unity.

Even though Nul'lus was of Lon'tus and not of At'Lann, the two governments shared their technology with one another freely. As a noble son of Lon'tus, Nul'lus might have had to complete the same mission on his home world should he have been there. Instead he was here. His being was just as primed as 'Lîna's. Normally, the King and Queen would undertake this defensive sanction but this day was for another generation. For a moment, 'Lîna and Nul'lus felt very timid of what was about to occur.

It was an experience akin to the feeling one gets before jumping from a high bridge to a great body of water. Their emotions found clarity in the liminal state of their situation. This would transform them, and give them a bond so strong it would never be avoided. This was the ultimate sacrifice and ultimate decadence of being, and 'Lîna felt honoured to share this with Nul'lus. Just as he was honoured to stand with her and defend her home as if it were his own. What was to be would set them apart, and set them above. This was the clouds before the rain and the lightning before the thunder of Zeus before he launched his storms. The pair activated the chamber.

It had begun. Like a spirally upward flowing mist, reality began to shift. Though 'Lîna and Nul'lus were quite powerful entities by their own genetic merits, the technology of this chamber would change their laws of cause and effect that encompassed their being. It was a talisman and a receptor that reshuffled their genetic structures being into forms beyond that which they had known. This shift in reality swirled about and above the pair. It grew larger. The shift also grew within the highest genetic structures of 'Lîna and Nul'lus.

This effect grew so large that the ocean flow of reality reached out across L'unn. Reality on L'unn had shifted so much that its entirety existed within, and apart from reality. 'Lîna and Nul'lus fuelled the effect and were enhanced by it. It was a tragic moment of ecstasy.

The attack by the force of doom was rendered useless as the weapons of the dark fleet no longer had anything to target, and if they did, they would find that At'Lann was in a state of continual phase variance. The L'unn phase generator had worked as it always had for those who entered with noble blood and pure hearts. L'unn, At'Lann, and 'Mura had submerged to a lower layer of reality but to this shadow of evil that had darkened her skies, At'Lann was erased from their murderous reality. They would not be herded away into Hades but Hades had already taken so much away.

They would have no choice but to move on. The fleet would be arriving soon to prevent any further damage to the system. Though they had caught At'Lann off-guard, and outnumbered them, the enemy still could not defeat them. At'Lann was still there.

The safety of At'Lann came with great cost to the pair, for their bodies, their minds, their souls both bore the scars and the smiles that this day brought and would bring until the end of time. It would be difficult especially for their genetic matrices to contain the energies unleashed from their psyogenetic genesis. Psyogenetics being high order telepathically designed and enhanced adaptive genetic structures. 'Lîna was the first to scream with orgiastic exhilaration that soared so far above what is primal. Her eyes were now wide open. The truth of it all was almost too much for her. Nul'lus was the first to fall to the ground, and like 'Lîna who fell beside him, they both had energy fires burning from their bodies burn like never before. Both were like a phoenix in the psionic flames. The fires above burned like those seen when one see when shuts their eyes after staring too long into a sun of expensive fires.

Their bodies lay sprawled about the floor. Their genetics were altered in, perhaps, a sinisterly vengeful and beautiful manner. 'Lîna and Nul'lus were forever changed like the way a rose would be when taken from her thorns to be displayed in some parlour. If not for the better, at least for the stronger, for these roses would not wilt away. These two were now like roses free to live unhindered by their being that once was lived in thorns. But this was not over yet. At'Lann still had to be purged of its roach infestation.

Nul'lus and 'Lîna came to their feet and they stood once again. Blood from internal wounds soaked out of their forcefully evolved flesh and dripped to the floor. Their sense of grogginess had faded and a mutual hatred towards a common foe grew to take its place. They dripped with a deflowering of warm sweat and blood that flowed down their bodies still burning as the beads of blood sweat fell to the ground.

As the fires of blood burned away into floating embers, 'Lîna and Nul'lus embraced with their hands again, and smiled a smile of gloating over surviving death. A dark magenta field of energy burned from their hands that were held in a gentle grasp. It gained concentrated momentum before it shot out to the sky like thunderbolts woven by a mathematically minded spider.

The pair decided it was time to launch their counterattack with an energy that would shatter the very genetic codes of the soldiers of the force of darkness. Across L'unn, the energy became one with the atmosphere. Within the vile walking dead bodies of the dark soldiers that lingered throughout L'unn, volcanic like explosions were erupting across their crackling and pus rotted skins. In the underground, 'Lîna and 'Nul'lus stood in their baptism of fire. They watched with their new and enhanced sight as the infesting agents had their basic double helixes collapsed like a poorly stacked house of cards.

This caused the bodies of the enemy soldiers to explode into a high velocity of decayed organic hale that burned itself away from reality. Where the great roads within At'Lann were now filled with the murdered innocent, these same grand roads were now flooded by the feculent blood of the enemy that smoked away and out of reality.

'Lîna and Nul'lus ascended to the surface using the gigantic lift of stone. As the sun hit their eyes, the pair finally saw the enormity of what they had done and what the dark storm brought to their existence. They looked at each other as comrades would but now with eyes for war and eyes that salivated for vengeance. They would not be forsaken if they would wage war in the inferno. Their innocence had been torn away from their sight like an unseen hymen left to fall away from their souls as they took their first steps to walk as warriors.

Her home lay burning, screaming, and almost broken. She watched the smoke billow and fill the phased azure skies. It was an eclipse of darkness that wounded 'Lîna to the point where she felt as violated as her world. Without a tear, 'Lîna vowed to have vengeance even in this moment this moment of defeated survival. A hole was in 'Lîna's heart for the lost innocence that bound her to her people once again. But this was not over yet, for the journey into war had only just begun.

11
Assemble The Fleet

'Lîna felt so different, yet so cold. Her parents were truly dead, and her life forever had been changed. She could no longer feel their guiding presence that always came over her when she came to exist on At'Lann. She could feel their loss from existence as a loss within her. It was consuming her. 'What would Kalu'ko say, she wondered as she drowned in grief. But before she could cry the scream of despair she erected a Haarlem dam to stop the tear filled waters of her mind from flooding her being.

The tears in her eyes swelled but they did not flow. 'Lîna buried the pain of the loss within her and reached even further into herself to find the darker emotions of vengeance, and she began to order her mind for the new state of war. For she would now become the Regent, and this was the order of things on her world. She was now enhanced. The task of eliminating this threat to life would become 'Lîna's. She vowed that this would be her action to control her sorrow and her loss. 'Lîna sacrificed her innocence to save her destiny and that of her people. It would be up to her to save existence from this scourge.

One could say 'Lîna gave into hatred to ignore her bereaved state. It was a terrible trade-off but she felt that she was left with no other option. It was, after all, her nature as an anchorite of exploration. She was solitary, and that too would be left behind. She was Regent now, and she would take her place amongst her people in the defence of life. Her natural curiosities would find a new home in the field of war even if her lone ways would find less time. Even love would wait. For she would become a warrior.

Those she gave her trust to would be given even more honour than felt before as she shut many of the gateways into her mind. She would only be free with her intimate relationships. As Regent, she would be alone by separation but not truly free to be alone. She became something more from this time on. Even her physical appearance began to change.

She appeared colder, and darkly more beautiful than ever before. Her youth would always be hers but the gaze of her eyes seemed shattered following the wisdom of trauma. As he stood beside her, Nul'lus could see the metamorphic changes taking place as he changed into something more as well. The changes had less of an impact upon Nul'lus immediately as he knew he did not lose his parents to the new war. But he did understand what impact so much loss had on 'Lîna.

Nul'lus watched as a ribbon of 'Lîna's hair turned snow white before his eyes. There was really nothing he could do for her, save offer his support, and the allegiance of his people against this menace. 'Lîna somehow even looked a few years older though she remained in the extreme blossom of the youthfulness of her soul.

'Lîna looked at Nul'lus with great purpose. The pursuit was to begin. Since 'Lîna preferred to communicate telepathically, Nul'lus already knew what was to occur. She motioned gently towards her friend, and as he stood beside her, she moved her hand back to expose her wrist. She looked to the sky. She had become so forged by the experience that she was easily able to twist spatial reality to bring the pair to the Royal At'Lann flagship, the Lis'talla. In spite of the dark cost, they were more powerful than ever.

The pair materialised in a large platinum hued stone chamber lit by soothing rose water light. There were hundreds of members of the Royal Court that had stood to greet the pairs' expected arrival. The elite ceremonial guard, the S'yana, was arranged in small twelve man phalanx arrangements. In between the six segments of their tidy order was a path to a large throne of teal and gold.

Awaiting the pair at the top of the elevated throne was Za'szu, much to 'Lîna's relief. 'Lîna's sister had a look of both loss and haste. Za'szu looked as if she wanted to direct something 'Lîna's way but for the purposes of state, she held her thoughts in for a later time of privacy. 'Lîna's thoughts let her sister know she returned home elated that she survived the siege of both war and evolution for war. Somehow, Za'szu was not surprised 'Lîna came through to stand at the promised time.

The lavender banners were unfurled, and above the throne the silk banners flowed around where the Royal coat of arms rested. It began to shine in rays of rubies. The tall triangular diamond adorning an onyx double helix: the symbol of strength in being, the proud emblem of At'Lann.

Za'szu stepped back and 'Zaya came before her eldest sister with a diagonally engraved cubic box which was about the size of a human head. 'Zaya bowed in a curtsey style before 'Lîna in a way that made one feel her moment, and all her moments to come were at hand. 'Lîna opened the elaborate trappings of power, the crown cut vanilla gold platinum box to find two immaculately composed emerald hued bracelets. 'Lîna felt like Pandora bent on redemption. Her path had converged once again, as it always had, onto the path of her people.

There was no time for 'Lîna to bid farewell to her parents for their journey that would take them beyond Death; the time at hand gave itself only towards coronation. Za'szu already had their genetic programs added to the central core of the At'Lann central interface. They refused cloning transfer and opted instead for their legacy to continue in the technological evolution of At'Lann as per their wishes for what was their consciousness in their final testament. Their genetic sequences would be infused into the At'Lann Interface. But even their dirge would fall in the shadow of 'Lîna's coronation. The path of war had begun and there was little time now to turn back.

At'Lann needed a Regent immediately, as the Regent is also the head of the At'Lann war effort. Her sovereign parents had known 'Lîna to be their daughter of peace and the pursuer of knowledge but they had also woven into 'Lîna a strong propensity to hold a spirit of ferociousness should she ever have to face battle. This spirit was awakened when 'Lîna and Nul'lus phased At'Lann to its new dimensional shift. Athena's prowess was ignited within her.

'Lîna reached into the box of bequeathment to seize her destiny. She smoothly slid the emerald jade bands onto her wrists with a momentary feeling of contentment. Za'szu, in her disciplined precision came around to 'Lîna's back and placed upon her shoulders a long, draping black sheer like cloak. 'Lîna raised her arms into the air to expose the ancient symbols of power to the court.

The emerald and the oxidised copper hue around her wrists began to glow and a fire of white light swirled about her arms. Those of her court assembled before her were a sea of light burgundy tunics and mauve violet soutane roared to life in adulation for their new Regent. 'Lîna motioned for her inner court to return to their duties. As the court left the coronation hall, a familiar face came before 'Lîna to have a brief moment with his luminary.

He was Commander Mu'tolma, a cousin to 'Lîna and a distant friend. He came before 'Lîna to request an address to the people. 'Lîna was still far from adjusted to her place in the new regime. Considering all that had happened, it was all happening all too hastily for her liking. 'Lîna linked her thoughts to her young cousin with ivory hair that it would wait.

Nul'lus rejoined 'Lîna's side. She placed her arm in his and they departed together towards her state room. Her sisters knew better than to go against 'Lîna's independent nature and they were escorted by Commander Mu'tolma back to the bridge of the Lis'talla. The ship had set a course to co-ordinates near the furthest planetary body in the At'Lann system, Nu'Ata. There they would join the At'Lann fleet that had survived the first wave of violence upon their existence. One wondered what shape the Lis'talla would find the At'Lann fleet, and if this would be further trauma for the new Regent to face.

Φ

'Lîna sat on the marble floor of night heron vividness of her Romanesque bath fountains. She let the pure waters shower her. After the molecules form automatically in the air, the waters poured like a monsoon down the smoky night heron marble ground. The waters steamed from their molecular fire but it was not enough to melt the sorrow in 'Lîna's heart. For she still shivered with chill. The sounds of peace seemed murdered by the invasion like the one that came on the first of September to end a volatile peace.

At the centre of the floor, 'Lîna's nakedness felt even more alone than ever before, and far more fragile. It was the sterile libations that made it all the more deplorable in her mind. She held her knees tight together with one hand and reached with her left towards the swirling, bright sage expanse of the bath's mist filled ceiling to catch the surging drops of falling water. She could see where the processing field was created. 'Lîna watched the hydrogen atoms combine with the oxygen and she could feel her tears falling only to be smothered by the fiery waters. 'Lîna had a look of contempt in her isolation. She could feel her emotions being drained away along with her tears.

'Lîna only felt bereaved loss for so many things. The love of her parents seemed lost, torn away from her soul, and she was left only with regret that she would never be able to take away their disappointment in her. 'Lîna never felt that she had ever proved herself to her mother and father. Like any child, 'Lîna wanted her parents to be proud of her existence. 'Lîna had always felt that she had not lived up to her genetic potential. She always wondered if her parents truly shared this opinion. She had always wanted to ask them but now 'Lîna would never know. And now she would follow the path of a *bodhisattva* to set the balance right.

After nearly two hours, 'Lîna brought herself to her small feet and went to the adjoining dressing room. The time was hers and for now, solitude remained a necessity. As she left her shower it automatically turned itself off and the air inside her baths became instantly dark and dry. 'Lîna found her clothes folded neatly on a short obsidian pillar before her. She used her own mind to dissipate the water from her skin. Her hair unfurled into long, functional twists of violet curls. She even placed a band of platinum around one of the locks of her hair that flowed to her left shoulder.

'Lîna always enjoyed her status as an aristocratic anchorite of exploration though only to a certain degree, and actually refused to keep a personal servant. She cherished her privacy as she dressed into her attire with her thoughts. She hardly thought a personal slave would be less burdensome than the pleasure of her sometime Spartan yet lavish path.

By 'Lîna's mindset, it would be most pathetic to have someone put on the pants of a young woman one leg at a time especially the pants of a young lady about to embark on a war of redemptive retribution. It was so much easier to dress one thought at a time as she had done since she was very little. She exhaled a mild breath and as she raised her soft arms, she twisted reality. Her clothes flowed in a funnelling brocade fashion unto her body. She had a strange realisation of being as she went about her conventional routine: she truly was forever changed.

At the very least, 'Lîna found not only a chance to prove her character to herself by this dire situation, and find some solace in knowing that this would somehow be passed along to her parents and they could judge her for themselves if she could find victory for her people. This extermination force, this force of degenification, would have war on their hands. 'Lîna made it her goal to become the fist of Ares. She would return the inferno of Hell to the dark enemy. She would die standing or not die at all but what she wanted was to crush her enemy with an equally dark fury of vengeance. The time for tears was at an end and the time to begin the crusade was upon 'Lîna. Whether or not she was unsure of herself, it did not matter now.

It was do or die, it was the dawn of Ragnarok and it would be this way for a long time to come. So there she stood in black leather, metallic mauve cut lines, skin clinging cashmere like leggings, a mauve metal waist belt of the same substance as on her legs, an onyx shoulder baring top of saffron with helix stitched straps that had two fist sized smooth rectangular gold broach clasps.

Above her left breast was the violet insignia of the Royal house of At'Lann: the tall, thin four-sided diamond covering a double helix. Her hair was like Medusa's; a tangled lotus blossom arrangement pulled back to unfurl into follicle twirls behind her tiara. So there she stood. The neophyte to what would become a violent war.

She hastily buried her feelings and clicked her way to fold herself to the main area of her quarters aboard her ship that she made her private orgia. Nul'lus awaited 'Lîna in her main living space. He had occupied his resting time with the solid photonic levitating At'Lann interface. Nul'lus had apparently begun to study the military reports on the enemy, the status of their estimated fleet size, and the build-up required by the alliance of all who would follow the At'Lann and the Lon'tus to defeat the onslaught. As 'Lîna came before Nul'lus, he rose to his feet and embraced his kindred friend.

Though 'Lîna rarely enjoyed being touched by those who found no meaning through sensation, her close friends, her family, and who she desired were her exceptions. She always did her best to fill her world with blissfully beautiful souls. Nul'lus then came to sit again on a plush dark navy leathery couch beside the interface display which hovered above a small deep black square table. On the table of seamlessly polished onyx like stone was a blue diamond serving tray adorned with a stack of freesia papered cigarettes. Nul'lus picked up the tray so that 'Lîna could partake in the therapeutic afters. 'Lîna took one then Nul'lus lit it for her with a Lon'tus hand lighter and its quick tawny flame.

As 'Lîna took her first puff, Nul'lus lit one up for himself. Her thoughts gave it all away. The justice of having to heal in the face of war seemed totally lacking. This tray had been brought in by her medical staff by Za'szu's order to subdue some of the effects of having activated the phase shift. Smoking these sticks of Caligula activated an ingredient in the genetic structure that balances matrix stability. Their genes were now enhanced with powers opened more wide open than before, yet hardly stable. Their bodies, in spite of their empowerment, still needed outside influences to sustain their volatile genetic sequences. They still needed to heal, and it was a problem compounded by the emotional carnage left by the contact point with the blitzkrieg that struck itself against the universe.

She sat beside her friend of the highest of Lon'tus peerage while the interface showed her the sanitised montage of visually graphic details of what she was about to face. War had at last broken their peace.

It was the ultimate siege, a horde, a force of carrion evil that had chosen a moment of apathetic distraction for their attack of lightning. All systems whether solar or galactic in reality, ones that teemed with life, were marked for death. The horde had attempted to eliminate as much as possible before moving on to the next killing fields. Once the universal siege had burned all there was to burn and scarred all there was to scar, and when having reached the ends of reality, would turnabout so the carnage may continue until no one would stand against pillage and death.

Their course trajectories indicated that, at this cardinal point circumspect, their wave of terror would swing back to purge the remaining elements of life in a far shorter time than they could presently be ready for. Sensor evidence suggested the warships of this sickness were difficult to target as the hulls of their warships and their crews possessed inverted life forces. This meant they were the constructs of a demonic being.

Science can easily be combined with the mystical but, unfortunately, the two can also be made into a perverted union. As Nul'lus and 'Lîna inhaled their cure, they read the terrible data of the status reports with eerie uneven disdain. Their attackers were automatons, yet their sentience and that which controlled them, was one of the purist of evils. A visual representation came on the screen of a corpse that once was the enemy before it had a portion of its calvarium vaporised by an At'Lann plasma rifle.

In charcoal brick like black garb, it had a humanoid structure but devoid of all goodness in now dead squinting eyes of a bitter cadaver. It was plain for the pair to see that these were creatures without souls. The void within their residue was filled by someone's powerful dark force. Nul'lus and 'Lîna had the genetic propensity to see beyond reality, and what they now saw only filled them with dread and disgust. There was not a single glimmer or ray of an aura around the corpse of a light that once served as a nest for a greater light within. The body had lived as it was: dead as an empty shell.

'Lîna and Nul'lus looked at each other while holding their mildly trembling cures, knowing what they faced was utter evil. The disgust, the repugnance of such a prospect, they could only feel their innocence was all the more quickly being torn away from their souls. Until eliminated, this plague of the darkest death would make their worlds homeless from the true spirit of home. Their insights and their instincts were in agreement, this threat had to be stopped at any cost.

A report came in from the Lon'tus Commonwealth data-link. The Lon'tus fleet was at half its strength. Nearly half of her ships had been obliterated in the first wave. Nul'lus's home world of the Rimisz'tii colony was spared most of the onslaught due to the valiant and the defiant strength of the Lon'tus military and fleet. However, Rimisz'tii's cities still burned, and their dead lay charred on their streets. The broadcast images estimated the loss of life in the millions. 'Lîna did not object to Nul'lus switching the interface back to alpha-numeric, and visual, graphical reports from other sources.

Their cigarettes burned and the room filled with a rouge hued frosty haze, yet the burning agent was so efficient that it left no ash. The two smoked their prescribed cigarettes and they began to relax as their enhanced genetic structures gained a stronger cohesion. It was a strange moment as 'Lîna and Nul'lus sunk into the chairs while preventing a serious health concern for themselves. They paid little thought to how important their existence was to the path for their peoples in war. The two sat transfixed watching planets burn on the mid-sized holo-screen before their eyes.

E'de had suffered greatly. Gaillard like cuts ravaged the surface like bloodied arms that protected a young E'de's face as she fell into the god-hooks of the wasteland. An estimated ninety seven percent of her living species that existed outside the home system had been obliterated and contact had been lost with the autonomous colonies of Hy'Bor with their inhabitants assumed to be all killed.

'Lîna's sight was unclear as to what remained. She had been distracted by her own selfishness. If I was not then what I am now...I could have saved them, thought 'Lîna. Though she felt sure some of their people lay scattered, alone but at least alive. She hoped for it to be. 'Lîna turned her attention away from the image of the burning E'de displayed on the holo-screen after lamenting for a moment of her time to the plight of her genetic cousins.

As Nul'lus and 'Lîna finished their first smoke, they lit up again to have every edge possible for when the two would return to the bridge. Their moments of repose were interrupted by a visual communication from Commander Mu'tolma. The interface lit up with his Roman centurion like features. He informed the pair that the Lis'talla had reached the rendezvous point with the fleet and the Royal flagship had come alongside the ships of her fleet. 'Lîna adjusted the interface with a finger touch on a holo-panel to have the image of her fleet brought on the screen. She could scarcely hide how very moving and tragic the image was. It was a terrible sadness but a sadness of future hope.

Though bloodied and battered they had remained as a testament to the strength of the At'Lann. Her ships had the appearance of being lain on a Weber's grill for far too long and without the joy of any taste that the walk across the bridge always brings. Some ships were barely holding their integrity fields together in the splintered metal beams that made them seem more like flying wounds than hulls of ships. But they had survived. They had survived the horde.

Some ships had the same design as 'Lîna's flag-ship with the majority of her fleet having a long cigar shaped craft of multiple solid metallic ellipses upon ellipses; a distinct framework like no other. Billows of dark mauve and emerald smoke blew into the spatial winds from where many ships incurred fresh battle damage. Some ships even tractor-beamed others to keep pace with holding the fleet's position.

In spite of the large size of 'Lîna's Lis'talla, what stood out to the eye was how unscathed her ship seemed to be, and how the smaller ships of the fleet had born the brunt of Hell's flames of genocide. Some of her destroyers were even smaller than that of some of the debris that remained from a lost dreadnought.

Though her fleet varied in size they did not vary in character, the gentilesse defiant nature remained in the crews that manned their fleet of plasma stream clawed vessels. In fact, it was a guilty pleasure for 'Lîna to be back in the lap of Luxor's caress on board the Lis'talla instead of the anchorite cramped voyaging that was exploring existence in her scout ship, the Kalu'ko.

It had been a long time since 'Lîna was in command of anyone other than herself. As a child, she commanded a division of ceremonial palace guards, the Sz'yana, before commanding a legion of the elite At'Lann guards, the S'yana, but rarely took a passion to it. She was too much a soul of freedom and 'Lîna's heart was always on the path of exploration. But in the today of her world, she had no choice: this was war, and At'Lann needed a leader. She had to give her gentry and her clan that followed a path like that for the clerisy, what they wanted. Uncomfortable with it or not, her people genetically had the desire to be led by an ancient Imperium line. 'Lîna was the genetic wisdom to lead, and it was her fate. Now was the time to use to its fullest her hidden potential that became the dogma of the At'Lann in war.

'Lîna tossed the smouldering end of the smoking roll onto the table for it to dematerialise into nothingness. She took another from the gilded tray and lit it up while still deep in thought. Nul'lus continued to pour over the combat reports. 'Lîna sat back, lightly crossing her legs, slid to rest her elbows onto the back of the couch, and then took in a long inhalation. She exhaled while at the same time waving away the hand that held the burning cure. She had a serious demeanour and seemed about to say something. 'Lîna stroked her violet flying willow hair, and twisted her locks into mauve with a curl of her slenderest finger. Then she spoke in a soft, gentle iris's way through her thoughts,

> 'Nul'lus. My years away. This siege. Death. Through all of it, I have missed you, our friendship. You are a kindred soul and though solace is now a precious commodity, I feel my last shred of peace knowing you share my path.'

Nul'lus smiled most humbly. He was every bit the genius loci of the mighty Lon'tus. He had too proud an aristocratic tradition to ever show openly the purest warmth of his heart but his face could not hide his happy feelings for what his friend 'Lîna thought of him. They were a kindred friendship. He bowed without boast as if he were saluting an equal. 'Lîna felt at ease having her ambassadorial friend here to fight alongside her. She passed him a cigarette and he lit another.

Nul'lus explained to 'Lîna that life had been quite uneventful without her on At'Lann. 'Lîna thought the forces of nature became the sardonic way to see things stirred up into cataclysmic proportions, to return home only to find war. Such a bitter pill swallowed so calmly. She wondered with him if peace had made them grow that weak for evil to unleash itself upon it.

She squeezed her friend's hand as she would for a brother. 'Lîna laughed a sad laugh and Nul'lus had a look of diligent attentiveness to procedure as his emotionally, passionately drawn masque of concern grew for her state of grief. But as quickly as 'Lîna almost lapsed into sorrow she found her way to regain concentration for the matters at hand. They both knew their optimum strength of their newly enhanced levels of power would take time to find and adapt to. Their genetic structures had been given little time to stabilize.

Nul'lus then showed 'Lîna a holo-display on the interface of their intelligence reports shared between their governments had estimated the weakest points on the warships of the enemy. He also showed her prototypes for stronger weapons that integrated aspects of both At'Lann and Lon'tus defence technologies. This was a joyous revelation for 'Lîna. She now had a slight bit of Pandora's hope.

At that moment, the bright yet subdued golden rays of the sun shone through the grand vertically rectangular windows of 'Lîna's vast conduct room as the pair looked out to see the remnants of the At'Lann fleet. Automatically, the contrast of the interface compensated for this moment of solar tangency. The room itself was set alight with the warm power that could never melt these wings of Icarus.

It was a sign before the At'Lann that would descend unto the breach, that at the very least, the true purity of their souls would survive this. 'Lîna asked Nul'lus to go to the main bridge of her ship and to contact his government to formalise an alliance for the impending war and to wait for her there. They both stood and held each other in their sanctuary of privacy before going to the business of governance. Nul'lus bowed to 'Lîna and left for the bridge.

As the hiss of the door tapered off into the silent run, 'Lîna sat down once again, took in a mild introspective breath and began to key in a rather complex sequence into her coffee table sized and placed interface. She activated the access point for the main data stream. The greatest wealth and bounty of the interface was now left in the righteous hands of Hebe jolted by blitzkrieg. But 'Lîna always lived by the laws that she was an equal shareholder to her people as she was the only shareholder. The only bounty sought by 'Lîna was freedom and this was the only path for At'Lann to head to. 'Lîna then began to speak in a soft and direct fashion,

'Interface Systems Flow. Implement the Imperium protocols. Authorization, 'Mura. 0 three, 0 three.'

A ravishingly succulent low choral electronic voice responded,

'Command Authorization Accepted. Proceed when ready.'

She pressed a large red square on the hovering holo-display of her interface.

She had been trained her whole life and designed so that duty preceded existence in times of war. Though a little frightened, she knew what to do. In lime green photonic sprouts, the fires of the data-stream flooding out of the interface flowed with an efficient fury. A sniper like shot of the lime flames flew towards 'Lîna. It struck her forehead without even a drizzling pain. However, her eyes became dilated from the gushes of this meld with new rivers of knowledge.

On the display of the interface terms such as "Spatial Folding Combat", 'Quantum Regeneration' and 'Tactical Warp Fold Alignments' in the spiriferous hieroglyphs that was the mauve pastel lit written language of those from 'Mura scrolled up the holo-display at an enhanced Johnson gold-jacked pace. Her form, a vessel of like that of Hebe and Sin, and her enhanced mind still walked the path as a neophyte to such matters in life. The data-stream extinguished itself in a wipeout whisper turbo thrust and the download cycle came to be complete.

'Lîna telekinetically reconfigured her tiara for even more of a razor-fest of angular edging and appearance. A fashion brought about by new specifications within her mind making one of her symbols of power an even greater talisman. She waved her tender hand into the air and a cloak of black sheer covered her once again. Tight black velvet gloves covered her hands and flowed underneath her emerald bracelets to her elbows. She could already feel the winds blowing from Hesperia foretelling a sliver of what was to come. It would be a venture into the valley of the most perilous of times. How pretty it seemed from the vista of one on the mountain path before it. 'Lîna composed herself into a mode of combat readiness. She was ready to go to the bridge and begin the business of war.

12
The Alliance Path

As she entered the main bridge, the crew stood to attention with an atmosphere of anticipation along with loyal faith and balanced devotion. They saw the configuration of 'Lîna's tiara under many draping of her black but now mauve bordered sheer and the crew knew what path she had chosen. The sheer end-tail trailed behind her like an evening summer's breeze over the wondrous Port Louis.

'Lîna swam in the tsunami of nervousness with the visage that was sculpted to the dynamics of one who returned home to lead. The hum of activity quietly lay sonically around her in this moment of circumstance. She walked with a confident stride, like one who was on the path Heraclitus could barely envision, towards the captain's chair. When she reached her throne of explorers, she sat as if she would for the slow easing of herself into a soothing hot bath. She crossed her smooth legs almost seductively before having a comfortable moment to see how the fleet had fared through the eye of the sensor scan displayed on the holo-screen. She waved her hand and tilted it lightly for the crew to be once again as they were.

The room still lay silent of chatter as the bridge crew resumed their posts on a plateau of high alter lit holo-displays of the Lis'talla's inter-link hyper-computational core. Even Nul'lus, sitting at a science station interface holo-display, waited to see what action the one who was now called herself Imperiatrix of the At'Lann Imperium would take. Like the rest of her crew and her people, he eagerly awaited her to carry out a command, speak, or even do anything to start a new chain of history. They all knew 'Lîna and what she could be for them through heritage and evolved genetic enhancement. As she had been trained to, 'Lîna had opened the Imperium protocols. With but the push of a button on the interface, At'Lann had become an empire, an imperium, with a young Imperiatrix taking her first steps on the path of war.

Nul'lus knew the At'Lann well, the soul of the people as it was but not of the feel of the At'Lann on the Imperium path. He did know of the specifics of the At'Lann Imperium protocols just as thoroughly as any of At'Lann would. It differed drastically from the imperial systems known by Nul'lus's Lon'tus Commonwealth. On his worlds, an imperial hierarchy, belief systems, and goals of acquisition existed in both times of peace and in times of war.

For the At'Lann, the differences in governance were drastic. When the At'Lann are only a speck on L'unn, they exist as a rather isolationist state of meditative existence and personal exploration and introspection. To the majority of the At'Lann, the exploration of the spatial wilderness seems fruitless as their belief is that home is only the reward of L'unn.

As an Imperium, the At'Lann spread their forces across the universe for its protection by any means necessary. Many worlds stepped upon by those of At'Lann in previous wars became part of At'Lann. Anywhere those of At'Lann walk can join in the holy allegiance towards the universal war effort. Their path in war was for the protection of life from what rises out of Death's mouth and the journey that is the march of war.

All would walk under the flag of At'Lann and the flags of her allies such as the Lon'tus Commonwealth for the cause of the Imperium. The At'Lann Imperium had always sought to find equals in her allies and gratitude from those too powerless to stand with the At'Lann in the cause of life and mutual understanding as allies in battle. These were the sole reasons the Imperium existed: to fight beside hyper-enlightened species or fight for the protection of all others. For the few who refuse to let those of At'Lann fly through their space, or walk on their worlds, would be left helpless to whatever threatened them, or they would be dealt with in a quick fashion but usually benevolently depending on the severity of the situation.

Historically and economically and depending upon the strategic value of whatever system they belonged to, the severity of the Imperium's actions were dictated by the necessary demands of the war efforts of the At'Lann.

For this had happened before. The hostile forces against the At'Lann have generally been found in the clouds of darkness that forges every heart of evil. And this is what draws the genetically divine species of purity of goodness into the fold of the Imperium's cause. Not only for the determination displayed by the At'Lann as they exist as a people in the Imperium but species are drawn to the At'Lann for their highly evolved spiritual, technological, and genetic unison of reality. Those factors play a key role in At'Lann leading the cause of those who flowed with the light from their ichor and this gave them the power to stand against the dark forces that wish to exterminate peace and freedom.

The Lon'tus Commonwealth's imperial system is set up to fully explore the games and theories of their permanent hierarchy, nobility, and civility. When At'Lann exists as an aspect of the Imperium, as Cincinnatus twice did, it is merely to facilitate a paradigm constructed for the defence of life threatened.

For the At'Lann, it was always drastic but never vicious. Even 'Lîna, like her At'Lann Imperium, would not rule with a fist of iron. Rather, she seemed intent on ruling with a tight velvet fist: soft and strong all at the same time. Sometimes their cause, their duty in war, is just like their own path which is to overwhelm existence until nature can be left to solitude again. It was this volunteered sacrifice of freedoms by lesser and sometimes equal species in the classic trade off that made the Imperium system work. Often, the most extreme cost of the lives given was for the protection of the Imperium. When their cause is complete, those of At'Lann, and those of the Imperium, return the autonomy and sovereignty to the regions they fought in or passed through, and simply return to L'unn. No strings ever attached.

When At'Lann only exist on L'unn they are the shining pearl floating along in the universe but as an Imperium they become another great link in the great chain of life called the Trinity links by the At'Lann. Their immortal and mortal path is to balance evil into its near extinction. It has happened before but never on such a scale as what was now facing the illuminated species of existence.

Historically, many others always rise to join the cause of the At'Lann as an Imperium. For it is the noblest honour to join the battles to protect life but many others also shed the most tender of tears for those who join the At'Lann and sacrifice their lives on the front lines for the continence of evolution and existence. This was Nul'lus's path as well. And for Nul'lus, there was not a more noble minded people that he could truly respect and stand with as he did for his own immaculately sculpted kinsmen. For Nul'lus, today was the day to be remembered as the first step on a great and perilous path. This was an occasion of fate and of vengeance driven pageantry.

Commander Mu'tolma, in his casual, near Tiberian diligence brought an updated status report to Lîna's attention. Apparently, A small but amply sized squadron of enemy ships had decayed itself away from the *horda* onslaught that had moved on. Their course trajectories suggested that they were on their way to the H'Raka home world to reinforce a leprous infestation that still was a siege around the warrior's dominion.

The H'Raka are a honed race of legendary and powerful hunters. Warriors of an ancient virtue, unique in the universe but had become an enemy of the At'Lann. Ever since 'Lîna's parents had revoked the exclusive charter and licences from the

Nordic etched beings of sword and soul, to hunt the macro-creatures of E'de, and sealed the borders of E'de and the At'Lann L'unn home solar system of Tr'Lann from all ships that belong to the H'Raka. The paths of the At'Lann and the H'Raka had remained separate for quite some time

It was a case of petty politics with a stink of something like rotting pomegranates that undermined the most minute and immense changes of circumstance, a decorum that led to a fall of an alliance barely remembered from the early time past At'Lann's inchoation. Long before their evolution toward maximized space exploration. A time long since past when their ships regularly travelled past one another to each of their respective ports to trade technologies and innovations. Relations between the two states were as frozen as being caught in the gaze of a bitter Medusa. And this was still the case for the At'Lann and the H'Raka.

In the early times, the two powers had fought as allies in many wars, a tag team to make the air of even N'Bira explode with supernovas, and together found many victories dreamed by Copernicus in the dreamlands of combat. 'Lîna surmised that the momentum towards unity fell to the winds of peace time, long past the days of early trading. Due in part to the At'Lann believing in a most rigid serenity which found itself unable to handle the gruff, aggressively efficient nature of a warrior race constantly visiting their world before going off to E'de to hunt worthy game.

The H'Raka seemed to remain an honourable people but the H'Raka could also be far too overbearing for the transcendent seeking At'Lann with their sometimes blood thirsting ways to find a true commonality with an At'Lann once in Imperia with H'Raka. In modern times, the two powers never went to war as neither government wished to offend their fellow mutual Imperium path walker but their respective ships always had their guns raised to one another if they passed by one another in deep space.

The Lon'tus Commonwealth still had relations with the H'Raka since their culture was far more tolerant of the ways of warrior races. The H'Raka were always proud to welcome those of Lon'tus as the H'Raka could be themselves without armour and battlements in the purist aristocratic serenity and diplomacy that are the Lon'tus are renowned for. 'Lîna in all her days of exploration, and even still, wished to visit H'Raka but never could due to the closed borders. 'Lîna had become inspired to take, perhaps, a different path. This information sent 'Lîna in search of what the next gambit would be.

'Commander Mu'tolma, display the astrometrical scan of the H'Raka home world on the main holo-screen.'

'Lîna's tone was both stern with only a slight tinge of sweetness as it was inquisitive. She could feel something was astir. The reality came to her eyes. The scan revealed in a Katyn like graphic detail that the H'Raka home world was surrounded by a swarm of enemy vessels. It would seem the dirty *horda* had singled out this world especially for the most damaging and most dastardly bombardments. Simply put, the H'Raka had offered the enemy too much resistance. One world out of the entire universe singled out by the invasion of the inferno that had garnered itself additional hellfire.

It more than piqued 'Lîna's interest as she studied the data. It fascinated her that the dark horde would save a greater brutality for what the enemy could only see as a powerful foe. This gave 'Lîna a great sense of hope and Pandora salvaged opportunity.

However, there was no mention of the continuing battle, in the skies or on the surface of H'Raka, or on any of the military reports. Nor was there mention of it in the report that Mu'tolma had given 'Lîna previously. 'Lîna had a wave of feelings of uneasiness wash over her. She could see by the nervous reaction in Commander Mu'tolma's face that he was unwilling to share his thoughts. His tanned saffron Aegean etched curls of short hair became puffed as the hairs on the back of his neck stood up.

'Lîna reacted with suspicion. 'Commander, why was I not informed of this earlier?'

'Lîna asked without the civility of hiding her accusative, comfortably toned anger and frustration. She did not hold back her displeasure. To have ultimate confidence 'Lîna expected nothing less than the essence of Myrmidon. As the empress, the Imperiatrix of At'Lann, she had to set a better standard of command. To 'Lîna, withholding esoteric knowledge and especially intelligence data, from an absolute ruler, was a heavy sin. 'Lîna's displeasure grew with each word out of the mouth of Mu'tolma.

'...Imperiatrix...they are our enemy, and have been for some time. I did not inform you as the H'Raka would probably betray us and use this incursion as an opportunity to attack our territory.'

The words seemed fit for the unenlightened hoi polloi through a media pitch. 'Lîna had never heard such a selfish and anxious statement from her cousin before but they had never interacted in the format of the military hierocracy and with her as ruler. 'Lîna found the stain of lies in his truth. She thought she knew her cousin well but perhaps she finally saw a side of her cousin for what he truly was: a young mind and soul. What angered her even more was that Mu'tolma would not have given such lacklustre loyalty to her father.

'Lîna could feel his thoughts, and felt her way in and out of his soul. She could see it as plainly as she could see the battle raging around the H'Raka home world: Mu'tolma was jealous of her rank that she had squandered her entire life. To him, her explorations bordered on heresy. It was not a malicious jealousy but it was a jealousy from a fate far better than Ixion's though just as perpetual, and denied lenity. It was obvious that Mu'tolma thought the line would end with her. She was incapable of victory in spite of her constantly refining form, strikingly dissimilar from his heritage. The blood flow of one like Ithun was far more unbending than

'Lîna's new evolutionary path.

As heir to the throne, she had been given the gift of command until this aspect of her lay restrained within in her after exploring the universe. Now, she returned to lead without a blink of time in the trenches. This offended Mu'tolma who fought in the last At'Lann war but returned unchanged from his simple creeds of temperance.

To 'Lîna, this was the disadvantage of what seemed to her an immature soul. Too young a soul to go beyond such things that 'Lîna began to know as the reality of dread that everything had become. 'Lîna was furious, the Imperiatrix could only see little depth before her. She could feel that Mu'tolma still cared for her but felt nearby to what was her should perhaps be his. For 'Lîna, at this moment before the defining undertaking, her pity could hardly stretch past a mere shrug of her shoulder.

It was a shame Mu'tolma seemed too young to comprehend that power is never truly enjoyed and that it is a responsibility not for all. What Fate thrusts upon is that which it does. The sweetest power is the delight of freedom. When one has to lead, their freedom is forsaken, when one lives, their life is truly their soul's desired reality. When one who comes to lead, theirs is the loss of true power since the greater good becomes united with ones' very path. 'Lîna's thoughts swirled as she shook her head in disappointment. She was slightly saddened by what she saw in Mu'tolma.

'Mu'tolma, I am quite displeased with your actions. Your cautious, near self-serving strategic decisions shall not be tolerated in the new order. Re-evaluate your thoughts. They are flawed. You are relieved of command.'

Mu'tolma was stunned as if he was just red-carded. He could not believe that he was being sent off. 'Lîna's pained blood ran icily with civil viciousness. She poured even more salt onto the wound,

'Return to your quarters and wait there for reassignment...That is all.'

'Lîna gazed and froze her thoughts into the expanse that souls find themselves in when in disagreement. "Yes, my Imperiatrix and Crown of the people." Mu'tolma said in his southern At'Lann military parlance in a tone that was taken completely aback and one wounded by her words. Mu'tolma had no idea 'Lîna would react this way. He gritted his teeth. Mu'tolma could not react with any measure of recourse. He could still feel 'Lîna's presence in his mind. Mu'tolma came to understand that even the slightest dissent was far too much for what 'Lîna knew as the highest of stakes. She hoped he would overcome this.

Commander Mu'tolma stood stiff, saluted the At'Lann salute, and 'Lîna nodded respectfully to her cousin as he left the bridge silently through a nave in the fourth wall of the bridge. At the very least, 'Lîna could feel in her heart that her cousin, a friend in the years before the transcendent genetic alteration, would have a measure of honour about the whole affair. 'He will overcome this. The war would be far too much for him once again as one had been quite enough for one of the few veterans of the last war. Though there is always a redemptive quality to fate,' 'Lîna thought.

As the doors hissed to seal themselves closed once again at the far left corner of the bridge, 'Lîna swung her captain's chair to confer with her friend Nul'lus. She raised her right eyebrow for a moment. Nul'lus returned the acknowledgement that this would be a very perilous path with a whimsical smile from one whose home could well have been Anfield. Somehow, he could feel what 'Lîna was to say far in advance of her mauve-violet lips. She seemed almost unsure of herself as her words entered the sonic land scape of a windhover.

'So it seems I need a new first officer for the Lis'talla, the flag-ship of my fleet. Would you like to join the sovereign errant by returning the Imperium to life?' 'Lîna asked without hesitation.

'Now, who was being selfish?', thought Nul'lus. To 'Lîna, who made honesty her way, often times far too directly, looked mystically to Nul'lus who with a smile back that responded to how ironic that thought was. She was merely impatient. 'Well, Ambassador?', 'Lîna asked again with a mild giggle of wisdom.

Many on At'Lann knew of the defining character of the Ambassador of Lon'tus and considered him and his Lon'tus refined ways, a soul of experience to be so akin to that of the At'Lann. There would be no opposition to her command decision but, in fact, it would be met with many cheers and grace. 'Ha! Ha! Ha!' Nul'lus' laugh of cultural brilliance filled their section of the bridge. He amusingly patted his right knee before taking her hand as if before to trek to the top of Kailas.

'Well, I suppose I could find myself in worse binds. Lets get to it,
and give it a good show',

'Lîna met his words with symphonic feelings of joyful pride. If this was not such a dark time, there would be high-fivery that she would be with her friend and they would share the excitement of going off on an adventure together. But alas, it was not the happiest of times and such behaviour was not befitting of a leader of an evolved people. In a station of play moment of command, 'Lîna spoke again. It was a voice that hardly wanted to order her friend about.

'Very well then. Commander Nul'lus. Signal the 'Verga and the Ki'Bur. They will be our escorts. Break off from the rest of the fleet. We will engage the enemy that remained behind in the H'Raka system and their reinforcements. Have the fleet deploy Imperium defensive protocols. Set a course.'

'Course set and laid in, Imperiatrix of At'Lann. We will arrive in twelve at'Lann cycles.'

It would seem Nul'lus played 'Lîna's game as well and was ready to play once more.

'What was the word from who might now be the Imperator of Lon'tus?', 'Lîna asked.

Nul'lus told her the words of support she wanted to hear.

'The Lon'tus fleet will reinforce the At'Lann fleet at a full Imperium fleet level by tomorrow.'

Comfortably, 'Lîna swiveled the centre seat to face the holo-screen. Its image shifted to show the magnification of the enemy vessel classifications they would encounter. Nearly four hundred smaller enemy ships, generally single fighter sized, jet-black scarabs of vessels, and a few warships close to the size of the Lis'talla. Her modified genetic structure seemed to thirst for the oncoming moment of battle. She could see it in Nul'lus as well.

What had changed them was beginning to shape them. The lust to battle the enemy would have to wait until they would reach the point of engagement, and to give a hint to her people of what will be the future. She was the holder of burdened privilege. It was her path to give At'Lann what the faithful craved: an enlightened honesty of being chosen as their leader of strength. 'Lîna, through autonomous psyogenic manipulation, was made the most enhanced of her species.

What was fast becoming her jaded innocence of being was exactly the spirit of the At'Lann gave their destiny to. What was becoming her reputation began in these days when it was thought the Imperiatrix bore suffering so well and returned from her time in the spatial wilderness so different from when she left as a younger girl. She felt guilty that she might not give them enough hope that goodness and balance of life would prevail.

'Lîna signaled a young brunette and peach skinned yeoman with lines like those of a Silesian princess, to begin transmitting her holo-image live from the main bridge to all communication inter-links across the At'Lann Imperium. She rose from her battle throne to face the eye of the holo-sensor. Her words came to her like the passionate Kalahari wind of providential felicity.
She was as laissez-faire as she was a believer in laissez-passer in her demeanour.

'People of At'Lann. This is your Imperiatrix, Za'Lîna 'Imiszi 'Mura'Lann. An enemy life-form has launched an onslaught against existence. There is murder upon the universe. We, the At'Lann and all those of the Imperium have declared formal war against the scourge. I will personally command our defence forces until this threat has been eliminated. Resource allocation will shift to the Imperium war model. Of those on L'unn, you will be protected from further bombardment by the L'unn phase generator, and by reinforcements to the L'unn defence force by the At'Lann Imperium fleet...However, be prepared to face further insurgencies as the enemy may still be able to counteract our defences.

Whatever the cost, I will protect you. I have personally taken command of our flagship, the Lis'talla. Along with the Ki'Bur and the 'Verga as sanctioned escorts, we are setting a course to join the fleet at what will be the front. The fleet will engage and counterattack the enemy.

With the Lon'tus Imperium at our side, we will liberate our universe from this spectre. Our military scientists have already adapted our targeting and weapon systems to find and destroy enemy ships. Our shields have been re-modulated. You

are my stakeholders and my own. I live to not forsake you. The vile nature
that is the enemy of forever shadows will be purged from our paradise of life. In
our defence of what is sacred, we shall not back down...I have returned to be your
crusader of all that shall remain immortal. I will rule
to return existence to peace and freedom.'

'Lîna elegantly raised her head, and let the hood of her cloak fall to her shoulders. The jet-black sheer fell from her face. Her face was still one of innocence yet her eyes reflected a heart that was forged into something stronger. Her darker than normal violet hair was tied tight past her tiara and her movements were just as fluidly flexed. She took a step forward from where she stood and finished her words to the people of the At'Lann Imperium,

'It will be a long time before I once again gaze upon the great ocean of K'mja Khonn and beauty of At'Lann, of 'Mura'Lann. The beauty I hold in my heart is what is worth fighting for. The oceans, the life flow, the people of At'Lann and all of the Imperium. Our purity of maximised enlightenment shall not fall to the darkness of what stands against us. My faith is all of At'Lann standing with me.

Be strength, be bravery, and stand tall. Though we are plunged into war, our soul of peace shall forever be immortal. Blessed are we who define existence.
Prosperity will remain continuous.'

'Lîna began to tremble as soon as the transmission was completed. Her words had come from her very soul. Though power had always been thrust upon her, she always hoped her people would accept her path. The enthusiasm on the bridge of the Lis'talla typified the total support given to the new order of the Imperiatrix. If one swam the emotions of those at her side, 'Lîna had infinitesimally very little to worry about.

As the commotion that is bridge became one of routine operations once again, ship life quickly returned after so much pomp, circumstance, and of officers standing at attention yet again. 'Lîna sat back down again in the captain's chair. She turned her attention to Nul'lus. She leaned over to him with the expression one has after a taxing situation. Nul'lus had a visage of halted amusement on his face. His tone was hushed but it was a sunrise of inquisitiveness.

'Are you of the At'Lann line no longer?'

'Lîna was playing a game that was all her own.

'I have my reasons. Besides, I am Imperiatrix. I can do what I please for the greater good.'

Her starkly delightful whisperings gave Nul'lus a head-shaking of amazement and a stifled thunderous gentleman's chuckle. She really wanted to make a mark. She was shifting the entire economy of her people to a catapult stream model. Nul'lus could also see beyond this to glimpse upon what she felt inside of herself was another matter altogether. Cocky moves were a dangerous motivational tool for a girl unsure of herself.

Φ

To keep optimism and morale constant, to have them gain confidence in their leader, 'Lîna took the path of burying herself in the work of war. As quickly as she had a moment of reflection, she went back to the business of preparing for the next leg of this baptism of hellfire. For all she was, she was afraid. For 'Lîna, there were no other options, her only option was to win. She did not want to let anyone down. She would have to be everything to all things. But 'Lîna always looked for opportunity amidst chaos. She would turn her fear into an outlet of near divine ambitious ferocity to use against the dark enemy. 'Lîna calculated the fiercer she was, the less she would have to fear from what is called evil.

She turned to face a young jade-azure skinned lieutenant with sea-foam hued hair manning the tactical systems interface array. 'Lîna instructed her lieutenant, a loyal youth primed model soldier, a model officer of the At'Lann military, to send engineering teams to reinforce the hull at specific co-ordinates chosen by her. By modifying the structural integrity of the Lis'talla, they would be ready to once again face an enemy that has a tendency towards suicide runs.

'Lîna could foresee it all too well. The dashing 'Valis Mir'hali Val'Damus, without hesitation, carried out the command with a crew pleasant 'Your will is ours, Captain and Imperiatrix.' 'Lîna felt well received for what was her due. This crew would voyage to peril and pleasure, through the gates of Hell and into the hurricane of the inferno. For one on the path of war, the juice is the action. Lt. Val'damus then signalled the Ki'Bur and the 'Verga to implement the same measures as he could see her will as thought intertwined with that which was the exactitude of what she wanted. And he soon completed what she wanted as well by transfiguring his interface to send the same order out across the fleet and had them also had them re-modulate their signal beacons to be cloaked from enemy scams as the Lis'talla crew had already done with theirs.

She sat back and began to reach deeply into her self. 'Lîna shot out her thoughts and telepathically, with her thoughts magnified into the At'Lann Interface data-flow, and began to give out orders across the fleet. From troop deployments, subspace mine grid areas, output levels, to duty hours, she designed an unorthodox paradigm of resource allocation. In fact, the fighter pilots on the Lis'talla, the Ki'Bur and the 'Verga were given new attack patterns directly from the Imperiatrix.

As the Imperium fleet was left in the wake of the Lis'talla, the fleet broke off and dispersed across the universe where their strength would be bolstered by allies and conscripts. She also sent a thousand of her warships ahead to the H'Raka border. 'Lîna was about to pour petrol onto an already raging fire. In the boldest of times, 'Lîna, of all people, walked the path to be the boldest.

With power re-routed from the space-folding drive shifted to the weapons batteries, the ship had to cruise along through quantum gates to their first battle. The vaunted counterattack awaited. A defence, a resistance, was taking form. This gave 'Lîna an empathic wave of confidence. She could feel it coming together. Indeed, she more than had the lust for it. It all seemed to fall into place so easily. It would be her first time going into battle, and as she made her way deeper into the path of war, she could hardly wait.

13
A Farewell To One

After a long shift on the Lis'talla's bridge, 'Lîna found herself once again in her main quarters. Weapons batteries, shield adaptations, attack patterns, tactical exercises, and ship logistics were all brought up to task. The Lis'talla's shields could now withstand multiple collisions with enemy ships. Using information gathered from enemy ship hull fragments found on L'unn, in At'Lann space and that of a Imperium member, the 'Tazi'ma, a quantum flux pattern, no longer in general usage, was found that could pierce enemy armour.

Feeling assured that her crew would be protected, 'Lîna now found time to better prepare herself for her role in the game of war that would become all too insipid all too fast. Her first chance to prove herself to her people that their trust in her was not misplaced. She wanted to honour them as only she could. After smoking a few gene stabilizing agents from her ample dispensary, 'Lîna began to place herself into a deep meditative state apart from the cellular balancing.

She had to rid herself of unwanted thoughts. She had to rid herself of the unwanted shame of what happened in the main corridor outside the bridge. It was kept restricted and, thus, deserted when had 'Lîna left the bridge for some private imperial solitude. She had pushed herself far too hard for herself for the first day of command as the Lis'talla etched itself ever closer to battle. As the lilac marble heavy door to the bridge shut behind her, 'Lîna had partially lost her genetic cohesion. She hoped no one saw her cringing with the skin of her face rippling like cyclone waters as her molecules came in and out of spatial phase.

'Would they have been horrified or would they have shed a tear for me?', 'Lîna thought in her moment of sudden, crippling pain. She thought she was becoming unbound and she especially had to rid herself of that particular thought. She fell deeper into the trance like a silent moonsault into a linn and deeper into the waters of the soul.

While her standing body remained softly still, in her room, 'Lîna shut her eyes and her physicality began to be variant. Flesh and bone were woven into mauve psionic energy. 'Lîna's form then entirely became an illuminating mist of mauve. She began to glow brighter and bright, as in a house throb of epileptic seizure inducing strobe energy. So much so that she filled the entire post-modern baroque sketched room with the self-divine light of her colour.

The ether around her danced itself into gravimetric, luminescing geometric parallel angles of light. The violet firelight drew into itself after one could say its touch was divinely lecherous. A lime green light of Eros eclipsed pushed itself out of 'Lîna. She stretched out across the reality of her room and beyond. She directed the emerald to intersect with the mauve at right angles.

As the surging energies intersected, they combined themselves to a perfect interlock. She found a precious moment of bliss now scarce to those who walk the heavens. Her light burned as brightly as her mind could allow in her joy of finding a diversion of peace. For a blink of time, community became unity. Somehow, 'Lîna found within herself the renewal of a more tolerable state of genetic cohesion. The wisdom of the Imperium protocols had been absorbed into every cell of hers. From within herself, she also found points beyond the extremes of the protocols. She wondered if she truly was something more.

'Lîna was in a state of optimal strength and genetic cohesion. Every piece of her seemed to be perfectly fitting into place after the trauma of having it all fall apart outside the bridge. Whether this would last was not known but 'Lîna, for this fractional blink of time, would enjoy the feeling of being complete in her transcendent meditation. This was to be savoured by her as an inspiration on the field of battle. Her essence seared everywhere beyond the beyond. This was nirvana, and it awaited. All became serene, solid, smooth, and penetrating. She was ready.

Like an end to a kestrel's search, the compulsion to return to the surface of all things came to her in the ether that was the fiercest depths of the ocean of her soul, 'Lîna called back the light of her being. It filled her until she was once again a slender Hebe like woman. Her post-orgasmic smile exhaled itself. 'Lîna's thoughts were structured for the mission yet they were also structured to gain the logic of peace in all flows of thought.

It was a good thing 'Lîna had this time to herself to compose herself from all the recent disasters as her sister, Za'szu, had come to see her.

If 'Lîna was not so distracted by the chime of her door, she might have felt a drop of blood trickle from her nose. Somehow, it no longer seemed important to her for that tiny blink of time. But as quickly as the few droplets of deep violet blood flowed out of her, the molecules of her ichor fell completely out of phase and dissipated into nothingness. With the luck of Fortuna, it went unnoticed. A deeper part of her wondered if Nul'lus had been affected as strongly by the enhancement but she was far too afraid to ask him now. After all, her sister had come her. 'Lîna signalled for her side-entrance to open. With a pneumatic sound of stone dragging across itself swiftly and smoothly, her door opened and magnificent Za'szu entered the state room.

Za'szu's demeanour was far below the warmth of pleasantry. She had come with gripes and caring anger, a result of 'Lîna's actions, and Za'szu felt more than justified in her beliefs. 'Lîna was, at times, reckless, and her younger sister could only take so much before she had broken her last straw. The results of such conflicts between them usually consisted of bruised egos and a further commitment to act as guide posts for one another in the path of life. But this day was different. Just by seeing the look on Za'szu's hyper-intellectually hyper-fashionable At'Lann female visage, 'Lîna was not sure if there ever would be a sisterly conciliation after this.

As 'Lîna changed her posture to a more defensive and defiant one, Za'szu came to a face down her maverick sister. The mauve metallic door shut, sealing the darkened room for the conflict of siblings to simmer to a boil.

'How dare you throw away an eternity of our history for your selfish whims. How could you?'

Za'szu's visage became moulded by the fires of angry logic.

'Do not even start, Za'szu. I have a war to fight.'

'Lîna's words were far sharper than were usual for her. She did not want to show her dear sister any weakness found in the strength of her new genetic structure and that she would lead the At'Lann on a proper course through this interval of time. But Za'szu was always able to dig into telepathic areas where 'Lîna did not defend well against her.

'Some preparation', quipped Za'szu.

'You expect to lead the war as head of the house of 'Mura and make it your house of 'Mura'Lann. Not At'Lann. Are you casting aside what you are? You have altered our arrangement and you use your highest of absolutes to zealously punish your cousin without thinking at all of your people. You *are* different now. I was wrong to think you would become anything more than a spoiled brat. What would Mother and Father say? What will be left of you?'

Za'szu's flood of thoughts almost put 'Lîna into a state akin to cardiac arrest. Za'szu was more than angered like a grizzly in a swarm of bees, she seemed to take this matter most personally. 'Lîna was even more coldly vicious with her words and thoughts.

'My reasons for what path I take are mine and mine alone, sister. Perhaps if you were not feeling so passed over, we would not be having this conversation. You knew this day would come and you have always known there are some traditions we can do without.

Do not act like you are burdened by disappointment. You are not taking the place of Mother and Father. I am. I will save our world by any means necessary. What would you have done? Anger the enemy with your logic until they would decide to kill you? You feel it is your place to lead, that you have earned this right, and it never should have been given to me.

Do you think your path of order will survive in such chaos? I draw upon the infinite wisdom of power that has been thrust upon me. Leave. You are nothing to me anymore.'

Ever since the psyogenetic change, 'Lîna's attitude became far too haughty for even tolerant Za'szu to stand, and Za'szu after hearing this wondered why she bothered coming at all. 'Lîna certainly did everything possible to fan the flames of disdain with her sister she once always competed with. By now Za'szu was clenching her teeth, and trembling as she restrained herself from striking 'Lîna. Most particularly, it was her tender yet strong, tiny fists that shook. 'Lîna had ignited all the rage in the heart of her steaming sister and like many conflicts past, 'Lîna had gone far beyond the line of proper etiquette.

Most of their sibling battles usually ended up being Pyrrhic victories for one or the other. Usually, 'Lîna would relent after going this far but she was so focused and obsessed with victory that she would not relent this time. So there she stood, letting the rage build in her sister. It all seemed so ridiculous but, sadly, there was nothing to laugh about.

'I can see what you are full of, 'Lîna. How safe will we be with you at the helm? Who are you anymore?'

With words of both love and seething pain, a disgruntled Za'szu turned her back to her sister and made way for the door. Nothing could be salvaged from the moment at hand and 'Lîna remained scathing in her viciousness, and raised her voice to stop her sister before she could open the door. Za'szu was dead in her tracks.

'Not so fast. If you want to leave my personal presence, fine. But I want you off my ship. You will not be part of our external military operations. Return to At'Lann using the secure subspace private corridor. You are the Regent-Governor of the domestic government. They will need your abilities more than I do.'

Then as the two faced each other for what could be the last time. 'Lîna twisted the long thorn all the way through as she spoke without any regard.

'Do as you are told, Za'szu!'

Za'szu had enough of this posturing. Time seemed to crawl incrementally slower as she furiously spit at her own sister with the strongest gales of emotional fury. Za'szu raised her fist and it glowed with a thick malachite fire before powering up to a level the three sisters called the opal cascade. Opal hued psionic energy fires burned from Za'szu's right hand.

Za'szu's inherent genetic structure allowed her to open micro-quantum fissures and direct them as controlled energy. The room was a frigid girandole display. Za'szu was formidable but she walked another path than 'Lîna after the L'unn phase shift.

Before the hurling 'Mura saliva could reach her cheek, 'Lîna vaporised the ballistic molecules with a trans-quantum energy blast from her right little finger, after which 'Lîna blew away the near aubergine phased smoke from that little finger that was the only one uncurled in her hand.

'Get out.'

As Za'szu left, she uttered the words to ensure the coffin like the over a year like that of 1795 would be nailed violently shut.

'I hope you never come back.'

The door shut again with the telepathic slamming of it, and with Za'szu gone, 'Lîna's heart was as empty as her immaculately arranged room. She had really done it this time. Some leader I am turning out to be, she thought. How could she run a war effort when her own House was not in order, she wondered. But 'Lîna was a resourceful anchorite, an ever more tormented creature of solitude.

She was once again in her own element, yet pushing away so rashly her sister's concerns out of the way to get where she would want to be. It was certainly something that did not please her. Perhaps, when the war was over she could reveal her weaknesses to Za'szu and be open to her about her true feelings that she was able to hide so well under the callous veneer of anger.

She had to shut out her sister but 'Lîna always seemed to find what sometimes seemed the hardest way of doing things and now only seemed to find the most difficult of paths. 'Lîna would have to try and bury her conscience as much as she could for the war. She was successful in isolating herself from Za'szu. And with the way things went, it would not matter to her if she lived or died. In the oddest of ways that is chaotic logic, 'Lîna was trying to protect her younger sister from whatever pain she would endure by having Za'szu filled with scorn for her. It was a strange and perverse path taken to leave her gentle sister in the safer hands of home. Hers was a most chaotic logic and it was a logic that did not want Za'szu to miss her if she perished on the front. If worse came to worse, 'Lîna wanted to see Za'szu outdo her as Imperiatrix if that became the case.

None of this would take away the pain in her heart but now she had nothing to lose and everything to gain. The ideal mind state for a warrior is one where there is nothing left to lose. At least 'Zaya still stands with me, 'Lîna thought. Not that she did not have strong feelings for 'Zaya, rather, they never argued, never competed, and never pushed one another to get under each other's skin. Theirs was a different bond, and the truth was, 'Lîna felt she would be helpless without her.

But 'Lîna felt more alone than had ever felt before. She no longer felt Za'szu's presence on board. She had indeed returned to At'Lann. 'Lîna was, at the very least, glad her people were in good hands. Za'szu would serve them well. Now there was nothing left for 'Lîna to do but think of all the emotions inspired by their private scandalous war of words. Her heart remained heavy, yet true to the task.

She sat alone, and smoked another cohesion stabiliser. Not that she needed to but this would be the last chance to work in any extra edge before the battle in the stars would commence. It was the only thing that passed the time while she sat alone in her own private limbo.

14
The Dankly Fermented Tastes of Battle

'Lîna was called to the main bridge as they neared the enemy's weapons range. They would soon engage the swarm that lay directly ahead. They were just past the Vu'latta system on the outskirts of H'Raka space. How their swarthy fleet polluted space; how the stench of the enemy was everywhere! So many natural wonders had been lain to waste. It was vile, 'Lîna thought. Only this time, the At'Lann were as ready as they could be for them. 'Lîna and Nul'lus had devised a strategy for this impediment.

'Lîna then walked from the captain's seat as the small fleet of locusts of doom came into perfect focus across the holo-screen in all their dark glory. She then took the fourth wall, an intra-ship spatial folding system, to the seventeenth cargo bay after giving the order to attack, commanding that the Lis'talla fire at will. Her youngest sister 'Zaya was there to take command of the bridge.

'Lîna left the bridge walking into a dive like that into the smoothly penetrating waters of a Muskoka lake as she phased through the sunset silver, iron cast looking fourth wall of the main bridge. Nul'lus followed her in but he had left for the main airlock on the lower level. For his noble role today he would not need a vessel or a ship. He would only need his enhanced forces of power.

'Lîna looked about the cargo bay, at the mandrake sketched rows of grid shelving filled to capacity with a simply gigantic number of black metal cubes, each the size of ottomans. In the dim gleam of this cargo bay came the first steps into the dank fermented world of war. She hoped her sister 'Zaya would leave her bridge as she had left it. The anticipation was cast aside as her mantic way blossomed from the very heart of her soul. Her bereavement at all that she had already lost was left to lament for another day.

She had her mind configure itself into a state of completeness. Her only regret being she would have less time allotted in their strategy to fight in a closer fashion alongside Nul'lus but she could feel the path of war would give her plenty of time.

Her curiosity still got the best of her as 'Lîna wanted to see Nul'lus in action with this being her first opportunity to following the psyogenetic enhancement. Then again, she thought, it would also be his first chance to see what 'Lîna is now made of.

Her eyes shifted to the style of a great predator, like those held by a resurrected phoenix whose gaze has fallen upon that which murders flight. 'Lîna felt as if she was nailed to the cross for far longer than three hours already, and it had only just begun.

She pressed down on an azure lined release button on a single control panel before her. Space and time fell silent for an instant. The offensive had begun. The cube shells faded away to reveal humming night train grey disc shaped devices that lay inside. They were slipstream splice mines, similar technologically to the output of their weapons systems.

The mines, when detonated, have the power to obliterate spatial and molecular linkages of most substances in such a destructive effect that the space the mines explode in cannot be traversed using even current hyper-flux drive technology for fifty At'Lann years. Spatial folding becomes all but impossible for generations unless a new innovation comes along.

'Lîna gave one last thought of her existential insights into all that is fate and passed them along to Nul'lus and 'Zaya in the fraction of Cronos's gaze before he would see action. The man of action would step up to the pitch of champions. Duty took on entirely new meanings.

'Lîna was being relied upon as much for her place at the throne of the At'Lann Imperium as she was for her new found enhanced powers. And for that, Nul'lus and 'Lîna were the crux of the mission, keystones of Imperium victory if it were to come. She did not want to be remembered as a ruler who merely watched battles.

'Lîna vowed to endure as much of the suffering of this dark chasm as she possibly could be able to. She wanted real memories of her to be made in action good or bad. Yet not everything was to be filmed and 'Lîna would not contradict herself. This was her fate, and she had begun to discover other sides of her nature. In this moment, she felt as if she had awakened to another truth of life.

She began to grow as if in light speed into herself. She not only went to a deep and powerful state known to those who swim the temporal surf, she became it. To the farthest reaches of existence her spirit reached out. And all the more quickly as she came to new thought flows, she left so many others behind. She had taken herself to a new path and crossed the threshold of reality. Temporal and spatial laws no longer applied to 'Lîna. She felt as if she was all things and existed within all things. She was so much more than she had ever been that it frightened her.

It was eerie for her. She never considered herself on the path of a god before, yet she felt as if she could be. 'Lîna refocused her thoughts as she had a mission to complete. She had gifts for the invading fleet. Though she probably would not be able to do this manoeuvre to effect the entire enemy force as she was not yet strong enough to, she could deal with this small fleet.

In her mobile trance state, 'Lîna came to exist in all spatial angles within frozen time, one temporally frozen state, and yet, moving existence. In this new state, all that moved for her was at a hyper-accelerated speed. She had all of eternity to simply feel a mine into her hand and place it on the engine core of each enemy warship. Time and reality no longer had meaning as she weaved her way throughout what was left. It was wondrous as she strolled the cargo bay in one reality segment while mining enemy engine cores in another aspect within 'Lîna's small dissection of time and space.

To the dismay that one like Fortuna would feel, the enemy became wise to this technique. Some influence rode ghastly from the dark void from which the enemy had been spawned and countered 'Lîna's move.

As the state of peace before war, akin to the stillness of walk on a briskly humid winter Ottawa day shattered into submission by the damning ferocity of the cold, 'Lîna weaved herself back into the reality before her. She shivered in from the humid cold. She found the jarring shift back to the linear temporal flow unnerving. 'Lîna regained her warmth by the satisfaction of watching one hundred and seventy nine enemy warships begin to explode.

Using her heightened perceptions, 'Lîna could see within the thorax like hulls of the enemy vessels to see the mines explode. Explosions of mezereon hued energy particles igniting to violently decimate their sinister containment cores, setting off a chain reaction in their power grids. The enemy warships then became the tar violets fragmentary fireballs. Their explosions tore the vacuum of space in their devastating thunder from tactics like those of the thunderous dreams of Kosciuszko.

'Lîna had multiplied and hyper-concentrated the mine's payloads, and from the lapping waves jarring the three ships of At'Lann sonically it showed. A hefty enough portion of the scourge before them was still exploding in fiery tortures. The heavens burned as 'Lîna steadied her essence that was jostled by her display of power. A grey mezereon smoke began to linger across space. It seemed like it would billow across the quadrant.

It was a further pollution to the universe but one mixed with the energy expended to eliminate it. At the very least, 'Lîna thought, it will blow with the winds of liberation.

'Lîna shifted herself to the stillness of space, away from the 'Lis'talla by about the same measure as L'unn's orbital distance to E'de. It was time to modify and adapt her battle strategies. From her vantage point, weightlessly aloft, she found Nul'lus in the distance. Her loyal friend, who with little persuasion, had championed the Lon'tus to stand by the benevolence driven At'Lann in the path of war. She felt blessed. She could see Nul'lus had already begun to move in for the kill.

Amidst the At'Lann war voyagers firing white ultra-luminescent spatial charges at the remaining enemy vessels, 'Lîna watched her gallant friend in his new powerful state. Like Hooper in perfection and Pele at his prime was the sheer beauty of their poetically moving forms. Instantly, her mind alerted her to her impending dangers. And she had other thoughts as well as the Lon'tus flame of azure with twists of red and white, the soul fire like that of St.George, burned dashingly around him.

'Lîna scanned her immediate environment, and placed herself in the portrait of war that painted itself around her. Fortified scalpel cut smooth beams of violet light sliced their way past her. Thousands of trolley sized cars singed violently past her. Her senses seemed slow as there was no fear with the At'Lann at her back. No, she was alerted of danger of the enemy reply; spiraling orange and ruby tar fires with the look of darkened tequila ballistic sunrises shooting towards her ships.

The enemy had succeeded in tearing through their defences as enemy fire and seven enemy hammerheads rammed the Lis'talla and two hit the 'Ki'Bur. The 'Verga became tangent to the At'Lann spatial attack runs to evade the spherical menaces and to shield themselves from having their ships rammed to death. Thankfully, only one enemy compromised the Lis'talla's thickly armoured hull. It was shocking piercing like a sword through Wallace in the most defeating of stab wounds.

'Lîna had no time to think of casualties in this moment of battle. Her participation fulfilled her drive to bring nothing but death to the enemy force. The battle intensified for her as she began to direct her new assault. She glanced over long enough to see Nul'lus transformed into a different state of being. As 'Lîna moved in for her attack on an enemy dreadnought, she caught a full view of Nul'lus in her distant field of fire. Like a stellar core, his body came to exist in the same state of heat. His physical form became the most concentrated azure hued white light and fire waters of the flesh.

Divine power came as simply to Nul'lus as it had to 'Lîna. His motion flashed like hypnotic poetry through the enemy ships, from fighters to carriers of the ultimate parasite, none were spared from his powerful state. He melted through them and they exploded in his wake, as stunningly as Fowler once thrashed the visitors to Anfield.

Their current defences could not stop him. Like a true aristocrat thrust into war; he gave the most and did not even have to dirty his hands on this first of these fields of battle. This was a superior being in action, and granting him a commission seemed only just, thought 'Lîna as she watched on. She was sweetly content that she made the right choice for placing her faith in Nul'lus.

The battle in the heavens of Vu'latta had progressed into a dissolution and was now fizzling away to the point of being in its end-state. Nul'lus had flown through just as many ships and knocked out six ramming vessels as well. Nul'lus had flown through them all in hyper-spatial lines of angular tangency and made the results speak for themselves. 'Lîna, the Lis'talla, and the escorts Ki'Bur, 'Verga, and their fighters took out the remaining enemy ships unceremoniously using At'Lann plasma bolts and basic psionic energies.

She employed a technique of firing freesia sketched temporally paradoxical energies in perfect geometric spirals through her hands. As she blew away the last of the enemy before her with her energies enveloping them, she brought each of them to the highest velocity, yet kept them at temporally stationary speeds. 'Lîna released the forces at one temporal polar end to shake apart the dark invaders' ships into the most violent outcome of twisted metal. Their humid frozen swarthy crews usually died a fragment of a second before their ships exploded as their inertial dalancers would overload.

In fact, a mere moment before the enemy ships did explode, their filth eroded crews would fly into their bulkheads at high quantum speeds. They were instant corpse puddles. Not very much was left of them except for a fleshy mush before their ships were destroyed. 'Lîna had a slight glee about it all. It was her perverse pleasure that only fed the grief of all she had lost.

Thankfully, thoughts of enlightened de Sade and of Theresa remained with her as her powers were diminished within her from going beyond their current limits. Even with all of her new found might, 'Lîna felt held back by the new path of circumstance. She also felt something in the debris remains of the enemy. Though space was now vacuum, the emptiness, the null in extreme, so divergent from her early path of explorer, was now etching its way throughout reality. She took in far too much of the stench of the inferno of death, the tragedy that became the new path of exploration.

The path of war was far too deviously twisted and disorientating that 'Lîna found herself in state of post traumatic anxiety. These beings truly were a long marching plague of death. Like the rotting stench of Stalin's corpse. Once again, 'Lîna felt a powerful presence other than that of the Imperium and the souls of H'Raka which the dark forces sought to eradicate. Like a cat-of-nine-tails, this darkest of hooks tried to lunge itself into 'Lîna's mind and soul. The burning bile spewing hooks tried to ooze their way almost infinitely into her but 'Lîna was the soul diamond beyond what was understood in Avila. Her soul would not be taken by this evil. Her soul was her fortress, and she strived to make sure it would never fall.

As she floated though the wreckage with a distracted mind, something came up behind her and gave her quite a stir. It was Nul'lus who flash-folded to her location. But as happy as 'Lîna was to link up with her friend of the same path on the field of battle, and to stand side by side once more, she was dismayed to see how visibly drained he was. When they each had the Janus vision, the sight of equality, the pair could now see in each the weariness from only a few mere steps. He seemed a little distracted as well but not with thoughts concerning whatever dark force controlled what was the enemy. Nul'lus was preoccupied with the last enigmatic piece of their current situation.

In the distance there was but one enemy ship remaining, hovering above the Imperium pair. The greying solar winds drifted past them as if it were the blowing dust over a cursed earth, and the warship seemed about to venomously strike. It was about to fire and the ship seemed ready to ram them. 'Lîna had not yet realised she had drifted into an area clogged by enemy wreckage that had been ignored by her senses or the sensors of her ships. This place has a variance about it, she thought. Perhaps, 'Lîna could barely see past Bosworth. She realised she had walked into a mirage. She chastised herself to make sure this would not happen again. Nul'lus seemed unworried about it all and that was enough for her.

Still, Vu'latta space had become murky from the Imperium flex of power. Even Nul'lus could not see beyond what was the murk. But 'Lîna could feel where to direct their fire. They could save themselves in spite of the Lis'talla being out of range. They were trapped and tired, yet the pair still had great strength in wait.

This was a moment where she found herself tested in her weaknesses and it was a moment she had waited for. Something haunted her but she was pure focus on the battlefield. After all, 'Lîna let herself get into this situation.

For 'Lîna had strange habits of testing death by placing herself in the most dire of straits. On countless systems she skimmed suns as an explorer in her scout ships. This day was no exception. She was a daredevil and Nul'lus had dared to join alongside her. It seemed a sunset farewell to bliss.

All at once her thoughts changed. She could smell a stench reeking through her psyche, and she felt ashamed for somehow wanting this from the path of purpose that she walked. She could sense such evil toying with her. Though she now felt much more powerful, she was not afraid as only a dark trickle dripped into her mind. She got a rush out of teasing death. She was concerned by what wrath Death might herald by this through its ever looming spectre. They were still mortal even if they were highly invulnerable. But 'Lîna became far more dangerous by it. She was walking towards the point of no returns. But she always had a way out and a way in.

She reached her hand out to the striking and duty attired man that is Nul'lus. They came to hold hands in their calm way to power. Within their clasped hands, an energy was created that was far stronger than their original efforts. Their shared power was a bounty. A brilliant light grew, of lights like those of the Vatican and the Vishnu in tandem. The light burned opaquely in the growing sphere that it became as their energies grew past their hands.

Rays of pure emotions radiated from their combined power as their energy converted itself into a more solid photonic unhinging. The strain became all too much as a gigantic blast was sheen out and ahead to the lurking enemy ship facing them. Their hands pulled away from one another with char and glowing violated violet and azure smoke lingering from them.

At a frightening speed, the enemy ship began to splash through its own dead to attack the pair as the output of their might hurled like an ivory spear toward it. And before it could, however, it was obliterated into Roman candle dust by something like a fire greater than that of Greece. For the Imperium pair, the moment seemed almost eternal. A snapshot in life always to be remembered as life constantly moves on. Kinsmen are the precious and the cherished. Theses were the days in the sun again always to be carried in the heart.

They could do anything and less than anything. No one had ever been this psyogenomically unbound though something was still out of flux. 'Lîna could feel something impeded them from further taking themselves to a level where their enhanced states could be used to end this war in an instant.

'Lîna wondered if she was not as complete as she might think. She looked to her hand that had fallen away from Nul'lus's and repaired it telekinetically. And then she just looked away to the smoke drifts veiling over the stellar bodies of Vu'latta.

She also saw and could feel the deaths, the loss of many of her own lying in space from pilots to never fly again and from personnel lost from the path of winds. 'Lîna felt as if she had not done enough for At'Lann to let this occur. She was just a girl that placed as much importance on her heart as she did with her image. Her actions with Za'szu weighed upon her as well.

In her first real outing of war, she had aided in destroying four hundred enemy vessels in a matter of minutes but 'Lîna as if it were her fleet lay strewn like floating seaweed in the ocean of space. She wondered what kept her from doing more. 'Lîna did not want to dampen Nul'lus's victory joy so she smiled back at him with her encrypted pale face.

Her skin colour had changed. It became much lighter in nature. Nul'lus assumed it to be from the fatigue of the first blood on this battlefield had affected 'Lîna and would quickly pass. So he said nothing of this to her, and 'Lîna herself viewed this to be the case. Besides, she thought, she would have plenty of time to rest up before they would have another go of it with those of darkness. Nul'lus's moments of introspection seemed saved for later as they headed back to the Lis'talla.

It was over for now. As the pair flew gracefully back to the Imperium flagship, 'Lîna had a sense that one segment of this war enigma would be answered soon and perhaps that would let 'Lîna gain a higher degree of confidence. She drowned in shame as she knew that she could not do more. And she was afraid; afraid of what was to come. After so many years away from At'Lann, she was out to make her presence known, and about to make her next move.

15
The Darkening Voyage To a Holy Allegiance

'Lîna was not pleased as she sat upon her throne which she had converted to couch form where she lounged near the backfield centre of the bridge. Though cheers and celebration continued to fill the air, 'Lîna still felt bothered by what she had experienced on the battlefield. The wind, like cold Georgian iron-wind, the wind of evil, remained with her following the battle. She felt as if one would while feeling the last ray of sun before an Arctic winter storm. This *morbus,* she thought, how it thrives, how it strangles. I already drown, she kept saying to herself inside her thoughts. And for 'Lîna this was only the beginning, the killing view before the path would become much thornier.

Truly, something was wrong. Something was terribly wrong. Thoughts of doom overwhelmed her. As she sat disturbed, looking to the holo-screen, out to the debris field left by the enemy carcasses, 'Lîna was a soul of worry amidst At'Lann's first victory. Thoughts of fear, of disaster, of apocalypse, took her, shook her, and nearly paralyzed her. She almost felt in fear of losing her genetic cohesion as she was overwhelmed by the spectre of this *morbus*. Then 'Lîna could take no more as she rose with anxious fury from her throne as the laughter and glee became stifling to her sanity that desperately clawed away at making sense of their predicament. It all became too much for her.

'SILENCE!'

The hammer of silence fell upon the main bridge with an Odin-worthy lightning swift thud. With 'Lîna's words, everything came to a halt.

'Something is amiss. Something more sinister has happened. Science officer Val'damus of 'Mura royal guard. Run the modified anomalous transpsionic detection program through the interface sensor system.'

'Lîna's tone was filled almost with fright superbly masqueraded by her supreme authority. At a sciences interface by 'Lîna's right side sat a glossy ivory skinned mesomorph, with raven hair and cut, and features both corvus in line and At'Lann in dignity, in a teal trimmed black uniform with mauve At'Lann crest embroidered above the heart, and the helix and sword, the symbol of the S'yana on the left forearm of his tunic. The young officer responded after the interface brought up the data.

'Nothing detected of significant scale, Imperiatrix.' Val'damus said with a look that attempted to allay 'Lîna's concerns. Unconvinced, 'Lîna issued a new command:

'Run a long-range scan to the maximum threshold of our sensor range.'

Val'damus punched into the interface the necessary decryption sequence to access the Imperium listening posts to perform the scan. It only took a few seconds before 'Lîna's dread and her fears were found to be true as she looked to Val'damus's look of utter astonishment. The totality of it all, he thought. 'Lîna motioned for him to bring the results up to the main holo-screen.

When the data stream solidified on the holo-screen and the data came up for all to see in its electronic form. It was all laid out in sweet rose graphics for the entire bridge crew to see. For Nul'lus's eyes, for Val'damus's eyes to what faced them fully shown to his compatriots, for the eyes of the two S'yana who stood guard by the fourth wall, and for the eyes of her six junior officers who manned various interface stations throughout the bridge. There before them was quantified doom. For the horrific nature of the data was enough to shock even the lowest rungs of those who lived to maximise the mind and souls of the life around them. But it was clear to see that the horror of it all would affect them soon enough.

The enemy was far more insidious, and far bolder than 'Lîna had first thought. This had gone beyond anything 'Lîna could have envisioned. She had to keep her composure for she thought fear may spread rapidly. Even Nul'lus looked at her that fathomed the near impossibility of this.

'Tell them how long we have, Val'damus.'

'Approximately ten years, Imperiatrix.'

The seriousness of their path of war became all the greater from their intelligence data. 'Lîna curled her right fist, and just as she was about to smash it down, she uncurled her fist to caress the arm of her throne couch.

'Lîna stood up and turned around in semicircle to look upon everyone on the bridge and raised in her hands before clenching her fist again.

'Do you hear that, officers of the Imperium? We have ten years to win what is now an all out war. A war to save existence itself', said 'Lîna with an impassioned shout before returning to her war throne.

Everything had changed, and everything was wrong. The path of war became one of sheer and utter survival. Her people and her reality, her universe, now had an expiration date. A time was set for their destruction. For the *morbus* that was the enemy had somehow manipulated the very nature of reality to invert and transform the expansion wave of the universe into one of contraction. Their universe itself would constrict itself to the point where all and everything would cease to exist. All life would cease to exist. The totality! The totality of it all! 'Lîna thought in hidden distress. Needless to say, there was near eternal air of silent pondering and jilted indecision across the main bridge of the Lis'talla.

Φ

'I cannot do this, 'Lus. I am far too weak. I do not have the power to set reality into balance.'

'Lîna's doubts became a confession of cynical truth to the one she considered a soul equal. In the respite that was 'Lîna's private quarters, the two souls on the Imperium path delved into the depths of each others thoughts. Her eyes were filled with tears like Cassandra's before sieges with the last of her sombre words becoming sound for her great friend. Conversation became thought and spoken word. Her hands shook as her fingers barely held her smoking cure.

It was a good thing for 'Lîna's pride that she left the bridge when she did. She kept a stiff upper lip until she gave the night watch to Val'damus. To 'Lîna, her fragility was not for her subjects to see, for their leader, at times, did fall to a state of shaken frustration and utter despair for what reality had become for all life across the universe. She saved her complete openness for the intimates of the soul.

On a positive note, both thought, if 'Lîna had not returned to lead the At'Lann in war she might already have ceased to exist as the first *horda* wave hit the Lit'vaa seconds after she returned to the At'Lann system. Sadly, her hopes were few that the Lit'vaa were left unmolested and had already fallen to the wave of death. 'Now', she went on, 'We have to face both the onslaught of our deadliest enemy in our history returning to annihilate us, and on top of that, the universe is imploding in what will be the extinction of forever.' Either way, it spelled doom.

'Lîna felt it rested upon her to figure a way out of the grip of the death over life where even death began to suffocate itself. In spite of Nul'lus offering all his support and his pledge to find a path to continued existence, 'Lîna stubbornly felt it was all up to her. Perhaps that was why she was so devastatingly hard on herself. She aspired too vigorously towards her own evolution with few ways to cope with her ongoing chrysalis. The impact of what war had begun to mean weighed her down. If not for Nul'lus she would only have 'Zaya to lean upon in times of crisis.

Even with Nul'lus's shoulder to heal her personal faith upon, his distinguished motivational consoling was not enough. 'Lîna exposed only the tip of the iceberg of her pain. Then came a ray of light to guide them on their first step into the descent into hell. 'Zaya came to call upon 'Lîna in her moment of need.

Nul'lus understood he could do no more for his friend that called upon him to stand at her side and take the enchanted path with her. He gentlemanly bowed his way out knowing their conversation would continue in a far more complex scope later. 'Zaya came to 'Lîna as she always had. 'Zaya was the special link of the daughters of the 'Mura house, the peacemaker and the soul balance of Libra between Za'szu and 'Lîna.

They embraced and held one another with the tenderness that sisters crave upon one another when things are at their worst. 'Lîna felt especially blessed by her existence and held on to her as she had not had the opportunity to for many years. And that was the truth of it all as 'Lîna, who had barely seen her other sister since she returned home, now had another moment with her. It almost felt long ago since the face of At'Lann changed with a mere piece of information. How quickly had At'Lann been plunged into the darkest shade of war.

For this time together, they decided to, for now, let go of what was to come. It was all pushed aside as much as would be possible for the serenity of each other's company. What truly mattered for this blink of time would be the understood peace of sisters having an occasion to catch up on the better times that seemed to fade and barely remain clung to before their dark precipice. 'Lîna welcomed her sister into her sitting room.

They never spoke even after they let go of each other as they looked into one another, impressed by what each soul had not gazed upon for a very long time. 'Lîna took her hand in silence to her living space. 'Lîna lit herself another medical smoke while 'Zaya fixed herself some drinks. 'Lîna altered her private interface to play music for them, and a tropical bliss seeking journey into the euphoria of trance was more than essential. The ethereal tone of heaven seeking filled the room as if it were the heart of the most precise atomic technique.

The room itself seemed afloat by the epiphanies of sound. The music touched their souls as their feelings danced into one another once again. Sounds like those of Ashtrax and 4Strings filled the air. This time, 'Zaya could tell something was off about 'Lîna. As one of At'Lann's leading geneticists, little could be hidden from

'Zaya. Though 'Lîna put up a brave front, the horror of what was the path of war compounded the mutagenic effect of facilitating the L'unn phase shift with Nul'lus. She could feel that 'Lîna was not as well as she looked. 'Zaya's hopes for At'Lann rested upon 'Lîna as she took on the burden of it. 'You have to survive this. You have to bring us out of this. I place my faith in you, sister. And now At'Lann Imperiatrix.' 'Zaya gave her thoughts to her sister. 'Lîna was their leader, and victory rested upon her shoulders for the At'Lann and all in existence, 'Zaya would do all that would be necessary to help her eldest sister out.

'Zaya's faith in 'Lîna had never wavered. She returned as promised and without hesitation threw herself into the inferno. 'Zaya understood it to be her way of looking out for them in a sometimes distant loving way. Their concern for each other created a precious bond always to be savoured. Their relationship was unconditional and impartial yet beautiful to even think of. And that is why she came to call upon her once more.

Every step taken upon the path of existence would be crucial turning points when erasure looms so near by. She needed 'Lîna at her best as much as 'Lîna needed to be at her best. She hoped Nul'lus was in better shape and made a mental note to herself to call upon him as soon as he would allow for it. She hoped that what ailed 'Lîna to the point where she could no longer hide it did not extend to him as well. He was on the path that would be their destiny, and Nul'lus was a high noble of the Lon'tus Imperium.

'Zaya was 'Lîna's youngest sister and one of the few in the At'Lann court that fully accepted 'Lîna's anchorite path of exploration of the universe and for her once solitary pursuit of knowledge. 'Lîna was so frowned upon by her family for choosing the path of spatial exploration. For they could not see the logic in leaving At'Lann, 'Zaya was one of the few who stood to reaffirm the heiress's freedom of choice that tipped the scales to not have her path be one of exile.

Za'szu was chastised for being too ambitious but she was never dealt with as harshly as 'Lîna was as her price for being the eldest. But 'Zaya was allowed and unanimously praised for her path. She was also the conciliator between the sisters of 'Mura, and Imperium Chief Medical Officer as her role continued within the new order. She was a listener and a princess endowed with the fairest of judgments. 'Zaya was exactly the type of soul 'Lîna needed in this trying time on her path.

'Zaya was an image of Za'szu in many ways and of 'Lîna as their genetics had been designed to make even Hebe envious. She carried a similar spirit of exploration but 'Zaya explored creation while 'Lîna tended to explore the path of creation. She was the special darling of both 'Lîna and Za'szu that bound the 'Mura trinity together and 'Zaya was the confidante to both. Like the Parcae, each sister possessed gifts of inner power, beauty, and masterful intellects, the equation of which would not have been complete without young 'Zaya.

She had a way with making emotions and secret truths pour out in moments of clarity. Though 'Lîna no longer had a thirst, 'Zaya, nonetheless, made her a drink. Something that was a serene chicory viscous aqua blue spirit was presented to her. The creatively designed beverage seemed to shimmer with glitter sparkles synthesised into a hand size lilac glass. 'Zaya handed 'Lîna her drink and she respectfully accepted it. 'Zaya took her glass and clinked it against 'Lîna's and made a small toast to their slain Mother and Father and to the new Imperium before they each sipped back the intriguing liquid.

'I call it 'Zaya's Ocean. What do you think?

'Zaya's voice was calm and reassuring as 'Lîna began to relax into an equal state of mind and thought. She always asked this of her sister when it was just the two of them as 'Zaya still liked to plug one of her earliest scientific achievements.

'Just like I remember them: sweet and deliciously gooey. One of L'unn's greatest oceans through and through', 'Lîna said with an intertwine of a certain romanticism for the past rolled into her gentle voice.

Such was a great tradition of theirs to begin their conversations in this way. But this day was the first exception of the many that would follow for a very long time afterward. The blade of Cronos had honed their souls into something quite different than the day 'Lîna left At'Lann. And now they were at war with an enemy out to rob them of existence itself. Still, all things considered, everything, for one brief shining moment, fit perfectly into the model frame of peacefulness.

The chorus of the most precise symphonic sounds of music shifted, like that heard in the early days of Moby, and swirled in a perpetual summer breeze of music. Sound earned from past duty like that of Nelson's swept inspirationally into their minds. Then after sitting back together, 'Zaya could not guard her thoughts any longer and she inquired about what was on her mind to begin their latest moment of confessional truth.

'You seem different, 'Imiszi. Not from your mutating psyogenomic phase
variating matrices but from your new powers as Imperiatrix.
As uncomfortable as you
feel ruling over subjects, you wear it well.
We've missed you.
Holo-communications aside.'

'Zaya was on the high path in her inquisitive yet honest pleasantries.
She was building up to seeing the truth of the moment unfold.

'I try. But I am glad you think so',
said 'Lîna with tone of innocent humbleness, a touch still unsure of herself, that
came out from time to time in front of her contemporaries.

'Lîna still had a strange belief that she was far more forgettable than most, and even around one the closest to her, a part of what was now her clan, sometimes she still did not realise how unique she truly was. The music, the ocean in a glass, the mauve smoke, all became the mood that softened 'Lîna's resolve to keep even that which she did not even confide to Nul'lus.

After an east side of 'Mura appetiser of nectar and small talk, and catching up on where their pursuits brought them, how so much had changed and how nothing had changed at all, the heart of the matter was about to come to her. The last barrier to fall before their policy of truth was 'Lîna checking to see if Za'szu was still not talking to her and if her administration of the domestic government was going well. 'Zaya relayed that she still was not talking to 'Lîna. She had fortified the defences of L'unn using an efficient construction productivity model to nearly restore the great cities to their former glory. Now 'Lîna was ready to bear part of her soul.

'So how bad is it, 'Imiszi? Let go of the fear. I will stand with you. I have become filled with knowledge like you.'

'Not like this, dear sister.'

From her most calm and concerned tone, 'Zaya came to find the secrets 'Lîna revealed.

'It is worse than you think. None of our present weapons or technology can presently prevent defeat. We could very easily drown in paranoia. At'Lann itself would not exist if the universe did not. So simplistic to comprehend and so final. This long march of the *morbus* cannot be stopped even with the combined strength of the forces of countless worlds, we will still not be able to vanquish the deadliest of enemies.'

'Zaya had the intellect to find accuracy with the expected conclusions of war and battlefield outcomes. She was taken aback by the near negativism of 'Lîna's mental stance. This was not the innocent or the strong soul that 'Zaya remembered. This was a soul that a had hard time existing after having the enlightenment to glimpse upon an extinction of the future; a hard truth that would be the sadness of the new darkening reality.

'But what of others like yourself? Like Nul'lus. They will come to us, and you will go to them. Our fate is yours. You are a visionary. You must be as strong as you are. What is our next step?'

'Zaya always looked to find solutions. Like 'Lîna, she was never one to give up and her optimistic words were the Osieck boost to 'Lîna's spirits as she smiled at her sister warmly.

'That is precisely what our next step is. We must gain enough strength from the combination of the unique abilities of our allies and our own to develop the technologies and strategies that will eliminate this darkest of threats. Victory will be life.'

Not the most optimistic of answers but it was the first step on the path to freedom. Then 'Lîna dived back into the murk of war. There was still the business of greater revelations to attend to.

'Have we gained any useful intelligence from the three surviving prisoners, 'Zaya?'

Only the sovereigns and the highest-ranking officers of the Imperium knew of this. In the back of both their minds was the ethics of At'Lann but for 'Lîna, the death of her parents pushed her to set ethics aside until the war was won. 'Zaya's military rank was equivalent to field marshal though all members of the royal house had all-inclusive access to military operations. 'Zaya had examined the enemy prisoners but until now 'Lîna had not even thought of the sludge that was imprisoned in her gallows since she had come back on board the Lis'talla. She had other concerns and hated the fact that her sister had to research such evils.

'Very little so far. Do you plan on taking over their interrogation and examination?'

'Oh, dear sister. I will get around to them soon enough but they are only puppets. It is the force that empowers them that worries me.'

'What do you mean?', 'Zaya asked with a little hesitation.

'During the battle I experienced sensing the strongest of evils that surrounds them and envelops them. This evil did not come from the enemy soldiers, or their warships. This evil merely drowned them. We can slay them all without slaying anything. The source of this darkness is the true threat.'

'Zaya was taken aback as she could almost feel it too. Beneath reality there was a dark humming like a shrike falling to the ground screaming as it plummeted, heard only by the enlightened. 'Zaya tried to comprehend this as best she could. Her mood seemed to dampen slightly as she asked,

'Do you know who or what exactly it is yet?'

'Lîna's reply was somewhat cryptic and somewhat lacking but it was their reality.

'Only that what we face is unlike any evil the At'Lann have ever faced. Time is also our enemy in conquering this dark enigma. Our fate rests in acquiring knowledge.'

All that was left to say was the crux of the real matter that brought them together. The consequential reality that 'Lîna was almost too afraid and too ashamed to speak of, that 'Zaya had already knew of. And like 'Lîna, she did not want to accept it either but it had to be brought out.

There was a moment of silence hardly enjoyed as 'Zaya touched a key on the interface that brought up a rotating holographic scan of 'Lîna's genetic structure. A rotating analysis in mint green with At'Lann script in mauve pointing to a stream of chromosomal sequences and teal map of sub-ribonucleic activity, forming a genetic alignment rarely seen.

At first glance, the genetic paradigm seemed perfect to the eye. But something was not right. On further inspection, one could see that the enhanced, near maximized structure, was losing cohesion as its subatomic bonds were disintegrating. The enhanced pattern was simply too strong to stabilize even with chemical adjustment and current matrix manipulation techniques.

'Lîna had not been prepared at all for the transformation and carrying out the L'unn phase shift. Her mind had not been properly honed enough beforehand. But she had accepted the burden and the risk, and accepted her fate.

She could only think of Nul'lus. 'Lîna was far too shy to ask Nul'lus if his Lon'tus genetics and philosophical beliefs had had a better effect of holding his enhanced genetic structure at a stronger level of stability. From fighting alongside him, she saw him either to be far more recovered, or was powerful enough to mask it from her as she had done. 'Lîna still was not sure. The admission to one another in this case, came without tears, or emotions of any great extent but with a quiet sense of acceptance.

'And that is what makes it even worse 'Zaya. I do not even have ten years to win this war. I have eight years to lose my own war. The one raging inside me. I will experience total genetic failure. Too much knowledge inside of me is making me sick! A genomic meltdown, in your parlance, at that time. The truth is, I will never know if I could have succeeded. Eight At'Lann years are all that remain, and no one will take my place. The true path of war is not for Za'szu. She shall stay in the safety of home. There is no cure for me, is there?'

'Lîna lit herself another smoke in spite of the fact that it was not enough. 'Zaya, without hesitation, took her sister's other hand and clenched it as tightly as she lovingly could. Without the mushiness that can crop out of situations like this, 'Zaya somehow knew just what to say to give a ray of hope to her sister's subdued distress. In the way that was only hers, she confidently and sweetly said,

'You will win the war. There's something about you that will make it happen. Genetics aside, you are the one...For At'Lann. For 'Mura…For 'Mura'Lann. Let me win your war as you win ours. This will be my gift to you for saving us all.'

They held each other tight in the musical temple that filled with the sounds of like those like Tiësto that brought joy back to their hearts. A moment to keep armoured and cherished for eternity. They sat back down. They drank and in a cathartic moment of peace in the lilac and mezereon smoke air of peppermint spice. Freedom for a blink of time was theirs.

'I have one favour to ask of you though. I want this kept a secret. For the time being no one will know but you. And I especially do not want Za'szu to know. Whether she is displeased with me or not, this is our path. Understood', 'Lîna said as she puffed away on her curative chemicals.

'Zaya nodded back without a hint she would do otherwise. She gave her sister an even tighter embrace as she got up to leave 'Lîna's sanctum of private peace and promised also to look in on Nul'lus though 'Zaya would not reveal his condition to her. 'Lîna more than accepted her protocol as she waved goodbye to her sister who disappeared into the fourth wall. 'Lîna was content and more than assured her secrets would remain safe.

After 'Zaya left, 'Lîna thought there was hope for herself after all. Such was her gift to her. She felt positively blessed as she pressed another key on the interface that restored a communication link with the main bridge. With a regained force of confidence, 'Lîna opened a channel and spoke once again to her great ally as she smoked.

'Commander Nul'lus. Be ready to practice your skills of diplomacy once again. We press on. Set a course for the H'Raka home world, and inform their leader the Imperiatrix of the At'Lann seeks an audience.'

Nul'lus's holographic form came up on the interface to replace the garnet geometric collage that was the interface communications link. His face had a certain curious excitement about it. It would seem, 'Lîna would give the effort and had the spirit to make for the most sporting of moves. With inspiration in his heart. Nul'lus carried out the request as he informed her with the first good news to come along since that which seeks to destroy them became part of their path. The H'Raka had successfully fought off the attack and it would be clear sailing to their world aside from H'Raka barring their entry.

'To H'Raka, we go, Imperiatrix', Nul'lus said with an enthusiastic smile.

Nul'lus's holo-image faded away into invisible photonic ether and the interface imaging systems returned to military reports, tactical analyses, and theorems that were now the cause.

'Lîna had nothing and everything to risk. She would make a fight of it. Her steps unto the path that was now her life seemed at first such a dark journey but rays of light always seemed to find their way to pierce through the bramble and maquis that obscured her ground from her azure skies. She could prevail. Could she? There was no turning back. Gambit after gambit, it was once again time to be bold.

16
H'Raka

The new direction became a tense one for 'Lîna. She could even feel it in her people. She had already broken one tradition by not taking the name of At'Lann but that of the Mura'Lann amalgam. One thing was sure, she was the At'Lann Imperiatrix and she ruled as justly as her soul was able. Now, she was about to break one more tradition. She had embarked upon her destiny.

'Lîna rarely conveyed her reasons behind her method of reasoning. For one who bathed so often in stellar showers, her face often was the reflection of the Arctic. For the Polar kingdom was often singing progressively through her heart. For those who truly knew her, she was what she conveyed: a soul whose compulsion was for that of the greater good of her people. Her choices were what she deemed to be the best choices for her kinsman. And sometimes those very paths took her down some very strange paths. This venture onto this path of war was about to take her down one of the strangest and most wondrous.

She would attempt to make a new ally from who was once a most legendary foe. 'Lîna had brought the Lis'talla and the Taurean holy sanction of her crew to the prime H'Raka system deep within their space to the seat of their empire. Tense was a most inefficient measure to describe the feelings on board the Lis'talla. Of course, the only exception being Nul'lus who respected and long awaited a return to such a place of dashingly inventive marvels of efficient technologies. 'Lîna too, long admired the same such things with a moderation inherited from her life on the splendour that was L'unn and throughout existence which she once adored to explore. 'Lîna looked upon him, the purity of that which is the aristocracy of Lon'tus.

Nul'lus had performed a rather significant ambassadorial miracle in spite of the spectre that loomed over all life in the universe. He had persuaded the lavishly reclusive, yet vastly powerful, K'or, or emperor of H'Raka, to grant an audience with the At'Lann Imperiatrix. Such was one of Nul'lus's many gifts was a divining might that raised the banner for equality of dialogue between that of all people both deserved and earned for such merits. He was a marvel.

When the Lis'talla entered the space of H'Raka, their defence grid did not activate as if their ship was not a target yet worthy of incedent. The grid of pocket dreadnought weapon platforms of night train iron hue just lay in H'Raka space like lions on far too hot a day. Nul'lus had anticipated 'Lîna's next step and conferred with her that the government of the H'Raka Empire had indeed deactivated their defence grid for their journey to H'Raka. Nul'lus's policy of truth was a blessing that made for a strengthening bond between them. He had cleared the path of what was to come.

The H'Raka were warriors that adhered to an intensive code of honour but like the hammerheads they were warriors above all else. 'Lîna never had a worry of deception. However, the rivers of diplomacy were rapid waters and ones that could be like those of Niagara and Victoria; ones that face great precipices. When four H'Raka warships came to escort the Lis'talla to the H'Raka home-world, their ships in a wide flight pattern of a diamond cube formation gelled closer together in flight. Two H'Raka warships came to cruise tightly along each side of the Lis'talla like a fierce smile from Bismarck.

The H'Raka warships were a far distance away from the Lis'talla and her escorts, which glided alongside in the lower phase underspace, and ran a course that was intimidatory in its parallel course with the At'Lann flagship. For the H'Raka were known to wield might that earned respect that was sometimes reinforced with fright; a delightful fright to those who walked a new path. That the H'Raka certainly were: sometimes frightening and sometimes glorious. And they proved it by the lead H'Raka ship on their port-side firing a shot of welcome towards the Lis'talla.

The white pulse fired was a torpedo of frenzied nova-particles of an intensity so severe that contact with the glowing crevice littered molecules would literally be like walking into a supernova. Being hit by one of these pulses would figuratively be like a lighter sailing directly into a floating mine at full speed. It was one of those times like that of Franz Ferdinand. Even with fully powered shields, the At'Lann defensive technologies would not be enough to sustain any direct bombardment from the H'Raka.

Many of the At'Lann's Tr'Lann class worships could more than survive under such conditions but even these vessels would last against such firepower for only a relatively short time. Comparatively, H'Raka warships when faced with the weapons of At'Lann would, for the most part, outlast the current At'Lann technologies.

For a moment, even 'Lîna almost flinched excitedly in the sights that was the target placed upon them for a small fraction of time. Ironically, the Lis'talla entered the H'Raka system with her shields down. 'Lîna, enthroned at the helm, regained her composure with a sudden insight. Her reaction to this realisation certainly put her bridge crew on their collective toes; she deactivated the main holo-screen, and switched the interface image to that of the Lis'talla's hull temperature readout.

All but Nul'lus could figure out what 'Lîna was up to. The standard mauve At'Lann *Imperiagrams* on the holo-screen were in stark contrast to some overactive imaginations. 'Lîna seemed amused by it all. As she swam through the minds so many of her crew, their only thought was that of the impending doom brought upon by a very brilliant, brisling sphere of hurling energy globules. She was most relaxed and expected it from all others who stood in her company. Her composure became serene.

Nul'lus turned and smile delightedly at 'Lîna. He thought it always proper and distinguished that honourable species hold alternative views of the path so that enlightened souls never have to resort to pettiness and especially petty thought. Even amid a few gasps, Nul'lus had little to worry about from this crew though he did have a good laugh from watching some of the less experienced bridge officers shudder with nervousness. They truly had no idea what to expect.

Val'damus, a son of the Obsidian House-nobles, merely accepted the reality of their path and thought only of attaining victory; yet Val'damus was smooth and had long ago broken free from the shackles of stress. So collected was he that he probably would not have noticed if the star shattering missile actually hit the ship. Such was his confidence that he was barely even curious as to what move would be made next though the nihilistic shadowed itself over a pint of his joy. His soul was in equilibrium with tranquillity and his intellectual drive made him a most impressive soldier. Val'damus looked back at 'Lîna and gave the Imperiatrix a 'show me the show' look.

'Lîna then pointed to the holo-screen with a sly smile as she sat back relaxed with her hands clasped behind her headrest on her touring throne. A throne many viewed as the compensating opulence for those with advanced order noesis derived from genetic enhancement. Happily, no At'Lann was offended by the maverick way 'Lîna carried herself. She sometimes wondered if she was thought of as anything less than a bold illuminated soul. And if anything, she wanted to be remembered as a crusader.

'Lîna, in other ways, wanted to be seen as a traditionalist in terms of how she carried out social, military duty. In the most polite ways would 'Lîna stir the aether to surround her crew with togetherness under her violet velvet gloved hand that yearned for peace and transcendence. 'Lîna took in one more L'unn calibrated atmospheric purifying inhales through her eye-drop tip tiny nostrils.

'Now watch this', she said with expert confidence.

'Lîna held out her violet velvet coated index finger with a mildly naïve exhilaration. As she held out her hand, her spiritual smile lit up as 'Lîna was assured she had the attention of everyone on her bridge. A few of her crew held a collective gasp. Then, for one of the longest of moments, the reading for the hull temperature spiked to one thousand times above normative readings found when orbiting the Tr'Lann sun. The deadly H'Raka torpedo flew swiftly past the Lis'talla on a no longer suspenseful heading and out into space.

If the Lis'talla had indeed been targeted, the bridge crew would be floating in space in pieces at this time. The H'Raka were artists of intimidation. For 'Lîna, an artist is never intimidated, and for that she held no fear as the H'Raka came up beside them. The H'Raka, were, however, dangerous, and 'Lîna reminded herself to treat them with the utmost respect. She was pleased her more anxious crew members breathed a sigh of relief. The H'Raka were still able to induce great fear, as only the greatest class of hunters can instill.

Even long ago when At'Lann and H'Raka were allies, the H'Raka constantly had jolted the At'Lann psyche to sends shivers even to the friends of the most might and professional of hunters. This was never done to be cruel or personal, the H'Raka too simply had an image to uphold, and enjoyed finding truth in others by getting under their skins. Their history, though many elements remain unheard by other species, was far more frightening than that of any posturing from their cut-throat exteriors. Perhaps it was far scarier than all their legends combined. The H'Raka also had a disposition like the Lon'tus and At'Lann draped over by the other spectrums of their reality that rarely was unveiled any more.

'Lîna was merely pleased to have the honour to actually be allowed to come to H'Raka. Even under the circumstances, it was still an honour to the Imperiatrix just to be there. She straightened out her back and gave the order to Nul'lus to fire three similarly measured missiles of gratitude. 'Lîna, in order to be taken seriously, wanted to singe the hull of the closest and most distant escorting vessels and one for the enemy. All to let the H'Raka know that the people of At'Lann may not be a warrior race but both their races were on the path of the greatest crusade.

She conferred with Nul'lus that she expected to be met on equal terms; to be met as a warrior. 'Lîna wanted them to see firsthand that even her gentle hand wields tremendous power. She was not about to come all this way for nothing. And instead of sitting idle before the lions, 'Lîna chose to react, to let it be known to the H'Raka that she was the crusade, that she was their faith and fate. And perhaps, she wanted the H'Raka to feel the yearning of her blossoming warrior's heart and of one who once was an innocent that cried for vengeance.

As the Lis'talla entered the orbit of H'Raka Prime, 'Lîna conjured a long, strand of tri-platinum and violet gold, a soul thread made from bold thoughts and cosmic desires brought into existence to mark historic days. 'Lîna's enhanced telekinesis tied her latest accessory to intertwine in an At'Lann braid with a lock of her mauve hair that had a touch of nightshade at the tips on the left side of her head.

'Lîna was a tireless worker of vanity, as an explorer she would sometimes be the only example of her people and she wanted the At'Lann to be well thought of across the universe for days like the ones that the Imperium now face. For all her primping, 'Lîna had no idea what to expect from the H'Raka on the path of war in spite of Nul'lus's nonchalant assurances.

'Lîna then decided to fashion herself the amethyst badge upon the side of her left biceps to adorn her armlet. Something to remember the first battle of war and the day I came to H'Raka, thought 'Lîna in the quiet frenzy that came to get ready to offer an invitation to fight alongside one another for the virtue of a thriving existence.

She looked to the holo-screen and marveled at seeing H'Raka for the very first time and this world's harsh, bloodstained skies. The subtle loudness of the H'Raka life-force pulse was almost sinister. This wounded force was enough to send a shiver through 'Lîna as she recalled that this H'Raka sky was not borne from the first wave of the enemy but arose from damage inflicted upon the atmosphere during a long ago H'Raka civil war, and was left that way to remind the H'Raka that, without unity, they would destroy themselves.

But in the modern day of 'Lîna, even few H'Raka cared to remember what made their peoples walk separate paths from each other. Such a perplexing world, she thought. 'Lîna was hoping to braid another lock with tri-platinum adornment fit for a kindly sensual muse. At the very least, she thought, Nul'lus would be along as the choice of the path taken would be influenced by his presence and by her very friendship with him.

Nul'lus was firstly 'Lîna's friend, a soul equal to her own and a soul of better calibre than all she had ever would meet, but today he gave the At'Lann the extra edge like invisible substitutes playing on a pitch unnoticed before the officials. And 'Lîna also had other hidden aces to play.

'Lîna would not shroud herself under a cloak of politics. Today, she would burn outwardly with the fires of the truth of her being. 'Lîna could only imagine how offended Za'szu would be by the next initiative of 'Lîna's reign.

And she wished to think that at another level, Za'szu would be proud of her once again. Even after all that happened, that was still what 'Lîna hoped for. 'Lîna's sisters, while not beside her, even in her days of exploration of space, were such an integral part of her reality, and even more so with the loss that still had yet to sink in. For her precious sisters, 'Lîna hoped that this day would bring some great reward for the At'Lann.

'Lîna looked to see beyond the blood drenched clouds that was the horizon of H'Raka. Her eyes glowed in a niveous brilliance unseen by her crew save Nul'lus. At last, she thought, as she first set her eyes on the monolithic cities of H'Raka that lay scattered across their world that once had a sky much like L'unn and that of Lon'tus. So here she was in the place that was once sanctioned as forbidden for her eyes until now.

The horizon of H'Raka, a numinous sky of garnet blood to ripe orange, was hers to see at last. The light of H'Raka's sun shot through the nimbus clouds far above the world of Hunters. So innovative were the H'Raka, and by the sophistication that their technology continued to be, that reverence for them spreads across many systems. The H'Raka were known to be able to slay any beast whether it be governments, armies, and game creatures of near infinite varieties. 'Lîna was about offer them the chance to slay the greatest beast of them all.

Such a unique planet, 'Lîna thought. The strange beauty of H'Raka was enough for 'Lîna to lay aside her worries about Za'szu, the way things were left between them had begun to eat away at her a little more now that time had grown between them. Looking a little closer, the devastation from the first attack from the dark soldiers gave her a slow stomach turning feeling of shock.

H'Raka's urban design was very similar to that of L'unn's, and just as clean. It was their law to carry themselves and keep their living space utterly free from filth.

'Lîna knew this from historical data, and was pleased that she could now see this world firsthand. Though amidst the splendour, many H'Raka cities were now looking as if they were Dresden at her most ravaged. Her shock dissipated into gratification that the H'Raka had already begun the task of rebuilding. 'Lîna had great affinity for fanatics of neatness of the most freakish degree. H'Raka seemed a fitting world for those who ascribed to be the veteran final option soldiers for the heavens. 'Lîna seemed confident what the H'Raka response to the threat of erasure would be, and she could feel part of herself in the ethereal soul waters of these fearsomely configured H'Raka. And even from orbit, this place frightened 'Lîna as much as its sight comforted her.

'Lîna felt the H'Raka were an essential, nobly trustworthy, and a much needed component of a strategic central command structure she envisioned and desired. Their souls were as alike the At'Lann's as they were dissimilar to them.

'Lîna did not require wisdom to see the H'Raka, bustling about under their garnet sky, were out for blood, and a peace which H'Raka sunsets would never provide until every enemy is slain beyond it. 'Lîna's mind could feel their souls readying themselves for war. And genetically few species could even claim to be superior warriors than those of H'Raka. For this was their path.

The At'Lann coat-of-arms which represents origin and existence, the diamond over the ancient double helix, the gateway symbol for the building blocks of a basic genetic construction. Certain species possess post-tri-helix intertwine bundled genetic structures, and three of the most powerful species past this genomic frontier were the Lon'tus, At'Lann, and without surprise, the H'Raka. These three species who all came from the same primal genetic origins, the separate freed path of the Origin species. 'Lîna felt somewhat relieved to walk a path that had taken her to world of evolved life not truly unlike her own and those of Lon'tus. Species who evolved beyond these three genetic strands working as one in the most harmonious symbiosis were species 'Lîna savoured the most to be around, politics aside.

The At'Lann, Lon'tus, and H'Raka did carry differences in animalized accentuation's of their humanoid form. The At'Lann, or her people 'Lîna called 'Mura'Lann due to a new chromosome insertion coinciding with the L'unn phase shift which had changed the mosaic of the At'Lann genomic structure. Their path had changed their species from an ursine edge to a ursine, aviary influenced combination. The Lon'tus were both aquatic and aviary, and the H'Raka were the prowl, the flash into just death, kingdom walkers and overseers by design. Their path was to bestow the gift of death from above, below, in between, and in whatever way would complete their hunt or mission. A flow of stone as lightning were the H'Raka. Together they could be the force over the land, sea, air, and space. For 'Lîna wanted this as she had come from the path to protect the sea and sky.

It was a simplistic logic but it was one force that compelled 'Lîna to come to H'Raka along with curiosity and desires of explorers to go to forbidden places. All else aside, 'Lîna was here to forge an alliance and create the strongest possible home army. She vowed that she would not fail. Fate would seem to be in her hands. Something told her, that in many ways, the H'Raka walk a path like that of the enemy and in every way they do not. For they were dragons as they had fought and slain so many.

'Lîna buried such disgraceful disrespectful thoughts though she kept them as she could telekinetically cut open, and she wanted the H'Raka to see through her mind in the most honest of ways. 'Lîna also knew the H'Raka to be able to, in some cases, trick their prey into thinking they were exactly like them. 'Lîna would give them the benefit of the doubt as she respected anyone who keeps a clean house. She had faith that their armour may be black, their heart remained protected underneath and strived to remain pure.

'Lîna needed a strong ally that could understand the enemy and challenge their soldiers enough to bring out the warrior within their being. 'Lîna's path was one now which would made her do nearly anything to get the H'Raka to stand beside her against the enemy. She was a traditionalist as much as she was progressive, and even though relations between the two powers were currently thawing, the H'Raka were the key ally sought by the At'Lann if they were to find victory against the siege of doom.

Yet since At'Lann only fights the most serious wars that rage across existence, and even with the wave of death passing through, it had been a long time since At'Lann fought beside H'Raka. And in spite of recent and historically high level of hostilities between them, 'Lîna was not about to let tradition be broken. The other more ancient ally had stood by At'Lann since a few centuries after their frontier crossing evolutionary inception were the Lon'tus who already joined the fight. She wanted the H'Raka to be with her and to stand with them.

The pungent looking luminance of orange and pomegranate coloured sunlight lit the bridge as the rays of their giant sun burned their way out of the holo-screen. It was a first time for many on the Lis'talla to gaze upon H'Raka in such a way. Such delicious once forbidden fruit was the visual banquet before them from one hundred story ziggurats to the greenest pastures where mint and tiger print poppies were growing, wildly aglow, in the light of their sturdy sun.

The H'Raka escort ships signaled their departure from the vessels of At'Lann with a chimed communications dispatches and disappeared with their warships, swirling off in separate directions into the blackness that was now space, like lions kings back into the grassy knolls. All to return back to the path of the hunt that even Nimrod could never take.

'Lîna stretched herself out of her throne and calmly exited the bridge with Nul'lus accompanying her. They space folded their way to the Lis'talla's main hanger via the flash-fold, and took what was now an Imperium class shuttle to transport them to the surface. For the pair, this was much more fun than the lift system of the Lis'talla. The two had begun to enjoy, to some level, their enhanced abilities.

Even in the more serious of times, both vowed to fully enjoy their new gifts as much as the burden it was to hold them. To 'Lîna, this was more reality than reality had ever offered her. Even in war, life was still ecstasy. She had a possible fate of death awaiting her that 'Lîna was as nonchalant about as Nul'lus savoured on his path. After all, it was still years away for her. Cronos was still a barely noticed consideration.

The pair both seemed to flow with a calling to enjoy and embrace all moments of life. They walked the path for those to be legends, a path where only duty to the path of the soul is the only soul stream. These were their autumn tactics. Unlike Nul'lus, who was happy to be here, 'Lîna came to relax into a mood, the ideal mood, for all to go well for At'Lann and herself as well.

'Lîna let Nul'lus take over the piloting controls from the assigned officer and flew the shuttle out of the rectangular hangar, toward the surface of H'Raka. 'Lîna sat back beside Nul'lus in the control room with two At'Lann pilots with her. She had her security personnel wait in the shuttle's ready room. As she sat back, she turned her thoughts to the Emperor of H'Raka.

The one who led H'Raka was their long time leader, Y'vis, rumoured by many to be immortal, and led their people to victory during the last great war where At'Lann was their ally, and unlike so many from At'Lann and Lon'tus, had remained unraveled by time. So deadly and powerful was he that he could live reclusively away from galactic affairs and rarely met with members of others species unless a large scale hunt or the greatest of perils presented themselves.

He would see only 'Lîna and Nul'lus. Her flight crew and security would remain on board. No others of At'Lann or even other Lon'tus citizens would set foot in the highest of Y'vis's palaces at this time. Not that many of At'Lann would want to anyway as the time away from interaction with the H'Raka made some fearful of them and their intentions. Some thought they may be killed and eaten for sport. The many years apart by the two cultures had led to some modern time twisted and mistaken beliefs. But in some ways the realities of Y'vis's world was far more frightfully fantastic than the myths about the H'Raka.

'Nul'lus and 'Lîna had the refined open and rational minds that such fears were baseless within them. 'Lîna was a little fretful as she was here to make the most excellent impression though that did not stop her from admiring H'Raka's ruby stone obelisk laden architecture as they flew into the atmosphere and over the great cities of H'Raka that lay sparsely across the planet.

Even with her high level of optimism, 'Lîna was still young enough to be unsure of herself. However, her knowledge of existence taught her the importance of sacrifice, and just to be on H'Raka, she knew and risked for what paths might offer themselves. Nul'lus appeared solely to be concentrating on the relaxed joy that is piloting the elongated, elliptical globule laden like structure that was the At'Lann shuttle en route to the throne city of 'Vanx. Nul'lus's thoughts, though allied with her in the greater cause, were altogether a world away form 'Lîna's.

Nul'lus had been many times to H'Raka before. In his youth, he visited 'Vanx with his father who signed a trade agreement between the Lon'tus and the H'Raka. During his time there, Nul'lus became friends with Y'vis's son, 'Iato H'Renn, and had continued to keep a correspondence with him even while he was posted on L'unn. Nul'lus, unashamedly, was happy to have the chance to see an old friend he respected. This fact, at the very least, bolstered 'Lîna's confidence in the mission, as a friend to Nul'lus was a friend indeed.

Nul'lus was as formal in his aristocratic appearance and noble Lon'tus military tunic as he was in his thoughts which were just as refined and in balance for what this day would require. Sometimes, it made for his emotions to be less than apparent in his pursuit of enlightened civility. It was his way and it was 'Lîna's way as well. He wrapped his feelings in the finest Lon'tus cashmere. He was a most enlightened being that 'Lîna found to be her most kindred confidant. The years and summers away from one another had not eroded their bond. He was just as pleased that he would aid 'Lîna's people heal a wrong that had kept the H'Raka and the At'Lann from formal relations for far too many centuries.

Nul'lus brought the shuttle into the lower H'Raka troposphere, through the red and orange fire clouds to the breathtaking skies above 'Vanx. The throne city had an air of both Byzantine and Kyoto embellishments in the sharp edged H'Raka architecture. Massive tar hued ziggurats were spread out in a spiral with Y'vis's palace at its centre: a dome with four equidistant towers at its base that stretched across an area larger than an At'Lann borough.

'Lîna was amazed that such a long lived civilisation wore none of the dust of its age like the At'Lann, it seemed almost illogical. However, she could barely contain her hidden excitement to be heard by one like Y'vis. This was a palace she knew from interface records to be much more inside its walls as the H'Raka, though uninterested in aesthetic exterior urban appeal, kept some of the most opulent homes in the galaxy. The H'Raka were not ones for avarice, they merely accepted the reality of high order economic systems, and were very profitable at what they did. Surpluses not put into weapons technologies were put into their worlds and layered their peoples under accumulated wealth. 'Vanx was definitely an auspicious place where weaker minds would fear to set foot upon.

'Lîna and Nul'lus enjoyed soaking in the purity of this place. It seemed to call to them as much as the path took them to the world of legendary hunters. They gazed upon one another knowing the promise of what would be would begin here. As they looked out the long and tall, pinched triangular window of the shuttle, their reflections were superimposed onto the backdrop of a city of guile and the living portrait of the fiery skies befitting of heaven fallen warriors. Today would truly be a momentous day.

Φ

The dark teal At'Lann shuttle hovered in a anti-gravity caress as they descended seamlessly. Its metal tip landing gear slid out of pneumatically out of enhanced conical projections at almost the same time that the ship was brought effortlessly down to the ground of the private landing pad of the royal house of Y'vis. Only a few paces away was a dreadnought of a palace. It was adorned, on closer inspection, with grey gothic styled lines running across the dome and bordering the many strategically placed grand balconies cut in and protruding throughout the structure. The domed castle was called S'linn and was many, many stories high. Both 'Lîna and Nul'lus could see the top of the great dome and its tower peaks piercing through the very clouds of H'Raka's seemingly burning sky.

The castle emerged in the sky as it were a concrete bridge with its pillars remaining above flood waters as deadly as ones seen over Bengal. Such skies seemed in trying times, where waters flow like corpses caught together in jams that constantly crack the mighty supports. On H'Raka, the imperial palace officially called S'linn K'jak (the highest house), had never cracked, and seemed unable to crumble to nature even. To 'Lîna, H'Raka was unlike any world in all her travels. Indeed, this was a powerful place.

Nul'lus opened the hatch past a single door that led to the ready room and deactivated the shuttle interface and left the shuttle in the hands of her small crew compliment. 'Lîna and Nul'lus left beside one another as their they left their window side vantage points behind. As they exited the shuttle they were greeted by the dry, warm air of H'Raka. A stair to the ground emerged from the tempered metal hull for the pair. So here they were. Here they were before the nexus to destiny.

An honour guard of two elite H'Raka soldiers awaited them. They wore a black H'Raka leather with strongly cut bayonet like edges and each diagonally held a golden staff with banner ribbons, and at arms length from their mighty chests. One flag of mauve and one of azure were blowing crisply in the dry air of H'Raka. The two stepped onto the ground and the hatch closed with a hiss behind them. With their backs to the shuttle, the two stood directly before Y'vis's stately house in a somewhat guarded stance.

The H'Raka guardsmen were not the most welcoming sight as they had not even seen a member of the At'Lann in such a long span of time. 'Lîna's empathic abilities saw the guardsmen who had come to view the At'Lann as a weak power though they were still respectful in their thoughts of what the path is for the At'Lann, and were as polite in their efficient diplomatic style as they could be with those of At'Lann. It must have been difficult thoughts concerning a land whose people had the gall to restrict them from hunting the great beasts of E'de who were now no more.

'Lîna also had to remember this invasion of nullity into their reality was just as painful to the H'Raka even if the faces of Y'vis's palatine only showed the balanced calm, and all the while their thoughts teemed with such utter ferocity. The H'Raka were passionate, the H'Raka were strong, and the H'Raka were fierce. She would not underestimate them. 'Lîna could almost taste their zeal as much she could taste their sorrow. For a genetically similar race, the H'Raka were unlike any on her path.

The stars in the blackness of space that now cast itself above them seemed countless over the backdrop of S'linn K'jak as the rouge sun set on this corner of H'Raka. 'Lîna tried not to think of how many points of light above H'Raka had already been extinguished from their horizon and if those left could truly be saved. Her nightmarish long run perceptions of what could be could not be avoided even now. With every day to pass, this most dire of situations would only grow worse.

So ‘Lîna once again buried her fears a little deeper into herself so that she still may find worthiness for this path.

‘Lîna shivered slightly with cold before turning to face Nul’lus. She put her hand on Nul’lus’s shoulder as he put his hand on hers as they sensitively and respectfully made their way on to see Y’vis. Time faltered to stand still. The two stared into each other’s eyes with a certain promised hope. With his usual panache, Nul’lus whispered encouragingly to her, ‘Well, my dear friend, fate rests with you.’

From his words, ‘Lîna sometimes empathic mind realigned itself into one of greater confidence; her weaknesses would control and hold some of her greatest strengths. For all her might, she was barely a woman who still thought as sparrows do over the bounty that was their forests. Only now she was the ethereally rising phoenix of war.

Time then began to move again and things on H’Raka were no longer still. Nul’lus told ‘Lîna he was off to see ‘Iato ‘Hrenn who had requested his company. He told ‘Lîna not to worry even though it was up to her to negotiate an alliance, and that she was, after all, an explorer. And an explorer of many systems, and one who B’Dak and her favourite son of Lon’tus had been taught the finer points of diplomacy. He assured her all would go well. Though ‘Lîna still felt unsure of it all as she would not stand with him before Y’vis, she knew as much as she would have to stand with others and on this path she had to stand on her own.

Nul’lus lit up an omega three curative agent as he escorted ‘Lîna to the monolithic sized entrance to the S’linn K’jak. ‘Lîna still could not measure the enhancement’s side effects on Nul’lus but she was pleased that while they were on H’Raka he could partake in what only looked like an aristocratic hobby.

‘Lîna could see that she was once again indebted to ‘Zaya. Since she kept her secrets from Za’szu, she vowed to herself the only thing she would keep from Y’vis was, perhaps, their genetically perpetuated death sentences. Her mind tossed all such thoughts into the winds of her soul to blow them far, far away. Today would be a day like no other indeed.

Φ

There were dark truths to existence, and ‘Lîna felt she learned of more of them with every step into the shaded olivine sepulchre hall that led into the centre of the palace. Knowing even more of them was an even greater burden than her delicate soul had ever had thrust upon it. Somehow with every escorted step, ‘Lîna the explorer, felt the burdens inflicted upon her soul become far more bearable, as her curiosity became assuaged by the splendour of this once forbidden place. It reminded her of why she chose the path of exploration in spite of this being a world where even Orion would be afraid to set foot upon.

During her youth, before she left At’Lann to seek her path, she had already sought out the truths of the path of being. 'Lîna learned to be a constant observer of reality. Her mind explored the truth of those in At'Lann who let her into theirs. And even then 'Lîna understood what was the great power and responsibility of possessing an ever adapting genetic nature of the At'Lann and what is faced by other species like hers.

Even now 'Lîna knew the secret truth of what she was, and sensed the same potential within her people, the Lon'tus, and the H'Raka. Perhaps, she pondered, even all life in existence flowed to the great path. Her elevated state of being had always been within her and would have been unleashed even without the technological assistance provided by the phase randomising chamber deep in the flesh of L'unn.

'Lîna like all others of noble genetic programming, and like all life for that matter, had the great genetic lode within her. She and others so enchanted could access their sub-genetic sequences to adapt or maintain their structure. With the enhancement she was able to open the gates even more so than most and suffered just as much for all she had gained.

'Lîna knew of only two other species as evolved as those of At'Lann, who were, of course, the Lon'tus and the H'Raka. Those of Lon'tus still kept a periodical program of genetic adaptation as the At'Lann continue to do. The H'Raka had maintained their genetic state for a thousand years after a heavy period of genetic enhancement which brought about a twelve fold increase in the state of their genetic predisposition. The blades of their chromosomes became far sharper and far more honed in a span of only a few years, and was still marginally higher in abilities and aptitudes than either the At'Lann or the Lon'tus combined. It made 'Lîna think of her own path and she wondered what price these people paid for their very advancement.

At the young age when 'Lîna learned to become an individual alongside Nul'lus and before the graceful, friendly taskmaster who was B'Dak, she also learned many ways and gained many insights into the ways of the Lon'tus. At that age 'Lîna's genetic substructures were far more empathic. She remembered the days when life was the atomic dance of findings the image of wondrous souls taking the great path together. From the well of life, there was so much adventure found on their path. So many of the sequences that abandoned truculence became her own, pieces of peace became an integral part of 'Lîna's being. She truly embraced the refined and especially the unique. Thinking back to and about it all, she barely imagined that she would be here on this path. Yet with every marker passed on the path, she felt more complete than ever before.

In fact, many of the networks of her mind were inspired by the eloquence that was Nul'lus's balanced way. She was one whose path is that of the Aristocracy's divine way. She chose what paths Nul'lus would sometimes choose. Her very template cast in part by the way of Lon'tus coursing through her, granted her the stronger perception to see beyond the razor-edged smoothness of their seamless edged faces of the hunt. She saw within the life-flow of all H'Raka that walked this planet were what she had hoped for. She saw the phoenix fires of grace where the highest of reasoning powers and evolved civilities that existed within them as well.

Nul'lus's grace affirmed the reality that she seek out all those who shared this greater flow of life. For these three peoples had all and would once again walk Excalibur's edge, and for those who would join them, 'Lîna would take the best of them to become her own; she would throw it all into the enhancement patterns.

'Lîna had the sight to see beyond the jewels that were the dark ruby pearl of H'Raka. The H'Raka once tempered the souls of her ancestors and 'Lîna would give them her purist of alliances. And for whatever way the path would go, she felt there was no other option.

And though others may come to enter the great path of war, the At'Lann would still stay beside Lon'tus, and H'Raka most intimately if they chose to join them. Somehow, in the palace built from the path of eternal killing fields it seemed more frightening that this place even now was in as much jeopardy as the solitude and paths of life and peace. And somehow, the H'Raka were also seen by 'Lîna as a beacon of grace. She could feel it in the seemingly empty state room of one like Sparta bathed in gold and platinum.

Even in the days of youth when 'Lîna and Nul'lus conversed on the subject of H'Raka and the H'Raka people, 'Lîna learned and listened well to her friend from Lon'tus as he answered many of her hefty inquiries into the lives of the great Hunters. 'Lîna came to respect and sought to one day seek the wisdom of a species that violently grew into its genetic order.

As she stretched out her thought searches into the seemingly silent, 'Lîna could feel the warmth of the flames of hearts of grace. Before it was to be, it already had been as if the H'Raka and the At'Lann already stood together in 'Lîna's heart. Still, with their past history and histories, she was fearful the H'Raka would find the At'Lann unworthy of respect. Their preference may be to hunt as warriors but she could feel by their life-flow the H'Raka were as balanced as this palace which was as much a trophy of commerce, of economic prowess, as it was of the hunt. It was a way that had kept H'Raka as one of the strongest of the strong for a very long time. They too were of the Origin Species.

Armed with her heart of grace and her tried and tested way of completely satisfying diplomacy, 'Lîna had walked a path deep into the pride of the Lion; she was in the deepest centre of Y'vis's spotless domain. Her mind returned once again to the now deserted hall that would take her to Y'vis's state room that she had already peaked into. She walked the path of Fate as much as she edged ever closer to the hefty trans-titanium, dark grey-teal doors.

At the end of the empty hall, the doors of the highly polished halls of conquest opened silently and sucked themselves into the walls. The room was all but dark except for an opal tiled gleaming floor. For such a blood sooted sky above, the S'linn palace was totally devoid of dirt and infectious agents and breathed with a lustre unknown to even the Pantheon. 'Lîna had walked the last few steps to where she would meet Y'vis, their great Hunter feared by many even within his noble house.

With the shackles of the previous generation cast aside, 'Lîna no longer had to carry the dark burden of political coldness. For one who has chosen the path of equality she was testing herself as the philosophies of the H'Raka were worlds vastly apart from those of At'Lann. She was still a neophyte and though on the divine path she still walked it as a neophyte. Yet even in the dark side of the truth, Fate had been dealt what there was to pursue; even if that truth was that 'Lîna could see there was nowhere else to turn.

The path was altering itself with every step. Psyogenetically and empathetically, she aligned her mind to remember sources of her essence, both old and new, the liquid Cronos flowed into new channels. She could almost imagine Nul'lus's deeply tanned jasmine form smiling in a supporting way to her. She was becoming more than Hebe, more than Ares, and more than Marduk.

More than that, 'Lîna could almost hear his encouraging whispers to her mild lavender form through the door before one of the grandest rooms of captured victory unlike the many others she had past to get here. Each room, like every wall, displayed a curiosity forever made the property of the H'Raka.

The polished floors of S'linn K'jak, for a moment, no longer had its hard fought silence broken by the heels of 'Lîna's boots until the sound of distant marching soldiers filled the air from elsewhere in the immense fortress palace.

'Lîna looked one last time down the hall into what was the various weapons, tools, technologies, biological matter, sculpture, frescoes, paintings, and even a few high spun perpetual cinema particle displays of perfect projection that gave the palace a museum like feel. Treasures abounded in all styles, stages of development, contrast, and opinion composed this gallery of capitulation to H'Raka. To 'Lîna, it was like a spring walk beside rows of amber tombstones shining in the sun. Such plunder, from many a species extinct as ones thriving, from creatures who had surrendered in their encounters with the H'Raka.

'Lîna could clearly see the irony of it all. Turning to the H'Raka was an option made despite the H'Raka having had rooted out a phenomenal number of species. But they had a purpose within life to continually push forward the partly Darwinian spirit of evolution. In a dark sense the H'Raka weeded out the weak, those who cannot stand in glory. The At'Lann found this a provocative, yet sometimes necessary, facet of existence and had indeed placed their faith and respect with them in the past.

As 'Lîna stood deep inside this place, her thoughts came to only think of re-establishing the honourable trust that the At'Lann and H'Raka once shared. Truly, this was a turning point. Everything old was new again, and sadly nothing had changed. The path of war stood waiting once more.

'Lîna had time to telekinetically manipulate the molecular structure of her attire slightly as she stood at the end of the hall, at the end of the displays of antiquities, from glories that could be theirs once again, and that which opened the nexus into destiny. L'unn gold accented her bracelets and her every line in a far more ceremonial fashion than even first contact situations required.

Her garb became a darker mauve and a stronger black. A long whisper trail of mulberry dyed sheer shimmered off in a trail emerging from behind the top of her left shoulder that fell to the ground a few steps behind her. She changed her features as well. 'Lîna tightly curled twists of hair into a slightly longer organised mess of harmonious violet, mauve, white and lilac. Her lips became a descending shade of mezereon. Her skin became a lighter, yet heavy violet tinged ivory. Like the path of Rama, this path would be one like no other.

The now dimly lit wall of the onyx teal hued state room had the most marvellous charred platinum tint H'Raka Yi'gra wood borders that neo-brutalists would love stretching across every angle. Golden dagger swirls were etched and sketched ever so cleverly across every surface with such detail that it could only be seen with enhanced vision. Like the den of a fer-de-lance and the palace over savannahs, this path of fate would have to go large or go home.

Her eyes tempered to harden into an intensely beautiful and never before explored lightened olivine that went well with her lilac eyelashes. So composed was 'Lîna she could slay Ravana with but a thought. 'Lîna entered the silent state room with logic and fortune at her side. The onyx teal door hissed in lightning speed and clanked itself closed. The state-room gradually began to become luminous as the spotlight rose ever higher above the room and ceased to produce any further overhead light. 'Lîna could feel it, Y'vis was awaiting her.

17

The New Direction Made in the Dark Country of Play

Y'vis was before 'Lîna. He was as immaculate, menacing, and as sensuously a delight as described. He could conquer the heart of any he chose. The H'Raka emperor, the K'or, as he was called by his people, had the appearance of a young, frighteningly handsome man who 'Lîna knew to be far older than even that of the age of her parents before they died.

His figure and panzer general tunic like garb were cut as precisely as Lon'tus diamonds, and with edges that became the sharpest of blades. His tanned platinum face and cropped lion mane of hair were equally cut sharp gems. The K'or's most striking feature was his, aeons on the path, hardened eyes forged from years of hard campaigns and ruthless sacrifices. Y'vis's eyes had cooled into the most rigorously cannon firing dark jade eyes of a predatory assessor of the highest of powers. In black, in his armchair, he truly was a dark angel of salvation.

Y'vis's strengths and powers made him able to eliminate virtually any target, threat, or prey, of both corporeal, ethereal, and those of economic natures. 'Lîna was in awe of his presence before her. It was if this powerful man always carried an aura of standing victoriously over the defeated bound into the entire planet beneath him. He was to be both feared and respected. He was an ultimate king over any jungle. For within him lay the strengths of a noble predator, and Y'vis's state room reflected his glories.

With the room growing more abundantly with light, 'Lîna could see in one corner, an overfilled pyramidal exhibition of glossy white-washed skulls of defeated enemies of the past forever clustered together by their varied doom. The scary thing was that set against the spotlessly sheared obsidian murals and skeletal displays, there was plenty of empty space left for more putrid droppings left behind by beheadings. Far more startling than that, 'Lîna took this as an injection of morale boosting confidence.

The state-room was quadruple the size of her own on At'Lann though the At'Lann were a far less boastful people. The largest of the skulls were partially phased into the end of each wall to form great white crosses of skulls. Many would tremble by the mere sight of it. S'linn K'jak was the house of the hunt.

Y'vis pierced his way out of his casual sitting throne to personally welcome 'Lîna to his world. His pace was deliberately and decidedly slow; moving like a jaguar surveying the kingdoms of its wilderness. His pace also was the hint of automatic warning: that he could strike with the fangs of an E'de forest viper. For he could be a snake if he chose.

'Lîna found it quite thought provoking to meet such a beautiful but sinisterly deadly man one would ever find on any path, and 'Lîna graciously felt honoured have her private meeting of nobilities carried through. She was usually, awkward and inexperienced in such matters even after performing them countless times but for this day she elevated herself into a stance that she hoped Y'vis would see as an aether they both shared, especially in the matters of kingdom and crown.

Y'vis gentlemanly escorted 'Lîna to an area of his conquest laden room where the two would find a place to properly converse as sovereigns. 'Lîna was given a finely crafted sitting chair made from a the satin like skin of a Ti'mat giant squid of H'Raka's saline oceans. A fitting throne of perfectly sculpted tourmaline colour and a glisten like a tequila sunrise over a frame of red H'Raka oak. Y'vis, in a hyper-blink, teleported away momentarily.

Across a long, hefty table of smoothed, crushed black pearls, sat Y'vis dominantly on a throne of thick carbon ash hued leather over the protruding end bones of an extinct Qus'na shark after rematerialising. The Qus'na had been a creature that swam in the few mercury oceans of this world that were some of the most coveted regions of H'Raka but had not swam in their oceans since H'Raka began to assert its presence in intergalactic space over fifty two of their generations ago. His throne may have been the sole remaining piece of H'Raka lower species heritage since the H'Raka found the cloned copies for sport and leisure rarely measured up to the original and had moved on to other markets.

For many ages, their departed prey were far too respectfully valued to hunt as mere imitations or ones enhanced of the original beast that could meltingly conceal its way through the heavy oceans. It was a beast said to be even able to evade sub-spatial targeting systems. It was a fitting throne for such an evolved immortal warrior; an ultimate warrior without the fashion faux pas.

'Welcome, Imperiatrix of At'Lann. Your assistance, though not required, is appreciated by the H'Raka'. She felt his soul presence jump across the table to coexist there as well. He paused and had, what felt like his cold hand, slide down her right cheek. 'You are far more different than what I expected for an inheritor of the At'Lann throne.' He laughed with a hunter's amusement like one who could out-hunt even the Spetsnaz.

> 'I know why you have come here but your fate will take you to another to state your case and share a path with if that is what is chosen.'

His words were as smoothly toned in their efficient gruffness as 'Lîna was mildly taken aback by them. A black android moulded as a salamander of servitude brought forth drinks for the Imperials before 'Lîna could even say a word. From a squarely cut polished onyx serving tray, Y'vis had his servant pass Lîna a Lon'tus whalebone chalice filled with Qa'lha (swirls of white and green adrenal extract derived from an extinct E'de beast that is served chilled), and had the same contraption bring his chalice over for himself. Totally unlike M'Goa Qal'latu, she thought. 'Lîna's hopes were at the point of shattering but she kept her composure as she took the chalice. The amphibious looking android servant silently left the room.

The imperials were alone again in the silent room that Death herself would find as a powerfully ruthless ecstasy of a place, where beneath its silence, it always pulsed with power. One thing was for certain: 'Lîna had not given up all hope. Realistically, she expected to gain, and did receive, an audience with Y'vis as she engaged an enemy shared and had extended the first olive branch. Optimistically, she hoped Y'vis would have enough gratitude in his heart to bring both the At'Lann and H'Raka onto a shared path of victory.

The strange pair raised their glasses to one another before heartily sampling the viscous extract. To 'Lîna, it had the taste of the sweetness of another kind of predator, that when faced with the moment of the instinctual and internal of that which was the beast. The taste was as if it were the feeling as it was about to be gourd open as it lunged to attack. But with the E'de beast still in a position of attack, the flavour was one of the rush felt before feasting on prey. The taste. The taste. It felt rather darkly sweet to 'Lîna.

'Where will my fate take me, Hunter of Hunters?'

'Lîna had finally worked up her reluctant courage up enough to see where this path would go and where she would find her equation of war. Y'vis let loose a piston like roar of amusement. He was impressed by the gall of the new leader of the At'Lann, and paradoxically, for one of peace, she was quite impetuous for battle and war itself. Though he could slither in the trenches like no other, Y'vis would not lead beside or lead 'Lîna into battles in pits of adders. Somehow, 'Lîna felt validated by wisely placing her fate on a path of promised risk.

'You are not as ephemeral as some might think in your government and what you seek in mine', Y'vis said bluntly with a tinge of reassurance under the near cathedral of white crosses. The skulls of yesterday seemed to gaze at her as tawdry examples of extinction yet examples of its ultimate severity. The life of this universe would be no ones trophy. It seemed a world away as Y'vis psionically seemed to surge with an even greater warrior's power in what was as much a meeting as it was an inquiry.

'Lîna felt something was about to happen and she was in as blunt a grip as the captive candour of what was fast becoming a silent storm of consensual inquisition. Like wild chain thrown blades, his astral hooks flew into 'Lîna's mind. The intrusions took her like awakening to something else as she felt her soul pull itself almost aback. Yet, even if she wanted to, she could not resist at all. Strangely, 'Lîna preferred this to the petty subterfuge of certain diplomatic situations she always did her best to avoid.

Their bodies seemed to stare at each other as if seen through a smoke filled looking glass. The corporeal fell silently away as the vision of what is telepathic inquisition swept 'Lîna like a water slide into a waterfall, and finally into a large fissure of what now became the astral menagerie. What started so slowly had now become a swift journey down the river of K'urszt; a river that flows to the heart of the Kem'ja K'honn forests of At'Lann once thought of by early At'Lann colonists as impenetrable. The game was afoot. For what would be the path was at stake.

That which is corporeal was cast aside as their thoughts became the heavy oil slick across the astral oceans ablaze and almost entirely consuming. The plane where their minds were taken was like a theme park for roman candles. This inquisition was far from exclusive as both minds could search through the other for the particular answers each sought. Y'vis already began to slash his way through 'Lîna's mindscape.

If nothing else, the enhanced experience was most unique. She became the ocean and 'Lîna had never before swam so far out of reality; the further she swam, the further Y'vis dove in ever more piercingly. Y'vis had not set out to drown her young enhanced mind but wondered how far she would go.

Despite the underlying political truths encountered in even the very best cultures which Y'vis selflessly pointed out, she no longer doubted her strengths, and she had a full grip as leader as she felt no shame about letting him see a part of her soul. Y'vis could now see her essence as clearly as he could see At'Lann's new order, and he could see she could not be cast aside.

Though slight, she was refined and constantly refining what would become Fate. In spite of her fragility, she held a warrior's soul as those who follow the path of peace fight without regard for restraining from the most utter reaches of viciousness in order to keep or restore peace in existence. 'Lîna burned with the fullness of strongest of commitments for the path of war. He could see in battle she would be bold, and that was enough for Y'vis.

He had simply kept his people waiting to sink their teeth into full scale war until the At'Lann would come to join them on the path of war. He could see it in 'Lîna that she would stop at nothing to be victorious over the enemy. Her innocence once more seemed to fall ever so slowly away from her as she filled herself with vengeance. She was the new generation for At'Lann, and Y'vis only had to see for himself if this inheritor of the Imperium was worthy of a formal allegiance. Like a phoenix coming to swim beside an enhanced great white, Y'vis would bring the H'Raka back into the latest Imperium. His exacting wisdom would have it no other way. It was now the merest of labours for their respective diplomatic corps.

The At'Lann, the Lon'tus, and now the H'Raka would stand as a triumvirate of integrated imperial systems, the masters of destiny set out to vanquish the *horda*. Though 'Lîna had found what she sought by coming to H'Raka, new matters arose during the time she linked minds with Y'vis. And she kicked herself for not asking who would lead H'Raka's war effort though Y'vis knew from the link that 'Lîna still waited for an answer despite his diversionary telepathic talents.

'Lîna knew from delving deeply into the Imperium interface what her larger court tried to cover up. The Imperium was splintering at its edges and could crumble without what necessary support they required to win the war before them. Many genetically immortal races actually desired their gift of life to be ended by the holocaust of ceasing to exist. Existence for them had become tiresome. Their gift had become the monotonous burden of an all too perpetual forever. With the majority of their historic allies coming from such races that conscript themselves into the Imperium and, in many instances, into the At'Lann aspect of the Imperium for their servitude of protecting life in times of war, everyone was needed in their unity.

Their telepathic conversations centred on the effects of this turn of events as the armies of At'Lann, H'Raka, and Lon'tus would be left with severe manpower shortages in the wake of such large desertions by minor but valued species that had fallen victim to mundane and benign paths. A few possessed great powers though most were genetically simplistic. What mattered now was compensating for their role in the production process. The Imperium would have to rely on even simpler species until their labour shortage would be eliminated by finding others as capable as their traditional allies for the construction of war materials such as warships, fighters, and ammunition. Their traditional services of the dead and deserting were already sadly missed and both hoped innovation would continue to be their salvation.

Both Imperials had known of this beforehand and already knew how this would affect their war effort: that even the combined fleets of At'Lann, H'Raka, Lon'tus and their current allies underneath them would not be enough to protect existence from what could be an all-consuming horde. They would fall to their sheer numbers. Their worlds faced a tactical disadvantage from the second wave that would herald the eternal holocaust. They would have to adapt or else they would fall to the enemy of the darkest doom.

Y'vis keyed with lightning speed an authorisation sequence into a H'Raka interface built into the executive table before them and it illuminated in crimson automatically with his touch. The dagger like H'Raka data-stream varied and transfigured with every keystroke. He had signalled for his fleet to spread across what was rapidly becoming less and less of a universe to protect and to reinforce the Imperium warships.

The military forces of H'Raka had already begun to conscript various worthy species to bolster their own. If species conquered by the H'Raka would be of better use to the At'Lann Imperium they would now be transferred to them. At least, they would find freedom with the At'Lann, 'Lîna thought. The At'Lann had been enslaved by a conquering species for three generations early in their free history and had no love for unethical economic policies. By bringing H'Raka into the Imperium along with their ways, 'Lîna, for the sake of the war, would have to condone it. 'Lîna had no choice but to agree and cast a few more of her ethics and purity aside for the greater good: the survival of existence. She was not proud of herself for casting aside so many principles she cherished and had lived so long by as she sacrificed a little more of herself in the ether shadow far beyond conscience.

Y'vis motioned for 'Lîna to link in as a panel powered before her. Within the link, within the interface inter-link, Y'vis showed 'Lîna a detailed schematic of that which could be their salvation. A blue-print for a device that would bring them victory was brought into 'Lîna's mind.

The difficult part of the equation was that some of the materials needed for the massive devices were supplied by the technology of higher ranking species which had lain themselves down to die and cut their trade ties to alien species as they closed their borders to await the inevitable, or in others still expected to be paid. The Imperium were left with two very diverse choices: either the materials needed would have to be bought (an absurd concept to 'Lîna for the most part but she respected the prerogative as she knew even at a time that could be so close to the end, markets still had to exist), or the materials would simply be taken by force, an option she did not prefer. The Lon'tus and the At'Lann would have to learn to stomach such activities as the course of the war depended upon it.

Aside from beginning the diplomatic process, the only action he would personally undertake would be to watch the war from the shadows. If he saw the need to enter into battle, Y'vis promised 'Lîna he would. He told her that this was the war for her generation and though 'Lîna would have liked to have fought beside Y'vis, she knew it to be of no other way. What was proposed was moral only by its ends for 'Lîna and her kind but she relented and gave her approval to Y'vis and not only wanted but needed the H'Raka to return to the Imperium fold. There was nothing she could do to intersect with Y'vis's pursuits. He would be everywhere for the H'Raka and the Imperium, and nowhere.

Even for those almost at the steps of godhood, the At'Lann still required paths of primitive simplicity into what had become for them lives of virtual labour of unravelling the soul. Strong races such as the At'Lann had evolved to no longer require the input of lesser workers in their economies and such practices of third party labour contracts were, for the most part, were pursued far less frequently than in their past. Now, 'Lîna had to accept old economy integration. At'Lann needed workers to build the structures shown to 'Lîna that she could clearly see would give the Imperium the best chance to win, and At'Lann would have to rely on labour markets supplied by the H'Raka.

'Lîna was uncomfortable with the sacrifices she had made but felt she had to do everything necessary to protect her people. She could forgive herself as she was now becoming ever more ingrained into the dark spectacle and strange menagerie that is the reality of war. She was long past the point of no return.

She was still unsure as to how she should take Y'vis standing alone in the war effort; either his contribution would be the greatest of all or one that made destiny possible for the neophytes to the path of war. 'Lîna had expected to walk in the wake of one even more powerful than her but now the war would become far more a part of her, and she did not know, even in the stateroom away from the halls of hunted truth, what path she would be placed upon next. The all but assured answer she sought was about to come as Y'vis broke the link with a seamless slash from his invulnerable will.

The young Imperiatrix's time in the H'Raka interface plane that seemed like a walk amongst jagged sepulchre came to a lightning flash like end. The psionic tethers between their minds broke themselves away. With so much data and so many thoughts absorbed, 'Lîna felt aged by the experience. Her mind felt chilled and seemed abruptly cohesive. Like icicles falling to the ground to break atop a melting Muskoka and Mariposa niveous snow, for a moment, everything made sense before everything once more became as uncertain as the weather. And the dark storm was still on the horizon. Even the war history of her people did not give her advantage of precedence for what would now be the current direction. If she did not remember what it was to sweat, 'Lîna certainly felt a little nervous for something that was all but guaranteed. She was still a little jarred from the data-load from the H'Raka interface but 'Lîna was able to face the next moment. Her thoughts seemed even more confused.

'I have proven myself and became what I am in taking the path of war for the H'Raka and the Imperium, and I have fought beside many generation of At'Lann. I am legend, I am ghost, and I now wage war in the shadows. My hands no longer dive into the waters of war. All that I am, I have already proven long ago. You are possibility, Imperiatrix of At'Lann, but you shall prove yourself and become what you are, not with me in the path ahead but with another... My son, 'Iato H'Renn, will place his hand in the fires of this path of war. It is his time to prove his worth and lead H'Raka. It is his time to succeed me. You shall fight beside him in the sacred cause. The strings of war that I pull shall be pulled from another place. This is your fate.'

With the last of Y'vis's words leaving his serrated lips, Y'vis turned about and disappeared into ether of the shadows with the smoothness of a regally sculpted jaguar returning to a rain soaked misty jungle as he phased himself out of existence. He left behind a few shakes of highland fog and a stateroom left empty but for a young Imperiatrix who had found her fate.

'Lîna knew that this would begin to get interesting as things would be not so simple as she would next meet the one who would share her path, and the one who would also lead At'Lann and the Imperium in war. Just like that, it was over only to begin again. And that which would be the true hurdle of her journey to H'Raka. Everything was unclear, everything was exciting, and everything bordered on frightening. Fate had found her way onto the path of the Hunter, and the true path to war.

18
H'Raka's Son

Y'vis was gone. To another plane and another path, and he had went like a silent Highland blade through a bluegrass of what was the unknown. 'Lîna was left to solitude once again. After returning to reality without Y'vis, she looked out and could feel the palace, on the whole, was as empty as this stateroom. After the enhancement, 'Lîna thought she had gone far. After meeting with Y'vis, she realised how far she had to go. But she was on the path of Fate, and with every step, reality was becoming more and more simplistic. Y'vis had given her a path to fight beside another who she could feel already to have a soul as advanced as that of her own and Nul'lus, and possibly more so.

'Lîna was swimming with sharks and her resolve seemed tested by bringing herself to the Hunters' world. She was, however, less afraid of the professionals she found on her path than she was of what she would become on the path of war. For anyone could rise to become a king of New York. When she first saw the darkness cover Lit'vaa and when she first saw war ravage At'Lann, her true innocence became loss. In her travels, she had seen only peace. Now, all that had been taken away from her. A few skirmishes between vessels but never with the utter brutality that had now spread across an erasing universe.

'Lîna was now a soldier of peace, and her desire to return peace to the universe was so strong that she had already begun to fight without regard to viciousness. She was a true soldier of peace and her warrior's flame came to arise in this, the worst of times that had become existence. And as fragile and gentle as she was, 'Lîna would not be remora in her alliance with the H'Raka.

She vowed to lead the At'Lann Imperium into war so that the H'Raka would once again remember why the great hunters respect the enlightened path of the At'Lann. She felt a hum of rumbling, unwilling silence whisk its way across the palace called K'jak S'linn. The momentum of destiny had curved her path into another. Her mind showed 'Lîna where to go as she exited Y'vis's vast and empty stateroom. She was anxious to meet with 'Iato H'Renn, the one Nul'lus shares his friendship with.

'Lîna could already feel the path ahead, and the path of war would be difficult and trying ones but like Kosciuszko and Pulaski, she would stand for her people. She vowed to not leave them with romantic tragedy. She had to let it all go for the war effort, and only then could she possibly succeed. 'Iato was an unknown element to her. 'Lîna felt she had lost any sense of control from the time taken with Y'vis in forging this alliance path, and making this war, her generations' trial.

The path ahead was dangerous and she could feel that the path she had chosen could easily take her through rifts into wastelands of uncertainty, to the nothingness of having everything lost to the nothingness that crept ever closer. If only Za'szu could see the price I am already beginning to pay to win this war, 'Lîna thought with a certain ironic reminiscence of their days of quarrel. And even in the now silent halls of this mammoth palace of Y'vis's, 'Lîna still took a moment to miss her sister. 'Lîna yearned to find peace with her once again but she knew with the demands of the war it would be some time before she would return to At'Lann.

'Lîna walked a seemingly endless hallway to where she thought she might find General H'Renn. After coming into his area within the great house of the hunt, she found it to be as deserted as the rest of the palace. As she wandered from hallway to room and back to hallway once again, she felt nothing of his presence. 'Lîna then came to be outside a sitting room adorned entirely with the skin and tusks of a Ram'sza (a gigantic beast of stone shingle armour that looks like a massive, gigantic, yet emaciated blowfish that swims through nebula gases). A frequently hunted creature of the H'Raka empire that made space its home. 'Lîna brushed her hand down the silky jade leather that was the skin before seeing an other being in the distance.

She came into contact with a member of the H'Raka elite royal guard, the 'Sonann 'Nor ('the North Blade'), who stood guard at the other entrance to the sitting room further down the hall. And this elder H'Raka, an obvious veteran of past campaigns, came to offer the At'Lann Imperiatrix some assistance like any ceremonial ornament of power but one who still could and still would fight like only the strongest few could on H'Raka. 'Lîna respectfully asked the high officer of H'Raka to escort her to where she would meet General H'Renn, a prince of H'Raka.

His highly polished shine of his black boots and leather accents of his uniform seemed to mollify 'Lîna as the sympathetic guard began to tell the At'Lann Imperiatrix his trained reiterations concerning the General's whereabouts. The majority of H'Raka nobles had left to command warships, yet he still stalled in telling her the whereabouts of General 'Iato H'Renn, the son of Y'vis and heir to the H'Raka Imperium. The burden of power on the path of war was now upon him.

At the very least, he was a H'Raka warrior used to dealing with the aristo-cratic likes of Nul'lus, sometimes on a daily basis, that made it easier for 'Lîna to insist on finding where 'Iato H'Renn was. He was a perfectly sculpted dog of war, of honesty, and to some measure, apologetically conceded, that he was under orders not to leave his post, and could not escort her to General H'Renn. His sole duty was to guard this central corridor that ran by his side of the sitting room.

She could feel his empathy as the footman almost winced as he told the young Imperiatrix that General H'Renn had already departed K'jak S'linn with Ambassador Nul'lus over an hour ago and was on board the Lis'talla. With his raised lip exposed as he raised his right eyebrow slightly, she could see the long H'Raka fangs of chrome and baking soda coloured teeth. Its sight helped calm her shock.

'Lîna, though restrained, almost gasped with surprise and anger before commenting to the guard with a tinge of chained anger. She was feeling slightly insulted. She was peacefully sardonic in her open thoughts on what an efficient leader their people had for a race renowned for its methodical efficiency. The black polished and galvanised soldier humbly and most understandably accepted the Imperiatrix's words as she had now become far too busy to toy with his words and thoughts.

The H'Raka liked to test and play 'games of truth' with other species in their company. Sometimes, to see if they can intimidate them, possibly into subordinate positions, or sometimes just to aggravate them enough to expose their true intentions. The H'Raka liked to see species constantly prove themselves to them but 'Lîna, annoyed and irritated, had nothing to hide and had no time on her path of war to play such silly games. With the violently foppish soldier before her, set apart by campaigns long since past but still distinctly part of H'Raka, even in the plundered artistry that is their sear of power, 'Lîna kept her composure as the guard pointed to the hallway that would take her back to her shuttle.

She waved farewell to him as she began the walk back to her ship. 'Lîna knew the H'Raka valued the virtue of truth above all others, even survival, and held truth as highly as the lusty excess that is the sweetest violence and the essence of being of the hunt. The H'Raka, by their very nature, possessed a perfect honesty and had the proper sense of order to fulfil it. The H'Raka are the eternal judges, yet their tact, left something to be desired.

'Lîna's feelings of personal insult would have to be lain aside as those emotions left her almost immediately as 'Lîna decided the best course lay in tugging at the same strings General H'Renn liked to pull. She would be the diamond of the mind and she would shine her thoughts into him. 'Lîna would see if he would prove himself to her as she thought for a moment of 'Iato H'Renn. Only time would tell.

The palace guard then gave her perfect directions back to the landing pad where her personal shuttle awaited her along with her flight crew and S'yana guards. 'Lîna courteously thanked the black garbed soldier that remained at his post for his assistance. And though she was not required to, 'Lîna created a psychokinetically sculpted opaque cubical ruby container as a form of gratuity that was the wrapping for her gift which she gave to him.

Inside, lain suspended in air at its centre, was a drop of blood, a genetic blueprint memorised from a worthy prey. It was the recipe for a reptilian predator, the Ersz'ta, that the H'Raka had hunted to extinction in the subterranean caverns of the Hy'Bor colonies. The guard's eyes lit up when his H'Raka sight was able to see the internalises of the blood drop's genetic makeup was altered by 'Lîna so that it may serve as the template for enhanced clones, thanks to At'Lann technology, that would make the hunt of such creatures far more challenging than the H'Raka ever could have done with this contained genetic universe. The H'Raka had no qualms, of course, about clones from other worlds. 'Lîna walked away from the startled elite guard with a sly smile. The guardsman graciously took the gift and bade the young face of At'Lann a farewell with a traditional H'Raka military salute that she saw through her mind as she walked back to her shuttle. He remembered.

Φ

'Lîna returned to the outside air of H'Raka and this world's crimson and carbon etched morning sky. She watched with a little wonder as the horizon became one of grey flurries but flurries that were falling upwards into space amidst a flame hued sunrise. She looked out to this Hunter's world to see a skyline like that of a Rome with the heart of Berlin and the raunchy piety of Constantinople.

As she looked closer into the sky, 'Lîna saw that it was actually filling with warships flying off to battle. It was an armada like no other as if they walked the path of Trafalgar before the storm. The sight before her was exactly why she came. 'Lîna had wanted this, and she now had it. With this sight before her, 'Lîna could almost forget about the, at times, snobbish H'Raka diplomacy as her mind and eyes watched the Imperium fleet grow. With the H'Raka returning to the Imperium, the combined At'Lann/Lon'tus/H'Raka became twice that of what it was before it became a trinity alliance. The enemy would still outnumber them but this would ensure that worlds in seventeen critically vital galactic systems would be adequately protected under the flag of the Imperium Trinity.

With the H'Raka merged into the Imperium, longer lines of defence could be established to phase shield as many galaxies for as long as possible through a satellite grid that held key systems and that of their homes. The independent satellite phase shield arrays could now be deployed in H'Raka subspace to bolster their reality and slow the rate of universal decrease that would follow the coming second incursion of the darkest horde.

From her psionic link to Y'vis, 'Lîna was given schematics for H'Raka technology that could create far more powerful phase shift generators, that when combined with At'Lann and Lon'tus technology, could theoretically be their salvation. 'Lîna believed it to be their salvation and would put up with any discourtesy in order to obtain victory for her people and all life throughout existence.

But if they were to build such devices, only 'Lîna, Nul'lus, and 'Iato H'Renn would be the only ones who could power them, and they would have to be built in the At'Lann home system as it lay in a central spiritual juncture. This was a juncture like few others which would enhance their combined power matrix. But with the satellite grid buying them so much time before the massive project, a Pax Fortuna project, could be completed, the subspace arrays would become more susceptible to failure, and especially at a time when they could be needed the most. The phased osmotic shield around L'unn, was a shield system which could also be expanded across existence to bring reality back into permanence. The protection of reality could only be temporary. She did not know. Time was also their battlefield and no one wanted an imposed reality of non-existence.

So here was a possibility that would protect them from the dark army that had a resonance like that of the invading evil that raped Katyn, raped Volhynia, and raped Kyzl Kum with victims but would protect them from the erasure to follow. At the very least, today would be remembered by 'Lîna as what she truly cared about: as a move towards liberation and escape from extinction.

'Lîna turned once again to think of her new ally aboard her ship and she watched as the skies continue to fill with the shark like warships of H'Raka ascend into spatial deployment; swimming towards space in search of enemy prey. Whatever the outcome and at the very least, this would be enough to inflict great damage upon the enemy. She could still feel from the link with Y'vis that 'Iato H'Renn, from what little she gleaned about him from the H'Raka Emperor, that this man was as firmly committed as her in finding victory. For she loved tackling almost as much as Ince.

She hoped that it would be enough, in spite of all the games, that with the proper technological integration and with their combined strength their peoples, they could defeat the enemy. From what she knew of 'Iato H'Renn, the son of H'Raka, he was genetically enhanced years before either Nul'lus or herself. He was like her in many respects as he had undertaken an extensive hunting expedition for decades in what is now the quadrant of the universe diagonally across from theirs. 'Lîna thought it ironic that H'Raka sensor signatures that she flew by in her youth could have been emitted by a vessel of the man she would meet today. Only time would tell how it would all go, and for 'Lîna even that river had finitely begun to shallow into a stream.

Φ

There was a silence of anticipation as 'Lîna made her way back to the Lis'talla aboard her ascending shuttle. She looked out a window to where H'Raka's horizon became space and wondered what type of soul lay in the heart of her new ally that challenged her with, in her opinion, such impudent acts of diplomatic truculence. 'Lîna almost felt ashamed by feeling amused that such a being could leave her, the Imperiatrix, on their planet emptying itself of warriors, going off with those of her flag along with Nul'lus's. And as her crew informed her 'Iato H'Renn and Nul'lus had used her shuttle, and had the perplexing courtesy to send the shuttle back to retrieve the daughter of the At'Lann. Perhaps implying, back to her throne of war.

From the very start, this ally had already left a trail of competitiveness that even rivalled Za'szu's, and a lure of curious that an explorer of existence that 'Lîna could not resist. She looked out again into what was still the vastness of space after glancing at her S'yana guards who stood as sentries by the shuttle entrance by the shuttle ready room. It was a room which was nothing more than a miniature version of her own little stadia-parlour that was her living space of her palace-pyramid back on 'Mura.

Her guards gripped their At'Lann pulse rifles with the same seriousness and dedication that the elite guards of K'jak S'linn did for Y'vis and the entire H'Raka imperial household. 'Lîna looked out to the stars, taking her mind off the war once more for a moment, yet she could only think of the one, the life, already missing from reality by erasure and from what she gazed out into.

Though Marley's sun was shining, there was far too much going on for what could be said. Thankfully, her flight crew and her guards could not see the erasure except by sensor reading, they knew enough of what was beginning. It was a wound upon balance that had become, in a way, the death of Death. There was far greater things to think about than my new ally's attempt to gain an advantage over her, 'Lîna thought. She had to believe he was the capable leader described by Y'vis that would bring the Imperium the most crucial of victories.

'Lîna kept looking to the glittering points of light that once gave her so much comfort when she used to fly though them. She was a long way away from Fiji. 'Lîna had little comfort left these days when she thought of how she would fly through them once again as a soldier of peace and as a soldier of death to the enemy. She would fly through all the placing, seeing beings remembered from better days along the way, and she would probably still think, as she did now, of how few of them still remained.

She knew she would risk a great deal and sacrifice beyond what she would think herself possible, and in spite of it all, would do the same for 'Iato H'Renn so that he may take his place in the Imperium. For 'Lîna, there was no other option.

Φ

In a routine pattern of perfection and with little ceremony, 'Lîna's Imperial shuttle landed in the Lis'talla's main hanger bay and 'Lîna was once again aboard her massive chariot that acted as her home while away from At'Lann until the war would be complete. She never spoke a word to her pilots or any of the S'yana during the flight or when she disembarked. Her flight crew and guards stood at attention on both sides of her as she quietly left them, yet she did not ignore them at all during her trip to the H'Raka home world. For 'Lîna reigned with both the enjoyable silence and power of a telepath. Her mind was always somewhere and everywhere. Her mind had adapted long ago. It was her time to be the gamemaster.

'Lîna, at times, rarely spoke but all her subjects felt her presence and knew she weaved the reality of their existence together for them. Her mind had the ability to reach out at a sub-astral level to give acknowledgement, communication, orders, empathy, benevolence, allegiance, and her soul reached out to her people to give them a small measure of peace. After the phase shift psyogenetic enhancement, this psionic symbiosis became far stronger than it ever had been before. It went nearly to the point where this embrace and rapture seemed to almost sculpt her into a living symbol for them and took their relationship beyond that of which genetically programmed loyalty could never inspire.

'Lîna felt that she had been transformed into a goddess of her people in spite of her intimacy with them where she relayed to them that she was no more than any other living thing. But if she was now a goddess of the soul, she would see for herself if she had any measure of it as she was about to meet General H'Renn, the son of H'Raka.

She passed a small phalanx of At'Lann soldiers standing in formation to greet their Imperiatrix as she arrived, beside the end of a long row of over one hundred At'Lann fighters also docked in the main hanger bay. She walked as a procession of one towards the fourth wall of the mica and iris hued metal polymer gigantic main hanger bay of the Lis'talla that was adorned with geometric, negatively sloped diagonally running thick amethyst trim.

'Lîna walked with the realisation she was becoming one with the aether as her people willed it. She was their innocent soul even though she now thought of herself as so damaged beyond what she was. Her private staff, selected by 'Zaya, from all walks of the At'Lann and 'Mura royal courts, came into the bay, and followed behind 'Lîna into the intra-ship spatial folding fourth wall.

With her every step, 'Lîna's appearance once again changed as it had before meeting Y'vis. It was as if she found her lost tribe. Her hair began to curl into longer, tighter spiralled trestles that darkened into a deeper, and darker violet, and mauve. Her darkest and brightest of mauves and lilacs and a subdued shine that was her cape began to trail and billow ever further behind her. Her skinned tanned into a more opaque mauve and ivory and the colours were far more noticeable and pronounced than they ever were before.

As she went through the fourth wall, her attire tightened and their lines became ever more militarised so that 'Lîna was better able to present herself to the ambitious and intriguing General 'Iato H'Renn. Sometimes image is everything and this day of pomp, circumstance, and near grand standing, it *was* everything. Due to its nature, it is unimportant in meetings of souls but 'Lîna wanted it overtly known that she would be every bit the warrior General H'Renn was.

And one of her arsenals like that of the Lon'tus, and the H'Raka, was luxury, and her garb became even more so to befit an Imperiatrix ready for battle. And she was ready for 'Iato H'Renn as she buried her insecurities. Though only an hour away from another medical inhalation, 'Lîna had composed herself, and felt to be in a perfect state of balance.

'Lîna knew exactly where to find Nul'lus and her gate-crashing ally awaited her in the cream fields of their thoughts. She stepped through the fourth wall of the main hanger bay and through the fourth wall of the Lis'talla's Imperial Strategic Operations Command Room. The fourth wall, of course, being part of every room and on every deck of the Lis'talla that, when activated through desire, becomes a fold-gate to any other part of the ship. 'Lîna stepped out of the fourth wall and into the strategic operations room.

The beautifully contoured room was of a midsize when compared to others on the ship. It consisted of three floors adorned with gothic style consoles and large brightly multicoloured galactic cartographic holo-projections of troop deployments placed throughout the space in a logically chaotic fashion. In the midst of this organised disorder that was governments at war, 'Lîna caught sight of Nul'lus and he who could only be Prince and General 'Iato H'Renn. The pair were co-ordinating command directives with a small gathering of H'Raka, Lon'tus, and At'Lann admiralty and senior military advisors who were either on board or who came aboard from H'Raka, as well as holographic images of a few of the battle front generals.

The cadre was conversing almost in unison about course corrections, and deployment, engagement strategies. And in it all, there he was; General H'Renn was indeed an imposing figure. He was handsomely young, looking physically only a few years older than 'Lîna though she knew him to be decades older than her. His features were precise; an explosion of sharp edges that were drawn perfectly below his long gold, almost white, ashen hair. He was like Thor after having taken too long a tour of Hel, and he was also one like a wandering Fenris. As the pair saw that 'Lîna had arrived, they ceased their activities, ordered the council in their company to work elsewhere, and the pair then turned to greet her.

'Iato H'Renn towered over 'Lîna and even Nul'lus was shorter in height than the son of H'Raka. He was muscular and he was fierce; a lion crocodile that danced a dance of the prowl. 'Lîna thought his fangs that were barely hidden by his lips were quite cute. His eyes, like his body, were hard from years of training and the price a soul pays for killing. His gaze already seemed ancient.

He was a handsome warrior but a most dangerous one and he seemed even more so as 'Lîna began to notice his aura. There could be no doubt that he was an enhanced being like herself and Nul'lus. She wondered what new sacrifices the son of H'Raka made in defence of his world, the extent of his evolution from an earlier time. 'Lîna could not be certain. So there he was. So there he was.

As she relaxed her thoughts, 'Lîna realised she was not afraid of him but she was a little fearful of him, and she did need him. Such a randomly unexpected ally; so much like Y'vis, so much his son, Lîna thought. She had her work cut out for her but she would gain equality with him, she vowed. 'Lîna made her gambit in this power game. And with Nul'lus, who had not lost any approval at all with 'Lîna, looking on, made her move.

'Welcome aboard, Prince 'Iato H'Renn. On behalf of the At'Lann
Imperium, I welcome the H'Raka to what is and what will be the Imperium
Trinity. May our lives end in victory and may we live again in peace.'

'Lîna's words were softly polite and she added to her sentiment with a gracious bow. She froze and buried her worst suspicions and left it to fate to see how their first meeting would play out. 'Lîna needed to see and paint the portrait of the man whose actions, thus far, remained unclear.

She held the palms of her hands outward as if in prayer before a high deity, and 'Iato H'Renn grasped her hands before taking her right hand to his lips.

'A pleasure to meet at last, Imperiatrix of At'Lann. May the new order of the Imperium Trinity restore balance to all things', he said reverently with the words befitting a perfect gentlemen though one forged of blood and iron of the day of

Jadwiga. How he moved with the soul of a poet, 'Lîna thought. He added, 'Come see for yourself what our compatriot and mutual friend from Lon'tus and I have been slicing together.'

To say the very least, he was impressive to 'Lîna. She could see it in his grey wolf blue eyes, the bright blue embers that they were, and that burned out his platinum hued skin. Though he may be a noble soul, 'Lîna could see that he was strong and fierce. Fate had made her prepared for the challenge ahead. For beneath 'Iato H'Renn's eyes, the fire-waters of Ran, his psionic sight had assumed a targeting position the moment 'Lîna had entered the room.

She had expected as much but she was bold and shot up her telepathic defences as quietly as she could. Surprisingly, her boldness impressed him. 'Iato did not foresee such bite from a soul came from such a spiritual people though he knew this war would have an effect like no other on existence. The music from one like Warren seemed to be the hymn of the technology around them.

'Iato H'Renn's towering presence undeterred 'Lîna in seeking an ideal equality with him and the more she thought about it the more she realised that his great size seemed almost diminished in the company of a reassured Nul'lus. Hopefully my aristocratic friend is not enjoying himself too much, 'Lîna thought to herself.

And she could see that she would meet the son of H'Raka in the astral plane. Though 'Lîna preferred rank being left at the door so that only courtesy and respect remain but this was a day like no other. The time would come for the one of Fate to see if she was worthy of the respect of the Hunter. Her fears shifted away for the moment as she knew there would be another time for her to get to know 'Iato H'Renn on a more singular basis. For now, she could see an atmosphere of precedence afoot.

General H'Renn outstretched his hand for her to fully join them.

'Oh 'Lîna, what thoughts you have!', H'Renn said in a most jovial tone. 'Together there will be no need for even the most morbid of optimisms. I should think we shall exist long after our victory...I suppose you are wondering why we came aboard without you. Please do not take offence, daughter of At'Lann and 'Mura. The efficiency of the H'Raka people is legendary. I hope you are not cross with us', he said in mollifying and sincere tone.

'On the contrary, 'Iato, son of H'Raka. All of the Imperium is ours to share and defend. In fact, it is that very trait that brings us together. After all, we have ten At'Lann years to win this war', 'Lîna said without any hint of being perturbed.

Nul'lus then entered the scene to part of the repartee. Nul'lus always had a dapper way of putting a soothing spin on any event, and this situation was merely a dusting off of the shoulder after a zephyr of a sand storm. Nul'lus definitely seemed far too pleased to have been a part of some impolite conspiracy. 'Lîna turned toward him with a foraging and forgiving smile, and shrugged casually to ask for an answer. He was more than glad to tell his friend from 'Mura what they all knew.

'As you already know, we have found a way to win this war.' Nul'lus's soothing Lon'tus accent was as resonant in its calming effect on 'Lîna as was his motion as he pressed a Liverpool red coloured key on the interface before him.

On the largest of the holo-screens before the three was displayed a map of the galaxy the Imperium Trinity would share. The home galaxies of the Imperium Trinity, called M'Plura, by each race was yet another marker that each species was always a part of one species. The path walked could be one, both of their own and of others, due to the commonality of certain genetic sub-matrix alignments. All life is interconnected.

Three siren red, blinking lights representing co-ordinates formed a triangular area that rivalled the size of the entire expanse of the M'Plura galactic inter-systems. Nul'lus hit a emerald green interface key that caused the holo-screen to zoom in on the top triangular co-ordinate. The galactic disappeared and a technical schematic came up in a lilac hued etching of a massive, planet-sized, and technologically combined and enhanced phase shift generator.

Indeed the H'Raka were very efficient. 'Lîna seemed to find faith in what she saw before her. She could see the promise of victory. The holo-screen zoomed in yet further to reveal the interior of the central core axle of the massive constructs.

A single room and platform were now displayed. 'Lîna could see the similarity to the phase generator on L'unn. Here was the design for a far more refined chamber to vessel the power of those in the burden of the prepared and unprepared enhancement. It was an option that would nuke their genetic composition to where they could enter other unknown realms. And this deadly option would become their sacrifice for existence. The Death of Death was strangling them with its presence, and the three knew the Death of Death was the puppeteer for the massacre of eternity.

'Lîna had begun to see where this all was going to go. For one who was the faith of Fate, it was difficult to grasp why such uncertainty always cast itself upon her. She secretly kept her fear of not surviving long enough to fulfil what could be her very sacrifice. For she knew she had to stand with them for as long and as strongly as she could. 'Lîna saw into the little harnessing sanctums and saw that this plan was perhaps their only solution to their plight.

Though General H'Renn expected resistance from 'Lîna regarding the pursuit of this all encompassing option, she nodded in endorsement of what many would consider a very risky option but the only option to be made. Too much rain over paradise, 'Lîna thought. For it had become part of her being to feel the burdening pain of a universe being devoured by erasure. 'Lîna felt obliged to take this path as it was for now their last and best option.

'If you, daughter of At'Lann, and what is to you 'Mura'Lann, General 'Iato H'Renn and I can open a gate into the realm of the invaders. We can then cross into this dark realm to slay its leader, the one with the reins over the Army of Two

Rings that torment us. The dark one who is already trying to invade our minds.

We must be victory or there shall be only a pillaged nothingness.

From the bio-readings taken from the necrotic enemy prisoners, we now have proof that these walking dead soldiers are controlled by the singular presence that is the Death of Death.'

'Cut the head off and the snake will perish.', 'Lîna quipped. 'Exactly. If we sever the sub-psionic fluid stream that binds the enemy at their source, they will perish en masse so that they shall never return to existence. All we must do is slay the dark beast. We can not only obliterate the enemy fleet but we can then reverse the infinity inversion', Nul'lus added in a decidedly serene enlightened confidence and surprisingly without a trickle of arrogance.

Loyal Nul'lus keyed in another sequence to bring up a bio-reading of an enemy soldier and the sub-psionic matrix resonance signature of what controls the Two Ring *horda*. The energy to splice open the enemy's reality would have to be acquired, and as enhanced as the three sovereigns were, they still would have to attain what was required. The holo-sceen displaying the zig-zagging, and frozen dark winding resonance signature progressed to revolve in its own seamless animation exposing and blinking up counterbalance points which revealed, theoretically, how all reality would be restored.

The thoughts of the three were united in the concern that the natural flow of existence be restored. Whether 'Lîna was an Imperium inheritor or not, her place here could not be denied. 'Lîna was reassured in her confidence as the blessed news was spoken aloud but an important question still needed to be asked:

'How long will it take to construct the macro-psionic phase generators, Nul'lus?'

No matter the answer, 'Lîna would have to find a way.

'The generators can become operational in nine years using the most efficient methods. However, we still need to purchase materials from three neutral worlds which had sealed their borders in the first wave. There will be little time for delay, and by following the path of this plan, we will be cutting it close to the end of what could be our extinction.'

'Lîna was appalled species sought to seek profit in this most dire of times though she remembered most of the universe operates using less evolved economic systems, and she was appalled she might not live to carry it all through. Nul'lus had the interface bring up a stellar map that superimposed itself over the technical schematics. The main holo-screen and two other large holo-units displayed the planetary positions of the three worlds and their co-ordinates in the now ovular universe. Thankfully, even the most outlying of the three worlds were safe from the erasure contraction of the second ring of the enemy for, at the very least another few years.

'Lîna looked to both Nul'lus and 'Iato H'Renn to find affirmation in how insulting it was to actually have to pay for essential war supplies though her nod was met with an expression that any price for victory must be paid, her two allies smiled back to agree. For they all knew, the demand for victory is always inelastic.

For a moment of time, her eyes became voyeuristic into that which is 'Iato H'Renn. For a brief instant, she stared into him. Past his sharp long canines of his smile, past his lightning strike and mainly platinum hair and past his eyes that were burning with the fires of a viper's strike. He was a wall of intimidation whose mind she could barely swim into. The soul core was too deep. But she had to trust him. 'Lîna needed him to stand at her side and protect their worlds and all others. Hopefully H'Renn realises that together we can be strong enough to seize the Death of Death by the throat and behead the darkest of beasts, she thought.

'Lîna, taking a moment of time for herself, had reached into the high psionic planes to discover the identity of the menace, the enemy puppeteer, and made the posturing between her and General H'Renn seem insignificant by comparison. Though from what she could see and feel, her mind had reached out enough to know that whatever was against them was the most evil of creations. She even personified it as the most evil of existence.

As 'Lîna quickly glanced over to General H'Renn once again, she sensed nothing of this within him which, for the most part, put her mind at ease except for the fact that the first wave of destruction had left a damning, dark psionic residue over all of reality. Reality now was a much murkier place. Though the Imperium was reborn and existence still remained for now, the damage inflicted upon reality became such a scarring part of it. But as 'Lîna fell into her own thoughts, she did her best to keep them flowing with hope. 'At least with H'Renn I will deal with this menace atop the great aether pillar. Together with Y'vis's heir to the greatest of hunts, and this heir to an empire has the soul of an avenging angel. He is sword and he is dark sonnets of justice. I knew it. My soul will find synergy with his.' 'Lîna's aside thoughts flowed into a momentary successive thought stream that began to see through the mask of the predator king that the son of H'Raka wore so well. She vowed that her day where she would swim deeply into his soul.

'Lîna turned to Nul'lus, who with the suave wave of his hand reconfigured the interface to display on the holo-screen the latest unified fleet positions throughout the universe. 'Lîna now knew something far more interesting had brought the pair to the Lis'talla without her. 'Lîna decided to investigate the matter.

'Anything else I should know, Nul'lus of the Lon'tus Imperium?, she said with a slyness that was all hers.

Rank was always too trying a thing sometimes for these friends of equal soul advancement and especially for friends like 'Lîna and Nul'lus to bother with. This day was no exception once again. Nul'lus's answer, though as exciting and elevating, was a sobering one, and this answer was one like many others in their shared experiences but one that would not take away their previous bond. 'Lîna had the faith of Fate in any event and complete trust in the Ambassador from the Lon'tus

Commonwealth that was now the Lon'tus Imperium.

'What you know in your heart is already true, 'Imiszi. The circle of truth is now complete. We returned so that I could respond to an urgent message from my home in Rimisz'tii. 'Iato H'Renn was merely trying to give it an element of surprise to one who rarely experiences it.'

H'Renn's lips slit themselves into an affirming smile.

'If it pleases you, I have decided to stay on board but I can no longer be your First Officer as I have been elected Imperator of the Lon'tus.

'I would have it no other way, Nul'lus. You will be found worthy of the path lain out for you by your people. Well done, my friend. Your worthiness has led to great power being thrust upon you.'

'Lîna's delighted response elated Nul'lus as she embraced him in all that she could convey in congratulations. Though only the path of war lay ahead, it had become their time.

As she held her friend in happiness for his new path, 'Lîna hoped the great responsibility of power would not be the continuous hurdle to overcome that it had become for her. 'Lîna had sacrificed her desires for duty, and her essence for her people, and even Nul'lus, on his own path, would sacrifice himself to the burden that is power.

However, she knew he would make the most of it. Besides, 'Lîna had already grown to dislike giving even the most minor of orders to her friend. She would work in tandem with him more so than she could have if he continued as her First Officer. She let go of her friend and held his hands for a moment of repose before Nul'lus revealed the final piece of the puzzle already alluded to by Y'vis.

'Furthermore, I will not be the only one at your side. Y'vis's final decree has been made official. General 'Iato H'Renn is now the Imperator of the H'Raka.'

'Lîna let go of her friend without being taken aback for even she could not stop the path of Fate. She saluted 'Iato H'Renn in the H'Raka style, a tight raised clenched left fist horizontal to his shoulders with her forarm held out in front of herself, to applaud his new status. Then 'Lîna felt it time to solidify the new direction of the At'Lann and their place in the Imperium Trinity. She would give the H'Raka what she would have given them in any circumstance. 'Iato H'Renn would lead at her side if he found her worthy. She looked to him to silence his predatory appetite.

'Lîna, telepathically, let the Imperator of H'Raka know she would meet him on the high astral plane when the opportunity would strike him. They would judge one another. But for now, duty was decorum. And 'Lîna would show the son of H'Raka she was bold and brave.

'Iato H'Renn, Imperator of H'Raka, and High General of your fatherland's armies, I transfer command to you, as was the ancient custom, for command of the unified Imperium fleet. I will ensure the fleet of At'Lann shall not falter.'

'As I will ensure the Lon'tus fleet shall fight as the Lon'tus always have', Nul'lus calmly interjected and reached out his hand to bequeath the Lon'tus fleet to the H'Raka.

She would leave the strategy to the H'Raka, as would Nul'lus, to continue the ancient tradition of what was always done in times of war. To have the H'Raka as your ally meant it was the only choice that could be made. 'Lîna placed her right hand on the interface panel, and had with only a short data stream inter-link, all At'Lann military command codes transferred to the H'Raka interface. As 'Lîna lifted away her hand, Nul'lus pressed a large teal interface key and the Lon'tus system became integrated with that of the H'Raka.

'Iato H'Renn looked at the pair who stood by his side: one a noble soul, and one who was not proven but one who was an ecclesiastic paradox. Her years of exploration made her so unlike her people, and yet she embodied them more than she realised. The son of H'Raka looked to those who would stand with him to lead the Imperium Trinity. 'I am beginning to understand why Nul'lus told me not to underestimate the daughter of 'Mura. Whether she knows it or not, she walks the path of Fate. She will be a most interesting hunt on the psionic plane', H'Renn thought. He then bowed to the pair and with the most noble of oaths uttered,

'May you find me worthy of honour.'

With that it was done and the Imperium Trinity was reborn, and the most holy of crusades could truly begin.

Φ

In the short time that passed after the alliance was formalised, 'Lîna had the time to make a live holo-address to the At'Lann people of what would be the new world order and what would be their path in the war. Her voice once one of such joyous innocence but on this day 'Lîna spoke to her people with stoic and brutal honesty. She respected her people too much to give them any less.

'Lîna also had time to oversee the new course direction of the Lis'talla alongside Nul'lus and 'Iato H'Renn. The son of H'Raka gave her quite a stir when he lit up a H'Raka hand rolled cigar and began to smoke on the bridge of her ship. He did not hide that he had been psyogenetically enhanced in the past and had recently undergone further enhancements. The chemical composition of the inhalant was similar to that created by 'Zaya and the At'Lann Medical Corps.

She wondered as he stood there unabashedly calm and triumphant if he knew more about her than he let on. What was for sure was that the son of H'Raka bore the burden of the sovereign affliction. But where 'Lîna and Nul'lus held their genetic affairs under a cloak of secrecy, 'Iato as he preferred to be called by them when not in the ecstasy of the hunt, openly flaunted his. 'Lîna looked across the bridge to see that Val'damus, surprisingly, found it all quite refreshing when the bridge crew became aware of what he was doing. 'Lîna shook her head with an inner smile. He was, after all, a gentleman like Nul'lus, and to 'Lîna he was not déclassé in his technique. 'Iato H'Renn still carries himself as any high officer should, 'Lîna thought to herself.

The Lis'talla was on a course for Armn'dallos in the H'Nua galaxy. Two Lon'tus Imperium armoured freighters would join the flag ship of the At'Lann Imperium at a rendezvous point on the outskirts of the Armn'dallos home system. With the enemy having sabotaged so many subspace corridors, it would take the Lis'talla a day to get there. The enemy was without mercy. This day lost was a result of the Army of Two Rings sabotaging lthe under-space in many regions withsome form of lower reality mines that made subspace folding far too dangerous for the Sovereigns of the Imperium Trinity and what would be their cargo.

Due to this fact, the Lis'talla's engines were adapted for multi-course correctional repositioning. The spatial repositioning technology allowed the Lis'talla to enter a liminal subspace phase and into a state of infinite particle warp. Hence the ship would travel by already being at their destination in another sub-spatial reality. Gradually, the ship would come to exist in randomised points throughout the existing universe with the Imperium interface compensating for the rate of erasure. As the particle warp slows, the Lis'talla would ever so minutely come to exist in the one point of her destination.

But a day was also gained by 'Lîna to turn into her mind and think of all the chain of events. As she sat smoking in her living space, her sanctum sanctorum, looking over 'Iato H'Renn's Imperium attack strategies and possible gambits displayed before her on her floating cubic holo-interface.

The Imperium fleet now had a plan for a major offensive to engage the enemy at their weakest possible points along the encroaching First Ring of the Death of Death in an attempt to slow what had become the implosion of existence. As the cranberry red light of Imperium warship positions reflected of 'Lîna's lilac soft cheeks, she could only think of what a keen eye her new ally had in finding any points susceptible to heavy bombardment from their weaponry at all. Though part of him seemed to stalk her waiting for the chance to roam her mind, the son of H'Raka seemed to gain more respect by 'Lîna with every moment they were together. Perhaps it was their fate to be comrades on the path of war. In any event, it was clear to each of the three that there was one thing they strongly shared in common: both had a thirst for victory that was just as ravenous in each of them.

She also thought of Nul'lus who she was elated for as she could now officially treat him as an equal of royal standing in her affairs as Imperiatrix of the At'Lann. She felt almost ashamed of her near Spice Boy exuberance that she let, for a brief moment, became unrestrained. 'Lîna reminded herself that she had already lost so much of herself from the very moment the Death of Death came to invade them.

She decided to cling to her empathy even if it wounded her more than all the death she already had surrounding her. She tried to think of herself as not being divorced from innocence though that was the way 'Lîna now thought of herself, and the more she thought, 'Lîna came to accept the way the war had already changed her.

With the enhancement, with every step, 'Lîna grew stronger as her psyogenetic matrices continued to evolve. Her command confidence grew as she could already see that she worked well in tandem with 'Iato H'Renn and Nul'lus, and it only made her feel a little happier that the Imperium fleet was a lot more empowered.

And she was especially glad that the son of H'Raka had set out on the path of war with so much to prove. For all she would sacrifice on the path ahead, she needed Y'vis's chosen one. She needed the highest of warriors at her side. They now shared the path of war whether he wanted her on it or not. He was what 'Lîna would aspire to be in her own way. She vowed to earn the respect of one so noble, so strong, and so fierce.

The people of At'Lann and 'Mura, she could feel that they felt uneasy by what their Imperiatrix had chosen for them. The At'Lann had always known 'Lîna chose her own path but the path she chose was always taken selflessly for her people. She had their faith and she was their fate and 'Lîna was given their full support. It was no longer rumour on the home world of 'Lunn that there was a silent cancer of apathy eating away at many within the universe, spreading its roots out, making the path At'Lann had chosen, sometimes the only path one could take. Most At'Lann knew this to be true.

Already this was a war like no other, and yet simply war nonetheless. Fate had seemed to lead to what seemed to be unavoidable choices. However, to 'Lîna, Fate was already made and yet always could be made. As 'Lîna cleared her thoughts to focus her mind, she decided to try a change of pace and fall into a sleep that could have been blessed by Morpheus.

'Lîna vaporised the last of her medical dispenser. With her genetic coherence lock stabilised for a few hours, she curled up in her violet silk and ivory silk covers of her bed, and began to sleep, thinking of how much she would have to adjust her mind and soul to be the fate of her people in the fields of war. The daughter of At'Lann, who left her sister behind to protect her by letting her sister's nurturing hands take care of the At'Lann on L'unn. She was alone in this war but more and more 'Lîna could see that she drew strength by sharing the path of war with the son of Lon'tus and the innovative son of H'Raka. The three were beginning to stand together. Still, much had to be done. For now, 'Lîna surrendered to the peace of sleep.

19
The Deflowering and Deflowered Totality That Awaits

During the day of waiting, life began to regain some semblance of order and normalcy for 'Lîna. 'Zaya had supplemented the inhalant curative so that her medical order of three hours of regenerative sleep a night would be enacted. 'Zaya had left a holo-message apologising for not telling her of the new course of treatment.

'Lîna could forgive this of her as she completely trusted her sister and knew her intentions were just. Considering time had become their enemy as well, 'Lîna knew she had no other choice. She thought it must be quite a powerful agent to induce sleep in one that does not require or desire it. But with the genetic instabilities that the enhancement had brought about, she now needed the regenerative and healing powers of physical sleep.

After she awoke from her rest, she got dressed and went into what would be her routine of taking a shift in command of the main bridge. It was becoming more of a ceremonial duty to her but one she took most seriously than anything else even her own pursuit of the Death of Death, yet she adhered to the more ancient traditions of her people.

'Lîna also transmitted another general message to the people of the At'Lann Imperium and began a tradition of her own by sending a brief message every day she spent on board the Lis'talla. Though she returned home only to see it plundered, 'Lîna knew Za'szu would return paradise to L'unn, and she began to miss home more than she ever had when she was in other ends of the universe.

The Imperiatrix of At'Lann even included Nul'lus and 'Iato H'Renn in her general broadcast so that her people could judge them for themselves. They were always enamoured with Nul'lus as he was the perfect facilitator of trade and was already recognised as an enlightened being. 'Iato H'Renn was an unknown variable altogether. Though the At'Lann can be potentially immortal like both the Lon'tus and H'Raka, few At'Lann lived to remember the last alliance with the H'Raka. But Nul'lus's backing caused many to see the logic behind 'Lîna's decision.

As well, in this day of waiting, 'Lîna spent a portion of her day on the main advanced technology research bay, inspecting weapon prototypes and experiments conducted on many different integrated technological components. 'Zaya fourth walled in to see how she was feeling after the rest. The treatment, to 'Zaya's delight, had thus far, been effective.

'Lîna spent her evening, as she would begin to spend most of them discussing military strategy with Nul'lus and 'Iato H'Renn and smoking the 'Mura'Lann Agent 27. Agent 27 was a hybrid of pharmaceutical solutions and compounds from At'Lann, Lon'tus, and a reserve supply of H'Raka substances that remained from the time before the embargo with them. And with their entry into the Imperium once more, such supplies were replenished, and access for 'Zaya to find the latest medical innovations.

The balancing agent, for the time being, had to be administered at least once a day. So in an effort to find unity and equality amongst the sovereigns of the Imperium Trinity, the three decided to meet nightly in order to bolster their alliance where they could administer to business of the Imperium and to what kept them alive. Such became 'Lîna's routine from the day the Imperium Trinity took form on H'Raka. She was not afraid of 'Iato H'Renn and she awaited their meeting on the astral and psionic plane. The reality was that there was no one else who was undergoing and experiencing such brave new states of existence. The three only had each other in this respect.

The Imperium military advisors even insisted that the three should not be involved in the war at all and should be kept safe until the phase generators could be built, yet the three went above and beyond what was asked of them. The three were risk-takers and each held the belief that fortune favours the bold, and each sovereign did not want to be coddled until they could open a gate through the phase generators into the arena of the Death of Death.

In what was the first of their many discussions, 'Lîna, Nul'lus, and 'Iato H'Renn all felt that laying in safe harbours was far too beneath their way. They would take on the path of war like no others before them ever could. They each vowed that they would lay down their lives hunting down the enemy and secure victory for all life.

The agenda of the day also covered the supplies that the Imperium would need from the three worlds that the Lis'talla was on course for. Their first evening session came an hour before they would orbit Armn'dallos and broke the ice a little more that stood between them. Though 'Iato H'Renn was quite personable towards the daughter of At'Lann, there was a shyness of uncertainty between them. Nul'lus did his best to provide a relaxed atmosphere to converse with one another, and he was kind enough to have brought some G'jhara, a rare Lon'tus spirit that had not been made for centuries.

Though none required drink any longer, the taste could still succulently permeate the senses. The G'jhara had a taste of island rum and sweetened cloves that was enjoyed by all in full complement to the curative inhalants. The G'jhara certainly made for a closer social setting in spite of the drawing of the three from such unique perspectives. Still, the taste was sweet, and perhaps, it was enough to put the three into a state of objective openness that could deal with the mission at hand.

Blessedly, the vibe, the atmosphere, was light on decorum and friendly in discourse. Barring an enemy raid, there was no cause for anxiety amongst the three. Nul'lus and 'Iato were even a little jovial about the whole thing. Though the task ahead was a sacred one, Nul'lus seemed to make the most of this difficult adventure, and Nul'lus made it an adventure as his way of putting the war into perspective. The tone on this night had a much lighter mood mainly brought about by Nul'lus telling those who he shared the path with, that his wife and his family were safe and had been well protected on Lon'tus during the first bombardment.

'Lîna realised she must have been away from home for a long time when Nul'lus married before her. 'Lîna had yet to meet her but wondered what powers this woman must possess to make her friend cast off a few of his Bondish ways.

'Iato H'Renn even went on to discuss his mate, his wife, at great length as well. 'Lîna almost felt out of place in their repartee as she had never found one to share herself with though she always knew there was one soul who would be for her. Besides, she thought, the At'Lann marry much later in life, it is pleasing to know my allies know a worthy joy in their lives. What made it even better was how inspiring it was in the way the one from H'Raka discussed love was a moment that captivated as much as Nul'lus's words of good news amidst the supply run mission.

'Iato had a philosophy that souls in love hunt for each other, and when they finally enter each others sights, they cast aside their armaments and embrace in an eternal union that transcends corporeal existence. 'Lîna found it almost a paradox that one who embodied the hunt for his people would carry such a view. Somehow, it warmed 'Lîna's heart to know the new K'or, the new Imperator of H'Raka, would place such a high value on the peace of love.

Of course, Nul'lus could not help point out how he noticed that 'Lîna had yet to find a mate even in all her travels. 'Lîna countered that she held to the belief that her travels had just begun and she winked at him and said, 'Just because I have spent so much time alone does not mean I have always been alone.' Both had the chance to have nudge each other in the 'Heh! Heh!' way.

Nul'lus always enjoyed playing and gently ribbing his life long friend whom spent far too much time in serious, ecclesiastical, and introspective states of mind. 'Lîna always enjoyed that Nul'lus would give her what she needed from time to time: a chance for her soul to remember the delights of being. He knew her to be playful. And Nul'lus always enjoyed the regal At'Lann way of responding to his ribbing that could always make each of them smile. 'I have yet to find what I am looking for, my aristocratic friend', 'Lîna thought smiling to herself.

'Iato H'Renn enjoyed all this banter and had a deep and hearty laugh. The roots of a unique rapport seemed to begin to be established in 'Lîna's living space that night between the sovereign tern even with 'Iato still waiting to evaluate the daughter of At'Lann and 'Mura. Rank was left at the door and the only hidden feeling was that of fate being fulfilled.

As the three casually began about the mission to Armn'dallos, the tone became one of confident readiness. The Three of the Imperium Trinity would transport to the planet and simply signal any member of their race to approve payment as they Armn'dallos were a cybernetic inter-linked species operating in a liberally modified command economy. Then the supply ships joining the Lis'talla would have the cargo folded aboard. It was as succinct as it could be.

The Armn'dallos are a telepathic species with a purpose that seemed strangely familiar to 'Lîna for the Armn'dallos explored existence through ultimate equality. Their collective consciousness had been so heavily interconnected into individual Armn'dallos minds that each was configured and conformed to be precisely identical in depth and structure in relation to the next.

Their corporeal bodies were nearly genetically identical and their evolution made them asexual making each member of this species appear the same to the next. Each mind becomes a grain of sand in its own Sahara. Their purpose, the way of their sirocco, became their collective being. Pleasingly, the price for their goods had not changed with the threat of erasure. All they requested was a new atmosphere for their world to cover their costs. Hardly a stiff price for the Imperium. The Armn'dallos found their present atmosphere possessed far too many variances for their liking. It would be a simple matter for the At'Lann engineers to create a planetary atmosphere which could be kept at a level of zero activity.

The Armn'dallos, ironically, found clouds, wind, and temperature variances to be too distracting for their society. So entrenched were they by their inter-link that their minds became far too cluttered with external perceptions to withstand seeing anything more than their solar body sliding slowly and seamlessly across a spotless sky in their day to day lives. Their planetary environmental controls were inadequate to prevent a few production days lost every year to meteorological variation.

Since visitors to their world was such a rarity for this species, 'Lîna felt it important to remind her allies assembled with her that it would be important to actually grab hold of a member of their species to get their attention, or else they would simply be left waiting for a reply, and left ignored. Nul'lus thought it quite churlish of them to become slaves to their own technology. 'Lîna thought it piteous. And 'Iato thought it diminished in all returns as compared to H'Raka efficiency. Despite Imperium civility, it was not considered rude to jar a Armn'dallos citizen from out of their routine; it was a necessity of proper diplomatic functioning with this species.

Nul'lus was still relishing his new status as Imperator and elected King of the Lon'tus seemed to think very little of the Armn'dallos. He recalled from previous visits to their world that they were creatures of a silly, contrived shyness that were far too absorbed with labour production to even come close to being considered remarkable as a species. If Nul'lus did not feel somewhat approving of them for their attempt to possess the civility of some of his stiffer gentry, he would think nothing of them at all other than that they had something to trade for.

'Iato H'Renn felt the Armn'dallos were a species lacking in any measure of greatness by their self-inflicted dissemination of the individual mind. Of course, 'Iato H'Renn's opinions were rather subjective as they were opinions based upon the perspective of the most intensive individualistically competitive cultures that liked to be noticed. Such were the mighty H'Raka. If not for what the Armn'dallos were exporting, they would be insignificant to him.

In the past, the H'Raka had generally ignored Armn'dallos in their economic dealings with a species one almost had to be condescending with in order to seal contracts with. But since they always left a wide berth for the H'Raka and had never gone against them in any way, 'Iato H'Renn had no ill feelings towards them. He had never been to their world before but had met with the few trade delegations that came to H'Raka, and were just as disconnected with reality there as they were on their world. 'Iato wondered why they bothered.

During her exploration days in the spatial wilderness, 'Lîna had been to their world only once before and that was only fifteen months into her trek across existence. 'Lîna, in between smoking, told her allies of how she had spent a day on their planet. She spent most her day there at one of their always empty rectangular, massive, natural reserve parks on their world in their global capital of Sl'ona. From the park she came to walk through, 'Lîna came to its highest treeless vantage point of a low rising foothill on a ground that rolled without diversity.

'Lîna for most of her time there decided to watch them, sometimes to see how their adherence to simplicity and conformity had failed their species in many ways. One could say that the Armn'dallos had imprisoned themselves from moksha, and did not desire to rise away from what they had created for themselves. 'Lîna did her best to study them and what path they had created for themselves. She could not help finding them simple and even now, she had about as much respect for them as she would for an ant colony. Still, all life mattered to her and she valued ant colonies as highly as some members of her own race. She always bore in mind, no society was perfect but 'Lîna realised how close hers was to perfection.

'Lîna always carried the egalitarian view that any living things that burned with the light of all light illuminating their existence was to be cherished, and even the Armn'dallos possessed it. And like all other life, the Armn'dallos were worthy of,at least, a small measure of respect. Such enchanted soul fires burn through all things but 'Lîna was dismayed that this light was a little obscured in this species by too much pointless toil. Work without merit does not set species free.

'Lîna might have thought nothing more of the Armn'dallos on her first visit to their world but during the course of that day on their world, she gained permission to enter their cybernetic and telepathic inter-link network and experienced first hand the paradigm of their collective order. Driven by the logic of the hoi polloi and ultimate parental government, 'Lîna came to find respect for the autarky the Armn'dallos came to find from the pursuit of their existence. For whatever advantages or disadvantages, the Armn'dallos lived in unity, and like the feeling of swimming in the data streams of the Imperium interface, 'Lîna could see how their inter-link became the crux of their existence.

But for the Three of the Imperium Trinity, the issue agreed upon was that there was no other choice than to deal with the Armn'dallos if work on the phase generator project could commence as soon as possible. For they had the compounds needed by the Imperium with no other known worlds possessing them. So it really did not matter what any of the Three thought of the Armn'dallos.

This mission was not, however, a simple and largely ceremonial affair. With the temporal constraint, the situation was tense. Even in this journey, there was still the underground reality that was dangerous to them in any state of travel. The Lis'talla pushed on in their quest with the Three searching for accomplishment. And that was the sole reason the Three took the path of war was to fulfil themselves. Their desires hinged on what sacrifices and victories they would return to their people. 'Iato H'Renn had already sent a thousand Imperium warships to strategic points on the ever shrinking front. The H'Raka heavy bombers would pound the enemy to weaken the Two Ring army of the Death of Death and to weaken their line as much as possible before the Imperium counteroffensive would be launched.

It became foreseeable that the Army of Two Rings would already be planning to retaliate against the Imperium for their resistance, and would retaliate by directly attacking the sovereigns of the Imperium alliance. But the Three would not take shelter. Wherever their paths would take them, 'Lîna knew they walked as marked for death by the enemy. The Three would have to remember to be on guard. Their good life would not come to an end to the abyss that is erasure. Then in their relaxing, things began to change.

'Lîna could feel the imbalance around her. Something had changed. Something had shifted. And something more was left empty. 'Lîna looked to 'Iato H'Renn and Nul'lus but they had not yet felt the admonitory air she now took in.

A bridge communications officer from Lon'tus, named Lu'va, who joined the Lis'talla by piloting her own ship to join the crew, alerted the Three through 'Lîna's coffee table sized structure before them. Ah, for an angel. The sight of her confirmed what 'Lîna had sensed. In her sweet Lon'tus accent she alerted them that all transmissions from Armn'dallos had ceased. Scans of their planet indicated all Armn'dallos life signs had ceased. The only communications noise coming from their world was the ghostly wind of silence.

After a pause, 'Lîna left it to H'Renn to order a contingent to accompany them on their fold to the surface. She insisted telepathically that the Three go; to see firsthand what had occurred. The Imperium would have to be shown what to prepare against, and what was the doom that could lay ahead. They would be living witnesses for their people. 'Lîna already knew they would stand before an atrocity. She could feel that it had the blood soaked hands of the Death of Death written all over it. This might be a trap. But if it were a trap, it was also an opportunity. H'Renn and Nul'lus readily agreed to go.

Perhaps the Three wanted to begin their enacted alliance in the war or whether the Three wanted to begin making a difference, it was time for the Three to begin to venture further along the path of war. When the Lis'talla arrived to orbit Armn'dallos, the Three folded their way to the surface along with their expedition and away team. In the same fashion as the *anime like* flash that brought the Lis'talla to this system, so too did it herald the Three before they stepped onto the ground of the Armn'dallos capital of Sl'ona. To a place that lay silent with death.

Φ

Sl'ona had become a capital where simultaneous death was everywhere. The lives of the Armn'dallos had ceased in the middle of their routines. The entire race had fallen to death in a single moment. There were queues of Armn'dallos, all laid out in orderly, tidy trains of one corpse fallen on top of another. The lines of bodies stretched from one building to the next across the planet, even those alone were not spared. Extinction was an ominous spectacle for the Three to see. Both disgusting and pristine was the sight of so many bodies.

Their city was just as 'Lîna had remembered its structure and appearance. Besides the corpses, Sl'ona had not changed in any way from the last time 'Lîna's travels had brought her to this world. Their slender and deep pink skinned bodies were so clean and still warm, she thought. Only their beluga like facial features had been laid silent and left empty. So cold they appeared after the hearth within them no longer burned, 'Lîna thought. For a moment, she imagined they would all stand up and continue with their lives, or would stand as the walking dead and attack them. But nothing happened. There was only the silence cast by extinction, for all Armn'dallos were dead across existence.

Nul'lus and H'Renn marvelled at the insidious power of the enemy. For there could be no other murderer of a people. Unless. Unless it was by their own hand. The Three would have to be sure. The truth would have to be found. 'Lîna then knelt by the corpse of a small, little girl and placed her hand on and caressed the child's lifeless forehead.

The youngling was so small and so still, and so unlike the particular line of death before the Three. She pulled the dead child by the arm out of the lined stack of corpses undergoing rigor mortis, and out from the lanky burial of Armn'dallos dead. She looked at the child while Nul'lus and 'Iato stood by her side, watched on.

'Lîna closed her eyes of ritual and opened them once more with a different sight behind them. She then placed the dead child back in the queue that the Three had come upon before 'Lîna had disturbed it. Something Hebe would do when handling her most precious possessions. She slid her right index finger down the cheek of the adult Armn'dallos that lay dead once again over top of the child that once stood ahead of him in the queue. 'Lîna then rose from the smooth, sanitised ground and turned to her allies. She revealed to them the truth of what had happened.

'It was suicide.'

There could be no other explanation as 'Lîna had come to this devoid conclusion from scanning the remnants of the Armn'dallos cyber-telepathic inter-link. Nul'lus, thought it was absurd, and that 'Lîna was only trying to humour them. But this was a Jonestown gone pandemic. He looked to her and saw she was the 'Lîna she had always been. She had a very small sense of humour and none at all when she saw the dead offerings that covered their silent planet. Like coming to a world where holocaust was everywhere. How it mirrored ours, she thought.

'Iato then scanned the Armn'dallos dead for as far as he could, and confirmed 'Lîna's words to be true. How weak and how brave of them, he thought. Nul'lus asked 'Lîna if there was a reason for their decision for he needed to know the intrinsic logic of their motives to cause their own extinction. He needed to know what made them choose to leave their world inhabited by fallen bodies that would eternally wait, and never get to wherever it was they were going.

Apparently, they died from a telepathic inter-link implosion; a self-destruct sequence activated en masse by the Armn'dallos. They had planned their own neural shutdown. All their bodily functions ceased as their collective mind collapsed upon itself. It seemed they had only lived long enough to gather the chemical compounds requested by the Imperium as if for no other reason than the obligation of doing so.

'Lîna looked over and past her shoulder to 'Iato H'Renn basking in the passively warm Armn'dallos sun that was lowering itself into sunset over the near perfect geometrically conformed jagged and curving skyline of Sl'ona. And he looked back at her with his Hunter's gaze that permitted the truth to be told.

'It would seem the Armn'dallos were a species that lacked any sort of faith at all. The Armn'dallos collectively decided upon a choice of suicide after their inter-link system calculated... the odds of our winning the war before us.'

'Lîna felt more shame than embarrassment as part of her somehow felt insulted that life would exist with no faith at all. The war, the enhancement, was changing her. Though their inter-link was a simpler version of the At'Lann and much larger Integrated Imperium Interface, even this simple species knew the odds were not in their favour. She was insulted that a species would act like a herd of buffalo pressing onward and off a knoll and precipice.

'They should have consulted our Interface. Then they would have known that in our findings, their probability of survival from erasure would have increased by 3.3%.', 'Lîna said sardonically.

'No need to worry, 'Imiszi. We are the Imperium after all. They should have placed their fate in the Imperium as the each of the Trinity has placed in each other', said Nul'lus as he unburied his aristocratic optimism. Though saddened, he had nothing but a smirk for those who had so little within themselves to believe in.

Less than H'Raka remora, the son of H'Raka thought.

The Three walked to a low wave electro-psionic relay station that had a queue of dead Armn'dallos going into what looked like a tan stack of metal cubes from each quadrant surrounding the building. How the Armn'dallos dead flowed from every corner past the Three. Nul'lus sat back in his dark navy tunic of his sovereignty over Lon'tus and he lit a curative cigarette.

As he began to smoke, his mood became ever more positive over the lessons of the empty loss of the Armn'dallos from existence. After he exhaled a huge cloud of panacea smoke into the once pristine, once pollution free air of Armn'dallos, Nul'lus began to laugh.

'Imagine for a moment, if they had waited until the Second Ring was just before them. If they had waited, perhaps their calculation for the greatest of wagers would have been altered.'

'Fate always seems to find a way, 'Lus.'

Nul'lus was now laughing so hard he could barely get a word out before the giggle-berry like laughter almost became all too much for him before snickering,

'What a silly species. They lacked patience. They should have at least waited for their trading partners to arrive before going through with their stunt'

'Then you should find it ironic that they did, 'Lus', 'Lîna said as she was now laughing as well while pointing out that which brought out a roar of laughter in 'Iato H'Renn.

'As evolved as the Armn'dallos were, they were never enlightened enough to understand even the Imperium's most basic scientific theories. I highly doubt the Armn'dallos had the proper ability to predict anything other than where their next queue would begin and end and how the Armn'dallos ahead of them would stand', H'Renn scoffed as he continued to laugh his hearty laugh. The Three had everything in common and nothing at all.

Nul'lus looked for as far as his eyes could reach across Sl'ona, across genocide, and across a world where life had been scorched away from its realm. 'Lîna then joined part of her mind to his and Nul'lus did the same with 'Iato. The enhancement had given her a sight that few possessed. She opened their minds so they may see the hidden truth they each could now see, the genetic make-up of the Armn'dallos had been splintered by the arrival of the horde of the Death of Death.

In his thoughts, the Aristocrat chastised this species for being so damaged by the descent of darkness that they felt they were left with no other option than to lay down in the embrace of the Death of Death for eternity. To the Hunter this was just another day. And to Fate, this was a day to sadly laugh at how perverse the battlefield of existence truly was.

It was only in times like these did 'Lîna feel foolish for what she strived to defend. Indeed, the Armn'dallos were quite silly. Far too dispassionate for 'Lîna's personal tastes. She felt that only a species that follows its heart would always bring them a step closer to the truth of their existence and that which is their soul. The Armn'dallos never had a chance to discover this. It was the greatest failing that the Armn'dallos thought system and why it was so backward in 'Lîna's eyes. For they had failed themselves.

Still, the Armn'dallos had a right to exist, and they chose not to. 'Lîna was saddened by their loss as much as she was angered and disappointed by it. But she did not want those she joined in the imperial triad to see delicate her soul had become from seeing all those dead bodies; an entire species left to extinction from their path. So she buried her tears for these people and had a good laugh along with 'Iato H'Renn and Nul'lus at the quiet folly before them. She kept her pity in her heart and refused to wear it, and hoped in wonder if her sovereign contemporaries had any pity for the dead across this still planet.

The Three said a brief cheer for the grace saving responsibility of the dead lying in queues about them and gathered their mission crew that became living witnesses along with them to the silent slaughter. In some way, it was best that nothing was said from that point on. Her sight had grown beyond what it was. 'Lîna was pleased not for the gift as the Three folded back to the Lis'talla but for what she could see inside the souls of her great allies. For they too felt pity for this lesser species within themselves. She could understand this of Nul'lus but she did not know what to think of what was felt by the son of H'Raka. The H'Raka had more to them than met the eye. As time worked against them it also seemed to bring the Three together.

Φ

Surprisingly, the Three returned to the Lis'talla in better spirits than when they first came to the Armn'dallos system. The subtle thrust was back upon them in their path. Nul'lus went off to oversee the Armn'dallos war materials transported to the Imperium war supply vessels, the K'Nang 'Soong and the Zun'oon that met the Lis'talla in orbit over the quiet world. 'Iato H'Renn left 'Lîna to her own devices as well. He proceeded to one of the Lis'talla's cargo bays to inspect some components of Armn'dallos technology folded over from the surface.

It was doubtful that anything of beneficial use could be salvaged from this world though 'Iato H'Renn still went ahead as sometimes lesser and more backward technologies hold a missing link in making new technologies work. And on the path of war, anything and everything is investigated for getting an extra edge against the enemy. The necessities of the day made even advanced species like those of the Imperium Trinity resort to the necessities of survival. One must do what one must do.

This lesson of the son of H'Raka was what persuaded 'Lîna to let him send a scout ship from her ship to scan and remove any relevant technology to the H'Raka cargo bays. 'Lîna felt touched that one she expected to challenge her authority actually had the courtesy to confer with her on command decisions. He even left additional currency on their world for what they acquired.

But courtesy and respect was the way of the Hunter as civility was the way of the Aristocrat. Though the war was the Hunter's to do with as he pleased, he seemed to want the Fate and the Aristocrat to share his path. The sweetness and bitterness of their victories would be earned and shared by the Three in spite of the path that awaited them on the psionic level.

'Lîna decided to go to the main bridge of her flag ship and make herself useful. They would be leaving soon for M'Gata. She made her way through the fourth wall to the bridge of the Lis'talla. When she arrived, 'Lîna activated a spatial fold and teleportational transport through her interface. She decided it was only fitting to leave payment for the dead of Armn'dallos. Bio-synthetic micro-particles were placed in the atmosphere of the Armn'dallos home world. Using her enhanced mind, she focused on these particles until they reacted by exploding in a mild sub-spatial intensity. And then, all at once, the dead of an extinct race had their perfect sky. Their corpses would be left to bask under spotless skies before the erasure of the Death of Death would come to consume them.

As she sat back in her bridge throne thinking of what she had done, 'Lîna heard the four words that no one likes to hear on the path of war. In fact, she heard these words in her mind uttered in the thoughts of Val'damus. Certainly he was worried about something to think, 'there is a problem'. 'Lîna looked at her officer with an exasperated expression but she was ready for the gruelling winds of war to blow on her shoulders once again.

20
The Truculent Breach Before Blind Obsession

'Status, 'Valis.'

'Lîna's tone expected the worst. On the path of war one needs to both find release and adherence to take nothing lightly, for anything could be a trap. Her imagination went awry with the most horrifying of thoughts. The shadow of the Two Rings had been cast upon them once again. The Triumvirate was revealed to the Death of Death.

There was no secrecy or any measure of privacy left in the universe. The At'Lann, the Lon'tus, and the H'Raka were marked for death and doom. The intensity of the campaign against them was beginning to build. But 'Lîna knew darkness, and it had changed her. Everything she foresaw became a curse worse than Cassandra's, and the path of war was all she could see. Val'damus did not sugar-coat their current dilemma.

'A sub-spatial breach is beginning to form before the Lis'talla and a graviton flux surrounds the ship. We cannot break free. Seven hundred enemy vessels inside subspace will descend upon our position. If we do not seal the breach in six minutes, we will be heavily outnumbered and unable to defend the supply ships.'

'Show me.'

'Valis Val'damus brought a rotating graphic model and magnification of the breach unto the main holo-screen. Damn, she thought. With all the damage to subspace the Lis'talla would have insufficient time to fold out of here before the enemy arrives. She was a long way from My House. The time came for a stand to be taken. Then 'Lîna noticed something strange and curious about the breach.

'Val'damus, analyse grid eight one seven.'

'Valis ran a standard scan of the region 'Lîna had requested through the main Imperium Interface Network. Seconds later, the results appeared before them on the holo-screen, and the results were disquieting. 'Valis's face was one of surprise and one the mostly searched for sense of the meaning of the data.

'A trans-metagenic scanning beam is piercing through?' Valis found the answer he sought as he ended his response. He found it as insidious as 'Lîna no doubt did. The enemy sought to exterminate the Triumvirate of the Imperium Trinity. What was still perplexing the enemy was their technology only all but covered their psyogenic signatures, and the tips of their icebergs lay visible above the psionic waters. 'Valis brought up more data to the holo-screen and pointed out there were similar scenarios taking place across existence wherever Imperium ships were deployed.

It would be a simple task for genetically enlightened beings such as 'Lîna, Nul'lus, or 'Iato H'Renn, to use their powers to seal the breach in space. The problem being the enemy would then know their position, and then could hunt them down and destroy them en masse should they leave their ship. Their true importance was still not known.

This was not something 'Lîna particularly relished as she wanted to be on the path that led to the enemy and not the path that led to being the prey of the enemy. Drastic action had to be taken. Like the rest of the Three, she wanted the upper hand. 'Lîna had to find an option that did not include the powers of the Three in sealing the breach. As well, she wanted to prove to Nul'lus and H'Renn that she could handle things, at times, on her own. She had to find another way.

Then 'Lîna turned to 'Valis and saw he followed the path of one like Nul'lus in treating graciousness and gentility as supreme. He had a calm patience as he waited for his Imperiatrix to speak.

'If we re-route power from our weapons, cloak, drive system, and communications, we can create a tri-anionic nova pulse to flash ignite subspace to seal the breach before us and those which threaten our forces. We can adapt the short range fold system to create the pulse'

'Imperiatrix, that will leave us cut off from the fleet and from home.'

'Lîna paused for a moment.

'What other options can you give me?'

'Though it will leave us vulnerable. It is our only option.'

'Do not be concerned with our safety while our power levels will be low. The Trinity of the Trinity shall keep our kinsman on this mission away from harm.'

'We give our faith freely, Imperiatrix.'

'Lîna bowed her head to her dashing science officer. 'Then proceed.'

' 'Valis then constructed the necessary data stream and entered it through his command console into the Lis'talla's interface. The automatic adaptation systems of the Lis'talla took care of the rest. The Lis'talla's shield generators, ironically, realigned to help create the tri-anionic pulse in tandem with the short-range fold system. In seconds, the process was complete and the Lis'talla began to be surrounded in a bath of the sandy orange and mauve tri-anionic energy that grew around the ship to form a nine-pointed star. A nine-pointed star grew to be slightly larger than Armn'dallos that loomed in the distance, a planet seven times the size of E'de.

The field created spiralled around them so rapidly that within moments the effect had moved beyond that of the light spectrum in many segments of luscious colour and into something beyond vivid. The swirling glow stick orange and violet colours became more brilliant with every second that passed. In the layers beneath space, a battle raged between lower particles. Collisions and explosions littered across all points of subspace as if crushed solar bodies were suddenly spread out and raped of their cohesion.

The hurling fiery bodies slowed to form a new pattern. A chain wall came to grow across the lower flow of space. As the energies around the Lis'talla crackled across the system, the tri-anionic energy reached its climactic point of intensity with a silent thunder quaking across the cosmos. At great cost, it was done. The pulse healed the wound left by the enemy and that which had pierced once more into the flow of life. The breaches were all sealed simultaneously. The enemy would only have their front this day.

'Lîna could see within herself that a few hundred enemy vessels did not have time to alter course before flying like rotten eggplant into the restored wall between spaces, a wall that became like iron for the enemy warships that had tried to fold their way through into Imperium space. What a happy mess. Smugly, 'Lîna thought, 'good riddance.'

'Valis congratulated his sovereign by raising the two fingers of peace to the sensor reading on the holo-screen fluttered back to normalcy as the breach sealed. In fact, everyone on the main bridge seemed as jubilant as 'Valis to see that the Imperium fleet would remain safe even though the Lis'talla was now operating with minimal power. For now, the Imperium would not be attacked within their own space even though their space receded with every moment.

'Lîna knew that she had placed her ship in a very precarious position and had done the same to the souls who shared her path. The path of war was fast becoming far more dangerous with every step. But she was their Fate. She would prevail. So she decided to let the bridge crew run with their excitement. Relaxation was very important to the spiritual At'Lann. They would need to be good spirits to put into perspective all they had seen and experienced.

The flawless crew had earned one more moment of joy before they would return to the routine of war. For the enemy would attempt to get through again. The presence of the Death of Death seemed everywhere. What they had bought was a moment to once again breathe freely like ascending into the hard sound of Savage.

As the spirits of those around her died down and her crew returned to their duties, 'Lîna smiled almost blessedly to 'Valis to grant him the respect due in continuing to do well in his service to the cause. 'Lîna tapped into his mind for a moment to tell him she was on her way to the largest power conversion generator on board. 'Valis by her pride in him, bowed without slight in acknowledgement of what she was about to do.

'Lîna then flash-folded herself into the central core of the main transformer that powered her ship. She found the crew had already set up the modifications she requested via thought to Valis as she exited the bridge.

With the breach sealed, the enemy could not strike directly at them and the Interface automatically instituted other Tr'Lann - class warships to spread false readings across Imperium space as a further countermeasure to conceal their exact location.

Lying beneath her feet were twelve hand-size, black, medically influenced designed attachments which had load bearing conductive cables tipped with L'unn silver running out of them. Telekinetically, she brought each to her body and straps formed from the end of the black techno tentacles. Three to each ankle and wrist joined her flesh. In the stadium sized chamber of corrugated turquoise advanced steel, ivory bio-gel conduits, and enhanced plastic piping, the daughter of 'Mura was the tiny speck of humanity amongst the underground world of their technology. 'Lîna flew, along with the cables, to the centre of the room. The origin of the cables came form both the ceiling and floor. Six formed from above her and six formed below her.

'Lîna felt too serious in her mission to even concern herself with the aesthetic dignity to being stretched out in a St. Andrew's cross so that she would infuse power into the ship. With the enhancement, though unstable she was growing far stronger than she ever had dreamed. She would sacrifice everything for her people and would give what was needed for the Lis'talla to return to her ship to full strength. And this method of power conversion seemed undetectable by enemy scans which made it all the better.

This was now her ship, where it once served those before her. She even cared for the ship that had become her home on the path of war as she did for all things that mattered on her path. And 'Lîna was more than ready to give her flag ship its much needed nourishment just as a mother would give her breast to her child. Though with genetic advancements, those days were in the ancient past of At'Lann.

Elsewhere on the ship, 'Iato H'Renn and Nul'lus watched on through the windows of the mind. 'Iato persuaded his aristocratic ally in this moment of subtle crisis to let this move play out. He wanted to see 'Lîna under the duress of a command situation. So far, she had handled herself well. For a spiritual people, the At'Lann seem far more vicious than I thought them to be, H'Renn thought. And then he reminded himself 'Mura was a place in the north affirming what he always knew.

He thought it admirable that the delicate angel of At'Lann would charm the warrior within him. He eagerly awaited seeing her drain herself of power for the sake of protecting all those aboard while leaving herself vulnerable. War was, after all, an exhausting business. H'Renn wondered if she would worry more about him or the enemy in spite of the fact she placed her faith in an alliance with him and the H'Raka.

Nul'lus began to see that this was 'Lîna's time to prove herself. He stayed aback from it all to let her do what she must do. He knew she would ask for his help if she required it, and so far she handled herself well. To the Aristocrat, this was just, 'Lîna being 'Lîna. She was the most unique and independent soul he knew of other than that of 'Iato H'Renn. He knew that if anything happened to her, his combined might with H'Renn's would be more than capable, and would be more than willing to keep up the fight. Nul'lus thought differently on this matter but he knew Fate was bold. He wished his friend luck. He hoped to share a night with her under the musical rays of the Fraser Sun when they get to what came after M'Gata: M'Goa, where their current mission would be complete.

'Lîna looked within herself to the very structure of her being as she was wired into the technology of her ship. She triggered the genetic catalyst to release the unrelenting raw energy of her power. She drained all the energy that she could within her and released it into her ship for the sake of the lives on board. Psionically, 'Lîna became explosions of raw power released from their genetic dams.

Like a phoenix soaring in flames in awakening to new life. 'Lîna brought forth all that she had. Violet and lavender flames streamed wildly, like lightning, across the chamber. The wiring that penetrated into her began to glow in a thick ultramarine. She became engulfed in the fiery whiplashes of her swirling energies. 'Lîna built it up inside herself and continued to grow with inner power until it could no longer be contained at any level.

Like releasing a dove into the summer air, 'Lîna brought out of her a near immeasurable burst of energy, and out it flowed into the energy conversion generator. Every last drop she gave freely that she could create with her mind. The hyper-charged conduits seemed to stretch 'Lîna into pulsating convulsions of energy absorption and conduction. She nearly shuddered from the display of her enhanced strength that Tesla could never have of dreamed of.

It became a spiritual release for 'Lîna as well. Never before had she given so much of herself. She was making a difference, and that brought with it a small measure of a peace, once not so scarce, once more across existence. It was a gracious relief for the now drained and depleted 'Lîna who began to fall to the ground as the cables loosened her to the ground. How the generator surged; overwhelmed with its empowerment. She was relieved as she could hear the rising hum of the Lis'talla's critical systems coming back on-line.

If she ever again had to feel the sensation of desiring sleep from utter exhaustion, now was one of those times. She gently fell to sleep as it became a biological necessity. But as suddenly as she did, 'Lîna forced herself to stay awake. She used thought commands to return for the Lis'talla to return to its course for M'Gata and to proceed there at best speed. Though she could get no sleep, 'Lîna strongly considered it her next best option after Nul'lus and 'Iato H'Renn flash-folded and found their way to her side.

Violet smoke of a luminescent nature still billowed and whispered around the Three as they reunited with one another. Like a phoenix arising from the ashes, the sounds of Chicane returned to them, and the silver sun was above them once more. Even the Lis'talla seemed to have been transformed back to life from Lîna's small battle that was yet another step away from her own spiritual and genetic ongoing chrysalis. Everyone was still looking ready for a set from the Dreem Teem. And though 'Lîna's transformation took on a slightly different state than either Nul'lus's or 'Iato H'Renn's, they saw, from a distance, what power their ally could wield.

'Lîna had the interface detach the power conversion cables off of herself in hisses as excess mauve hued psionic energy dutily blew away from her. Disconnected from the generator, she grasped Nul'lus's arm to raise herself to her feet. Telepathically, she hoped her allies did not worry for her, but what was plain to see was that they did not need to have bothered lending her their assistance. 'Lîna felt more than capable, and surprisingly, 'Iato H'Renn had no qualms about her taking command of the situation. To that, Nul'lus told her that had made a 'good show' of it.

'Iato H'Renn with a smile even bowed his head to her for he recognised the logic behind her strategy chosen. Imperator H'Renn also noticed something his Hunter's eye had never seen before on his new ally.

For a microsecond, probably without 'Lîna first realising it, her body rippled out of phase as her genetic sequence momentarily destabilised especially surging into large gashes across the subspace within her. She was in pain from the ordeal but chose to conceal it from her allies as 'Lîna thought it would only make her look weak.

'Thirty two percent of her musculature has been ripped apart internally from defending and re-powering the ship in stealth from the enemy. She must be in excruciating pain yet she tries to hide it from both of us. I wondered if she is trying to impress me,' thought 'Iato to himself. The Hunter hoped she would have time to heal up before their next encounter with the enemy and the intersection of her path with his on the psionic realm.

Bringing the Lis'talla's key systems back on-line also cost 'Lîna a marginal amount of her own weight though that left her figure to have a dash more muscular definition which looked good on her slender frame. Like the Three, with every step on the path of Fate, 'Lîna evolved, and she was another step closer to being Fate.

Through shared thought, the Three agreed to have a private meeting to confer as to their own paths towards the enemy and to learn more about what they faced. It would be a week until they would reach M'Gata, the next supply point, and the last place they would have to go to before M'Goa. The Lis'talla was returned to normal operations, and the Three decided to part company once again, now that the minor danger was abated, to return to their current personal concerns.

'Lîna took the fourth wall intra-fold system to her quarters and collapsed in a pool of dark mauve blood that flowed from the vivisected places on her body that was the damage of coming genetically out of phase with reality. Everything fell to silence before the lone daughter of 'Mura was able to muster the strength to light a curative agent that began to repair the latest damage to her genetic structure. She had little concern that 'Iato H'Renn saw her genetic essence degrade slightly but she did worry that he still thought less of her as an ally. 'Lîna had enough to deal with already and this latest skirmish with the enemy just made things far too interesting.

Nul'lus and 'Iato H'Renn fourth-walled to Nul'lus's quarters for a smoke before returning to their investigative pursuits. It was Nul'lus, who on the astral and psionic planes, convinced H'Renn to not intercede as their thoughts were one on that path. Both were able to watch the one who still remained far too much on the path alone. And indeed, she was an independent soul in action and in suffering. As they smoked, 'Iato H'Renn asked his aristocratic friend how he knew 'Lîna would succeed. 'She is Fate', he told her. Privately, Nul'lus was impressed whatever her motivation. Soon would be the time to truly judge her.

Φ

As 'Lîna slowly returned to a better level of genetic cohesiveness, she became aware something awaited her attention from a fist size aquamarine square silently flashing on the main interface on her living space was. She watched its rhythmic, trance like pulse as her body restored itself with every puff and every drag of the 'Mura'Lann Agent 27. At the very least, only twenty-two of her tendons and ligature were vaporised throughout her body, and thankfully was rapidly regenerating.

Her very being fell apart for one brief moment, and was only now reforming. She found that 'Zaya had left her a visual message on the interface.

'Lîna activated the file to find that 'Zaya had found a way to further stabilise her genetic structure using a newly created bio-gel the other daughter of 'Mura called triketracel-9. Sadly, this would not be a true cure for 'Lîna or any of the Three but it would reinforce the healing effects of the Imperium inhalants. For now, no more could be done. 'Lîna had injured herself, badly, and even she realised she had injured herself almost gravely defending the ship. She was in no shape to do anything other than to rest and heal.

'Zaya even told her seemingly splintering and evolving sister that she made a data stream of her research into the data-flow of the Imperium Interface. She had it freely given to both Nul'lus and 'Iato H'Renn so they too would have one additional option in their treatment. 'Zaya ended the message by stating how she wished she could do more but this was the best she could do for now.

Truly, 'Lîna felt blessed, and even more so to know she still had a home to return to at all. So much had changed so fast. One moment exploring the universe, the next fighting for its very survival. If not for the pain, it would seem surreal.

Though things remained strained towards Za'szu, she felt fortunate their sibling trinity remained. In times where her soul seemed to shatter even more from all the death she had surveyed: the murder and the loss of her parents, those like the Armn'dallos, and perhaps, those like the Three Imperia, 'Lîna had already lost more than most soon would or already had. She would sacrifice everything for liberation. Now she would let the path of her sister that, at times, was just the peaceful shoulder of the path of war have the faith of Fate.

As an added benefit, the triketracel-A (the merging of 'Mura'Lann Agent 27 and tri-ketracel 9 as a therapy), as the message indicated in graphics and holo-text, would increase her healing factor by six fold, and would reduce her recharge time on her advanced abilities by a third. In order to have the proper concentration of the compound, 'Lîna would have to flood her quarters with it every night and to regenerate in it by floating in the hot, watery, *kisiel* like compound as well as inhaling it. 'Zaya also thought to leave a pre-configured activation panel on her interface so that she could flood and purge the agent with but the flick of a switch.

'Truly, 'Lîna cherished what little family she had left and continued in her vow to avenge the deaths of the sovereigns that came before her and the lives lost and the ones that continued to be lost, to be cut down in a bloody trail left by one like Vishinski. Though her family extensions were vast, only Za'szu and 'Zaya remained from a world she once hoped to return to and no longer could. How she cherished the work of her youngest sister as if they healed and transformed the path of the other into something more. The daughters of 'Mura, no matter the path, would rise up together.

As 'Lîna sat back reclining under the bright, luminous sour candy purple hued tri-ketracel waters that began to stream in, she relaxed her mind as she felt she finally could. She puffed on the last of her new agent 27 as the bio-gel came to rise to her waist. The interface saw to the room being sealed. The room was locked as 'Lîna would have no visitors after the bio-gel release. Hints of black mauve lightning seemed to find their way across what appeared only to be watery, yet gooey and glowing gelatine.

'Lîna tossed away the last of her smoke and dimmed the lights in her quarters as the roomed filled to the ceiling with the tri-ketracel agent. She did not worry about her belongings as her quarters tidied themselves. She floated to the centre of the room like a child though the Aegis. Though her body was still battered, her mind seemed more powerful than ever. And so she closed her eyes and continued on another path and the search to find a way to bring peace back to existence, and to fight the Death of Death on the highest psionic levels of the mind, towards the path of a liberated future of all existence.

21
The Strangest Dance

'Lîna found the new therapy quite refreshing, and she came to feel less exhausted in her days leading up to the next supply point. Initially, she did not feel so fulfilled as her mind was still in pursuit of the enemy. After the first night of bio-gel aether rest, something still weighed upon her soul. She had been awake in her nightmares. Yet she was Fate, and these were more than dark dreams, these were her visions. For her dreams were also her path of war.

Though the experience had been muddled and confusing: she had seen At'Lann under siege, the face of the enemy, a glimpse of the battle on the front, and so many of the dead. The dead lay everywhere in her visions: her family, her people, the Armn'dallos, and thousands of members of other species seen only once before, and never again from the erasure. 'Lîna felt asphyxiated by her dreams that left her without breath in the only freedom she had left: her private time. The enemy had taken away so much, and now even her very soul felt invaded by the great darkness that covered the universe.

The burden left by the enemy upon 'Lîna's shoulders had encumbered her to the point where she could, at times, think of nothing else. She could hardly wait for M'Goa where the gathering of spirit and celebration had already begun as their way of combating what their existence had become, and word was received that their contribution was ready to be purchased by the Imperium for the war effort. Her burden seemed a double edge sword as her condition was now necessitated with the importance of entering a relaxing meditative state to infuse upon herself the maximum regenerative effect, and in her restlessness she could not.

Beneath it all, 'Lîna could still hear the laughter of the evil one she sought to kill; to end the unwanted destruction of existence. As best she could, she tried not to think of her dream time, her new therapy, one created by the hands of her sister, as being time spent in a chamber filled with the blood of those she could not save. Rather, she would not let her dark dreams fragment her anymore than her genetic structure was already becoming. She would avenge them all, for there would be no time to mourn them. And if she did not have the time to properly mourn the loss of her own parents, she would have little need to continuing to reflect upon the extinction of a growing number of species.

After Armn'dallos, she realised how strongly her very empathy could tear away at her on the path of war. She would not let the enemy have the perverted satisfaction of victimising her as it had to so many others on this path and the path of Fate had become the path of war. She needed to be at her best; for her best was needed for war.

From the first night spent in liquid suspension, 'Lîna attempted to numb herself from the evil her mind sought out to destroy. 'Zaya's latest curative enhancements was all that kept her pure from the evil pollution her mind became infested with every night she lay to rest and was, for the most part, cleansed away. 'Lîna was confident she could provide closure to her emotional wounds by turning to pure logic and boldness as that too could be her strength in the battlefield of dreams. And her reign as Imperiatrix began to already take a coldly logical direction though few could blame her after all At'Lann and 'Mura had lost. What was important was that she remain alive.

The next day she conferred with Nul'lus and 'Iato H'Renn. One thing on board took away a large measure of her peace, and she was about to do something about it. 'Lîna decided and was granted licence for the morning of the next day. She would have done what she was about to do anyway but knew that her fellow sovereigns were only too willing to let her indulge on the path of war.

Staying true to her polite respectful nature, 'Lîna in her standard At'Lann Imperium tunic, fourth-walled to her where she wanted to be the next morning that came to pass. Indeed, she thought. Her allies would enjoy watching. As she arrived to the room, she was greeted by her clerics who informed her that the science and military branches of all governments had completed their analyses. Nothing further remained, and the dead weight of dead weight was what would not be left to remain. So 'Lîna had the usz'Shn, or enemy prisoners, brought before her in a isolated military science brig of the Lis'talla. 'Lîna had one of her S'yana guards hand her his rifle after motioning as if she were Rourke wating for a metal pipe.

After glancing over the usz'Shn one by one, she realised how pathetic these necrotic drones were when cut off from the rest of the swarm. How pathetic that which stood chained and held in force fields in front of her. Pathetic and weak, she thought. If not for their countless number, they could be easily crushed.

'Lîna wondered the depths of depravity of the true face of the enemy as she studied with her own eyes in ways she could not before; the moulded inherent bitterness towards life that was displayed in the construction of the verminous army of parasitic nihilism, the greatest plague to lay waste to existence. 'Lîna could see through the usz'Shn to where their strings came to find themselves around the Death of Death who awaited within the two rings of doom. What was for certain was the Death of Death's laughter was fuelled by the onslaught inflicted by his lethal puppets.

They were nothing to 'Lîna as she began to execute them. If there was dirt beneath their feet, she wondered if she would have had them dig their own graves first. But an evil such as this did not deserve burial. One by one she began to go through the assembled lot of them. Taking aim each time, she shot the usz'Shn through their heads at a range where their rotting stench permeated the air around them as their cranial matter vaporised.

A small and perhaps empty measure of peace returned to her, and as fleeting as it was for 'Lîna, she felt better than she had before. She had peace of mind to share with her companions on the path of war. She left two other cells of usz'Shn alive on board the Lis'talla. She tossed the rifle to Nul'lus and said to him without any hint of emotion, 'Here, my friend. I have left you something you can consider a belated present for your new path. Perhaps you feel as I do, and may consider sharing your gift, and to share it with the K'or of H'Raka.'

One of her S'yana officer promptly gave 'Iato H'Renn a rifle so as to not dirty his hands by having to waste the powers of their enhancements on such filth as Nul'lus would not. Nul'lus took the weapon and found 'Lîna's invitation quite a civilised way to deal with the most fowl of refuse on board an Imperium flag ship, and he especially did not want to squander his powers on the usz'Shn. He was also a little saddened that the war had pushed 'Lîna to acts a soul that only feels like flying that should never know. A few hours on a hill like Calvary would be nothing to her. So much continued to change on the path of war.

Though 'Iato H'Renn preferred the traditional H'Raka direct approach, his soul thought the prisoners lacked any measure of worth to die in any honourable H'Raka way. Even he was not oblivious to the damage the war was already doing to one that Nul'lus only spoke of as gentle, kind, and innocent.

And 'Iato noticed how much the daughter of 'Mura seemed to compete with him. 'Is it out of a desire for respect or is she out to challenge to me?' he wondered. Whatever the case, there was no argument that their souls had observed far too much needless suffering.

Before leaving, 'Lîna instructed her S'yana officer that the remains of the usz'Shn were to be purged from existence. As 'Lîna fourth-walled away and left the brig and science labs. She entered the spatial fold energy stream, and used her mind to observe what she left behind when she had walked casually away.

Without remark or any measure of flamboyance, she watched Nul'lus and 'Iato H'Renn execute the last of the prisoners. From this moment on, the Imperium would keep no enemy prisoners for study. All that could have been learned had been discovered by the Imperium Trinity. And she also watched from a distance as her crewmen sub-atomically incinerated whatever remained of the usz'Shn bodies.

For a long time after this, 'Lîna's only distress at night would not come under the roof of her own house. As far as she was concerned, the usz'Shn no longer existed. However, her actions taken on this day did not mean she would find peace in rest, only that she would find a little more rest.

Φ

As the tension seemed to ease in the days that followed, 'Lîna returned to being relaxed as she prepared for the next transaction the Imperium Trinity would be a part of. The Lis'talla would arrive in the M'Gata system in two days, and 'Lîna came to savour the last of her routine filled days that followed the emptiness of leaving Armn'dallos.

The enemy had not, as yet, attacked her ship again at this time but activities along the ever-reducing front had intensified. As well, newly encountered species pledged themselves to the cause of the Imperia. The 'Xo and the 'Raanu being the most notable, in terms of economic, technological, cultural, and spiritual advancement piqued 'Lîna's particular interest as the newest members of the At'Lann Imperium. Their ships were now engaged in deploying mines in strategic areas of space to hinder the enemy advancement of erasure for as long as possible. Soon, 'Lîna thought, soon. For it shall all come to be as 'Lîna edged ever closer to the ever more finite front line. So eager she was to prove her worth.

During her nights floating in the thickness of viscous bio-gel, 'Lîna had now begun to hone the other edge of the highland sword of war. She sacrificed even the most treasured parts of herself as she combined her love of exploration and her pious zeal to win the war through a path taken that she could not turn back upon. Now she pressed on long past the point of no return as 'Lîna had begun to construct and alter the highest psyogenetically accessed psionic plane she could find within herself.

It was fast becoming clear to 'Lîna that she would walk the darkest of paths to find the true face of the enemy, the Death of Death. She created and found a realm to find her way. If not for the chaos of war, it was possible for 'Lîna to wage war entirely from this new place as an oneiromancer. Luckily, and for now, she had time for both. The paradox was that she found peace in not separating war from her time alone though M'Goa would give her, at the very least, one opportunity to relax.

She spent part of her nights in the psionic realm weaving temporal spindles so that she could make further incisions though the psionic barriers. Ridding her ship of the usz'Shn had resolved a lot of the guilt that she had. And so far, it had done so little to avenge the deaths of her parents. The twisted laughter of the dark one, the great *morbus,* still slithered in the winds of her soul. She did not enjoy it. Perhaps the only reason her soul permitted it was to motivate her emotions and her being to find victory on the path of war. But the war in the psionic realm was, for now, hers alone.

For the time being, she wanted this to be her private little war that she would keep from Nul'lus and 'Iato H'Renn. She bound her suffering to her heart alone. This was the path to take; a yearning that seemed unlikely to be assuaged and one that was no longer ignored. 'Lîna would not deny herself.

But this night on the psionic plane was one where her secret truths would be brutally exposed and would come into certain jeopardy. 'Lîna became startled. Something strong and fierce entered this place. Using her natural skills, she immediately made a psionically cast cloak around the spindles she had been weaving together.

There was an intruder in her mind and soul that was the Hunter; an intruder she expected to would come. H'Renn still considered her prey and came to judge her worthiness as a way to truly see her inner being. He was hunting her down, and he remained hidden, pursuing her from within. It seemed the Hunter would make a game of this. But she would be like Owen and step up to the pitch.

'Lîna knew only too well that the Hunter thought of her as prey, and she would play along. For beneath her passiveness lay a force of will that she hoped 'Iato would see as worthy. The world before 'Lîna's eyes transformed into the gauntlet cast down by the Hunter. He had altered the psionic level with his every step into her soul and 'Lîna found herself in an astral Hy'Bor jungle valley far from the cities of the colony. He was as succinct as he was direct. The strangest dance had begun.

'Lîna never figured 'Iato H'Renn to be such an exceptionally high ordered telepath but she had never ruled it out as he had been part of existence for such a long time. It seemed he was experienced with manipulating the psionic realm, as she could feel that it came easily to him. She awaited his opening salvo in meditative stillness as the psionic environment spun around her.

'What a lord of his land in mine', 'Lîna thought beneath her stoic battle facade. She made her way through the both leafy and large leafed jungle to the centre of a valley made of thought that was more than likely was a recreation of a reality destroyed in the first wave from the enemy. She was startled, rattled, and before 'Lîna were giant iron emerald statues of her parents cast in an almost Minoan way. Apparently, 'Iato H'Renn liked to throw salt in wounds. The memorial even rusted with gold. She paused and looked to the faces that it seemed she had not seen in a lifetime, and looked to once more see their faces she left behind for the path of war.

Indeed, 'Iato H'Renn had disturbed the most blessed and sacred silt. A tsunami formed from the great stone cast into the oceans of 'Lîna's mind. The artist's hand of the Hunter captured the perfect image of their emotions in a vine strangled tribute in the heart of the jungle. Things were becoming haunted as much so as the sharpest of images before her. She felt it time to end the pursuit.

With a slightly louder than mild raising of her voice and external thoughts, she engaged the Hunter with her succinct query,

'Is there a point to this, 'Iato?'

A voice that came both from a great distance and close enough to whisper to 'Lîna answered.

'I want to see what you are capable of. I want to see how you will react to various stimuli. Defend yourself.'

The aether sucked itself away from her an instant before a huge thrust of malachite and ruby hued psionic energy zoomed past her and into her. 'Lîna parried the blow like she would have done with a photonic body in space. On one plane they circled each other like great whites with disciplined blood thirsts. He was Ares, he was Thor. He had magic and so much more.

Strikes into her soul came from every telepathic vector. 'Lîna anticipated them and grabbed onto their approach and contact points on a near infinite number of thought planes. She counterattacked with three times as many softer techniques of multi-spectral soul-fire. The silver and mauve flames of L'unn began to burn brighter within her soul. She tried to find more angles of thought and psionic paths of energy to use as thought strike de-stabilisers.

She succeeded in finding other realities in thought. This was the dream time as much as it was an arena for thought flows. 'Lîna's counterbalance produced weariness in 'Iato H'Renn's astral and psionic forms. So much so that he almost dissipated out of her mind and soul while psionically trying to reassert himself. He seemed certain to return to himself and to his state room on the starboard side of the Lis'talla.

As her consciousness drifted in the various streams of psionic energy, 'Lîna found a thought filament that had been brushed off his astral form from beneath his telepathic armour. She had found access conduit into his memories and presence on board. She watched as he screamed in agony as he lay restrained on a operating table as a H'Raka field physician began to implement a regime of blood mineral vapour following his first and battlefield enhancement in a memory from a time long since past. She was beginning to see within him as he came to be in her mind and soul. How they circled one another in the salt waters.

'Lîna could see into him and through his eyes as he sat back at his bureau and to his H'Raka modified quarters. She could feel the temperature there was thirty-eight degrees higher than anyone else on the ship. Seems his attendants had adjusted the environmental controls for him, and the room was now able to self-adjust for typical At'Lann visitors.

Her eyes returned to the psionic plane, and reality continued to swirl. 'Lîna never realised 'Iato H'Renn, so filled by the gifts and power of psyogenetic enhancement also paid equally for it in what was needed of him in the path of war. He too was the virtues of sacrifice. Truly, they both shared the greatest and highest affliction but one well worth what each was and would become.

Their astral *kumite* continued into a tussle of cross-face headlocks up across the stratosphere of thinning psionic planes flying faster than the light of their thoughts; a psionic battle of two minds that seemed to go nowhere and everywhere. The uncertain conflict seemed to move with near ultimate speed, and the psionic reality slowed into a bored purgatory twiddling down into the deadness of no time at all.

The psionic reality changed its dynamic once more. Things came to remain on fewer levels. Questions formed and answers were to be had. The strangest dance of souls became an inquisition. This was to be a battle more evolved than most by its very nature but it was one that was just as fierce as any. The battle became a frenetic carousel of vertigo where so much became exposed. It made one feel like flying, and it made one feel like falling.

The secret truths transferred through each of them like spears thrown to impale each of them, across the Hy'Bor jungle which they remained in and left behind. The carousel became more and more an ecclesiastical one as 'Lîna regained her sense of self. The soulscape seemed plentiful of hunted noble beasts that once traversed the great lands of the Imperium.

Psionic reality also became a court of judgement of being. The realm of truth was unleashed.

'Do you truly consider me prey, 'Iato?'

'I see now that I never could. Remember, 'Imiszi, predation and prey are only limited perspectives.'

The swirl had become a face-off.

'Tell me why you did this to yourself? This enhancement, this path. Would you have followed it if not for tradition? Are you a false prophet?'

'I follow the path of Fate. I am Fate, and I stand at your side in the path of war.'

'Really.'

'Yes. Really. No matter the path. This is my fate, and I wanted it. I will bear the burden and penance of my path, and I will find peace again. Do you not want peace, 'Iato?'

His soul hid it well beneath the armour of H'Raka.

'I live to find victory for my people and all life.'

'Just as I do.'

'Why is what you have chosen a punishment? Do you believe suffering will bring you worthiness, 'Imiszi.'

'No, I chose to be worthy but I also chose to suffer for it. For I am Fate, and I choose to bury my happiness the day darkness descended across existence.'

'You live with a psyogenetic matrix you can barely contain, yet you are ashamed and too selfish to share the state of your health with your allies. Do you not have your full faith behind me?'

'It was not my intention to deceive you, 'Iato. So many of my years have been spent alone in the isolation of deep space journeying to other worlds that I still choose to be alone and bear my pain alone that I sometimes act like I still am. There is no slight involved though I feel I have done everything I can to prove myself worthy of sharing and not made a slave to following you on the path of war.'

'We will see, 'Imiszi. Your force of will is strong.'

'I want to earn my rewards. If we are victorious, that will suffice.'

'Did you enjoy killing the usz'Shn, 'Imiszi?', H'Renn's thoughts asked; almost sexually.

'I felt nothing and I felt the rush. But they were constructs. A theft of our dead as the Death of Death steals our existence. The only lives that matter are our own in this existence. Your people, my people, 'Lus's people, and all living things. The only guilt I feel is that I could not prevent the lives already lost to the invasion.'

'Or it all a lie? Is it only that you only wish to avenge the deaths of your parents, and earn your inheritance.'

'I sacrifice my soul of peace for them but I also do it to walk the path of war. For without war there is no peace in the same way there would be no At'Lann sun without L'unn. I have always felt a disappointment to them. I never wanted to lead At'Lann and 'Mura, and I could always feel they felt less of me for it. The war is the only thing that brings me to power. I live to show what became of their souls that I have it within me to save our species. And I will do so by any means necessary.'

'Is that the one reason why you came to H'Raka?'

'No but it was my only path.'

'I also came because I wanted to see if our peoples could find a new understanding after so much time apart. It is our fate to walk together as one once again.'

'Do you find me worthy, 'Iato?'

Time became still in the bliss of trance of one like Van Buuren.

'Yes.'

'Lîna felt a brief return to peace that she had been without since her return to At'Lann. She needed this validation if she was ever to heal her shattered soul. She thought she would never find such things in the Hunter but she did.

'Do you see the future, 'Imiszi?'

'Yes.'

'What do you see?'

'We are being drawn into the mouth of the Death of Death.'

'Can we escape its vile thirst?'

'Possibly. It is still unclear if our combined strengths will be enough. But I do know this: only the Trinity can defeat the Death of Death. It watches us.

'The enemy?'

'Their master. I can feel it. The Death of Death is an embodied pure state of evil in its finality.'

'What is its purpose, 'Imiszi.'

'It grew from our very universe, our very existence. This evil is a final judgement. This evil was made from our own weaknesses, and we have grown weak by not seeing it coming, 'Iato H'Renn.'

'Perhaps our species, yours and mine, have grown weak. Never before have the H'Raka been caught so off-guard. We have become bored with existence for there is little but this war to challenge our species. For even the universe had begun to offer only wonders lacking uniqueness. We have fallen from our path and we must return greatness to our imperia. Once again we have found purpose... thanks to the Trinity.

'Then you feel as I do, 'Iato?'

'I do. I too have not forgotten hope. These are the time where we will exist between hope and fear.'

'Do you fear me, 'Imiszi?'

'No. I have no reason to.'

'Now that is why I find you worthy. Like 'Lus, you possess an advanced soul as well as an evolved genetic design.'

He added, 'You are compassion and empathy but you also have courage. Your path has been a difficult one but we shall carry on, and you shall bear the road ahead.'

'Do you also see into the future, 'Iato?'

'Rarely. But when I do see it is as perfect as capturing all that remains elusive.'

'Why do you choose to make your path one to be taken alone? Do you remain an anchorite? Why do you exist here in your time of rest?'

'I mean to find the being driving our reality into erasure. I mean to kill...to kill the Death of Death. Sometimes I feel, this path is one to be taken alone and taken with the Trinity.'

A revelation seemed to come to 'Iato H'Renn.

'Was it once like us?'

'I can only see the shell, the guise. But it is almost as empty as its puppets, and definitely more 'it' than he, she, or any other known combination.'

'Do you accept what I wish to do, 'Iato?'

'Yes, but I will watch over you in case you come into trouble. Was it not your wish to show me that our fate is to need each other?'

'You fought well, 'Imiszi. Your parents would be proud.'

''Imiszi.'

'Yes.'

'Your fate is to stand at my side.'

Φ

The vertigo carousel came to a stop in what seemed only a moment before that it had begun. 'Iato H'Renn and 'Lîna returned to themselves in their rooms. It was not a night of long knives but it was.

Now even 'Iato H'Renn could truly see how far 'Lîna was willing to go. She would give up everything for the cause. Respect was once again earned in the arena of secret and sheer truth. The path of Fate had become her. Her soul became the path. The powerful psionic link between herself and such a noble mind had infused great confidence in her. She felt she had found and made balance and brought equality to the Trinity.

After what she experienced, 'Lîna came to think of 'Iato as a brother she always and had not had; much in the same way she had always thought of Nul'lus. 'Lîna did not have feel alone as she once had. How the saltwater danced beneath her feet.

Φ

'Lîna returned to the psionic plane, a midnight garden of her soul. She left herself to float in the suspension of bio-gel as her room remained in its regenerative mode as quickly as her mind and soul returned to her body. Thinking of all the things exchanged between herself and 'Iato, 'Lîna now began to feel some of the weight had been lifted from her Atlas burdened shoulders. She had no misgivings about entrusting 'Iato with so many secret truths. Otherwise 'Lîna would not have joined him on her path. She had sought 'Iato H'Renn out after all. It was all coming together.

The purpose of the Trinity arose from the path of war but there was no other path for the three souls to take. And only together could 'Lîna, Nul'lus, and 'Iato H'Renn, survive. Their purpose went beyond everything and they existed as in their here and now. But they were the visions of the future for the Imperium. The war against the Army of the Two Rings was beginning to heat up.

'Lîna returned to her weaving in the hope that everything the Trinity is working towards would soon shift the balance of the war. She worked away diligently. She was getting close to her objective: the darkness that she called the Death of Death.

22
To See The Fallen Who May Never Rise To Stand

It was early in the At'Lann morning when the Lis'talla arrived to the M'Gata system. Far too early to return to sovereign duties for 'Lîna's liking even if it was her people's standard time. The Three were to be given an audience with the M'Gata world operator, Gn'rys P'rynn, in one of their hours. The Imperial shuttle of the Trinity of the Trinity had already disembarked from the Lis'talla and was en route to the systems juncture world capital city of M'Gata, 'Ea'tel'som.

Escorting their shuttle was a unified Imperium squadron of fighters that would protect them along the way. The vanilla and sierra hued ships of At'Lann design flew in loose four pointed diamond slot formations that streamed their way across M'Gata space along with the Three. Time seemed to move with the slowest of cruelties. Even 'Iato and Nul'lus were as groggy today as 'Lîna felt. Finding balance in such trying times was a most difficult path.

Thanks to 'Zaya's work and support and by the urging of the senates of each Imperium for each of the Three to undergo bio-gel therapy, their restlessness seemed ready to abate for the day ahead. As their conditions became more and more matters of Imperium defence and a little more of their privacy fell away, intense regimes of preventative and stabilising treatments became mandatory in the days that passed. The classified became the unclassified as unity needed to be maintained. The new state of rest, now made a habit of by each of the Three, became essential. And no one amongst the Three was thrilled to have their rest cut short to conform to slavish early morning obsolete creeds that cut thickly into their essential trance of finding cohesion in themselves.

The Three went about spending their time watching their focus return to themselves while they watched the latest casualty reports come in from the front over the interface in the cosiness of the shuttle's ready and state room. The stark statistics, the field footage, the visual, the audio, the horror, the totality, beamed itself though the rotating and hovering holo-interface. The S'yana were unseen as the Three had their small by Lon'tus standards shuttle state room all to themselves. The only other crew on board were at the command controls two decks above.

The Spartan like ready room was composed of emerald panelling and four L-shaped black Rimisz'tii leather couches in each corner along with a mauve and jade marble diamond shaped, interface protruding, table in the centre of the room. The only other thing worth noticing in the ready room was the three throne chairs which the sovereigns of the Imperium had seated themselves in to analyse the current state of the continuing atrocities being inflicted upon them.

'Lîna sat back and became more alert with every name and place on the hyper-scrolling interface data-stream as did Nul'lus and 'Iato as their eyes chanced to see the records and reports for such horrors that kept flowing into the interface at a more than exponential rate. They could feel the path would soon take them to the battlefield that 'Iato had already sent a great many of the Imperium military to for the sake of the survival of existence. 'Lîna also noticed that a cousin of hers and Mu'tolma's had died in the fighting. M'Skoto's ship, the Mer'ka, had been destroyed by enemy fighters at the fringe of erasure.

It made 'Lîna reconsider how harsh she was with her cousin Mu'tolma though she knew by her ruling that she probably saved his life. He was the near same age as 'Lîna and another spiritual brother in his own dynamic with her. She hoped Mu'tolma could bear the burden without him. But 'Lîna was a realist for she knew many beloved souls of the Imperium would be cut down by the rancid blade of the Death of Death.

H'Renn and Nul'lus had luck on their sides this day as no one of their immediate relations were on the latest casualty list. Though each of the Three knew that would not last much longer. 'Lîna hoped M'Skoto's soul found a path to freedom at his last moment. And somehow, even with the penetrating darkness of nothingness surrounding existence, she knew he did. She had to stay strong for her people. 'Lîna had no time to grieve for anyone. What concerned her as equally as it concerned Nul'lus and H'Renn was the high number of At'Lann, Lon'tus, and H'Raka dead and slaughtered. So much would be lost for the sake of victory. One is left to wonder whether it would truly be worth it. But they had to strive on.

What was done was done, and nothing seemed able to change this. Yet little more could be said of the matter so the Three returned to mild morning conversations, and discussing their preparations for the upcoming audience. Each felt as if they were covered in remora. For there was no doubt their business partners had survived the first invasion while so many others were slain fighting back.

'Lîna modified the colour of her top to a mint sea green, and put up her hair to let her violet curls fall down the nape of her neck in the prettiest of ways. And she adorned herself with the latest symbol of the cause upon the top of her left breast. It was the amalgamated symbol of the Imperium alliance: the tall thin diamond from the At'Lann, overlaid by the sharp-edged perfection of the Lon'tus X, overlaid by the H'Raka cross of white swords. 'Iato and Nul'lus also added the seemingly platinum cast new symbol of their alliance to their attire. Each leader was now a citizen of the realm of the other. Their territory was theirs to protect. The Trinity was fast becoming an enlightened noble unit.

Their focus returned to their thoughts on the M'Gata, a people that take the name of their leader as their own. Hence the M'Gata called themselves the P'rynn after their World Systems Operator. When 'Lîna had last flown by their world, they were called the I'occ. It would seem the M'Gata species had re-engineered their collective management. Quite a confusing people, thought 'Lîna.

She had never even bothered to land on their world when she explored their section of space during her first years on the paths of discovery. And with good reason, for some of the P'rynn, were as plastic in their practices as they were in their competitive ones. Few gems of creation sparkled on this world. Even the enemy seemed bored enough by them as to not scathe their world with the agonies of Tartarus.

Though 'Lîna could see, there was indeed a method behind the madness of the onslaught of the enemy. It appeared the Death of Death spared worlds that were already destroying themselves in a mocking stroke of sardonic efficiency that could even sicken those from H'Raka. All in the same fashion that let the Armn'dallos befall to their own hand. 'Lîna cautiously wondered what she would find on M'Gata.

The P'rynn were notorious commodities traders that relied on technology, similar to that of the Imperium Interface, the M'Gata High Network, which co-ordinated their markets. A obsolete technology of the Lon'tus acquired at bargain basement prices by the merchants of M'Gata. The exclusive domain for all meta-economic data transfers that extended to other systems as well.

On the surface the P'rynn are yet another simpler people, thought the Aristocrat. H'Renn gruffly thought of their advanced trade negotiation techniques inherent in each member of this species as the only thing that gave the P'rynn any real measure of worthiness.

And 'Lîna, at first, thought M'Gata unremarkable from her first telepathic glance of this world. For far too many P'rynn had their lives governed by the ethic of greed, emotion buried under a veneer of temperance, corporeal fantasies of simple compartmentalised avarice, overburdening and inefficient labour structures, thoughts consumed in a thick soup of plastic platitudes. A species still measuring their wealth in lower order commodities. A culture of consumer and nothing more and a species that the Trinity felt had far too many members of the P'rynn flocking to having their lives ruled by stress driven ambitions.

It is a pity such a species could impose such constraining burdens upon themselves, 'Lîna thought to herself. Still, the P'rynn had now become a middle power simply by what they possessed for sale. The Imperium could easily conquer but the way of the Imperium was not the way of the enemy. The Trinity had no qualms with negotiation, and though diplomatic relations with the P'rynn were mainly dry affairs, the Imperium would honour their agreements.

What was agreed upon by the Trinity was that the P'rynn, for all their detractions, were a species only a few generations away from being as competitive as the Lon'tus Commonwealth was before it became integrated into the Imperium. And perhaps this was the sole reason the Three journeyed to this world. Indeed, the P'rynn were resourceful as they had unearthed a trans-temporal carrier generator that the Imperium had come to this world for.

Thanks to treaties with previous governments of the Imperium Trinity, the P'rynn were able to access, under Imperium war measures, the retrieval of artefacts for the war effort from the galactic museum of the Origin species. It has licence that few neutral worlds could ever dream of being granted.

The galactic museum being the ruins of the first fully settled galaxy by the Origin species that was rumoured to have transcended reality. 'Lîna saw her path one day taking her there. She thought it beneficial for the P'rynn to even venture to a space of a people that they could one day be. She wondered if they took a chance to look around and think of the lives once lived there.

In the past, the P'rynn had been awarded commercial contracts with the At'Lann and Lon'tus going back five of their generations. Though the Imperium tried to keep their practices competitive, it was those of M'Gata who were the tacticians who continued to be chosen. Even lesser species than the P'rynn advanced by their sheer example. 'Lîna found their path lacking, she decided upon the slim possibility that those of M'Gata could take the shining path of the ways of the At'Lann.

The P'rynn had within themselves the potential for a higher evolution; their tenacity was empowered in the extreme in their drive to succeed as was shown by their crucial find. For it was they who found the monumental find, and it was the P'rynn that would be awarded a most expensive payment.

After great deliberation by the Imperium Senate, and with the approval of the Trinity, the Imperium agreed to constructing a fold-gate for the M'Gata home world that would bring their world into the At'Lann system in six months time. They would take their place in the At'Lann home system in exchange for the technology the P'rynn had salvaged. An ancient, yet both contemporary and superior technology the P'rynn would deliver upon sealing the war contract.

'Lîna was unsure of their worthiness but considered the potential of some of those from M'Gata to pursue higher drives. Though their conduct was for the most part stale, the P'rynn certainly had passion even if it seemed contrived. But for far too many M'Gata, it remained a passion for banality.

Initially, 'Iato was bitterly opposed to the trade deal as the P'rynn demanded too steep a price but he came to agree after Nul'lus convinced him that this was the path set by Fate. Ironically it was Nul'lus who thought it would lower the value of the Imperium state. A streak of the old Lon'tus ways came back in that they should only pay them through their submission to the Imperium.

They were like the Lon'tus once were, and the P'rynn, were simply less civilised and did not understand what they possessed on their path. But even he understood that 'Lîna would make them earn any measure of paradise. She would take them into her fold but they would bear the burden of their own elevation by ceding the P'rynn the most distant orbit around the Tr'Lann sun almost beyond N'Bith and far beyond Nv'Ata.

Those from M'Gata had a lot to learn. Their lifestyle had been one of expropriating technologies and soon they would begin to follow a different path. Though the price paid for a crucial component of the Imperium war effort would be high, their contract and treaty with the Imperium would be full of compromise.

The At'Lann Imperium would change as a result, and 'Lîna especially knew Za'szu was not exactly thrilled to pay such a high price but their way was to be selfless in many of their affairs. 'Lîna had to bear with it once again and rose to the occasion to do what had to be done; for she had become the logic of Fate. She had to consider the losses from the front. It was a difficult decision to share her space with a species that sacrificed so many of the wrong things but she would show them sacrifice, and would become their guide. It's the least I can do, 'Lîna thought as she tantalised her mind with the lessons she would teach them.

Considering that the Imperium was an engine of perpetual economic growth arising from their path as the newest masters of creation, if not for the cultural pollution this was, in essence, a small price to pay for what could bring the Imperium a step closer to victory. If not for their eventual close proximity to the At'Lann throne this would not even be a concern for 'Lîna.

Besides, the Tr'Lann system had plenty of room created by the gravitational steppes of the At'Lann sun. The At'Lann Imperium could accommodate the P'rynn as they knew this was the highest of gifts that may become a permanent provision. The Imperium vessels, Ki'Bur and 'Verga, in fact, had the required technological components on board, and had also arrived to M'Gata, to proceed with the transfer. The agreement was to be signed by the Trinity on this day that was yet another day of dreary beginnings on the path of war.

The barely aroused thoughts on the P'rynn came to a hasty end as their shuttle touched the ground with a mental jolt that was felt by those who can perceive and are a part of the collision and course of particles. The silent landing was made upon the immaculate fluoride hued marble that flowed into the grey spires that towered over the main M'Gata landing field. The Trinity disembarked and set foot upon the sanitised ground of 'Ea'tel'som, the P'rynn's world and financial nexus.

'Lîna noticed the spires of the world capital of M'Gata were nearly identical to the ecclesiastically inspired spires of At'Lann and 'Mura, and far too similar to be a coincidence. Then she remembered the M'Gata, under T'Moda, had purchased older At'Lann architectural schematics from her paternal grandfather, King S'lanu, for what was first their early capital Eyat'sia.

As beautiful as it was because it reminded her of home, the lines of each spire seemed out of sync with this world and its nature. It seemed a world of obsessive compulsive *feng shui*. Their technology seemed without passion. The At'Lann jade spires were far more beautiful to 'Lîna's eyes. Still, she thought, it was almost flattering for lesser beings to seek the beauty of those who exist in greatness.

The Trinity were greeted by the P'rynn's official greeting ceremony which consisted of stolid, contrived marching music along with choreographed mime like dancers that were at the side of the P'rynn functionaries and dignitaries who bowed before the Three in their garish grey adornments. Yet, Gn'rys P'rynn was not amongst them. The Three were not impressed by the frivolous waste of their time; which also had the stink of being a delaying tactic.

'Iato H'Renn grabbed one of these automatons, a so-called member of their constabulary guards by the scruff of his neck and ordered to know where their world operator was. Nul'lus read his thoughts and knew the way for the Three who were already eager to leave the muscular and nonemotive smiles behind. 'Iato H'Renn commandeered an ashen hued puffed rice shaped monorail car to take the Three to the top of the spire of Gn'rys P'rynn's financial cathedral.

Apparently, Gn'rys P'rynn was conducting government activities that he viewed as far too important to put aside for the Trinity of the Imperium to greet them upon their arrival. Such utter disrespect made what was a trying situation even worse. For he would find himself facing three near omnipotent and annoyed beings that had the same sternest way that a rigid elder feels when before a mewling child who has disobeyed.

His lack of regard for proper etiquette left the world operator of M'Gata in the dimmest of views held by the Trinity even before their first meeting with this truant world facilitator. It all seemed so low and pathetic that an entire species would enslave themselves to the pursuit of consumerism at its lowest extent.

As the Three arrived in the executive office of Gn'rys P'rynn, they were greeted by its ramshackle nature. Amidst the light of the pleasant citrian stencilled skies, their world leader seemed to lead without a clear direction. P'rynn data crystal currency and portrait art of galactic figures lay scattered and strewn about the executive office of the World Systems Operator.

Piles of material wealth were littered everywhere around even Gn'rys P'rynn's crescent shaped elephant size desk, grown over with M'Gata inter-link terminals whose screens were filled with P'rynn financial data, which went whizzing across the screen in a sea under a violent storm of red and green ups and down. But this storm of data made for a blood red sea. Everything was wrong. Everything was unorganised and stressfully chaotic.

The walrus like and aspic like Gn'rys P'rynn was in a panic before the Trinity. Yellow warning lights stretched across the fear driven blood-sea of markets plummeting that overwhelmed every inter-link screen. The Trinity watched as a helpless Gn'rys P'rynn watched market after market disappear. As a crushed pace of data jaggedly stormed in a zig-zag across the P'rynn inter-link, it was plain to see the P'rynn were losing everything other than what they offered for trade to the Imperium.

Their financial empire was collapsing. Their commodities exchange market, the driving force of their economy had dropped to 9.6% of its pre-war value before all trade halted as the inter-link screen faded to black in front of a broken leader and the rudely treated Trinity that offered M'Gata its only salvation. Apparently, barely 25% of their trading partners remained following the invasion of existence by the Death of Death.

Gn'rys P'rynn slammed his fists on his desk before his dandy lion yellow wheel barrow body fell despondently into his swivel chair. His face became green olive in complexion as it took the expression of a squirrel in anguish. His face filled with shock as he saw the Trinity had let themselves in instead of waiting for his arrival. The Three glared at him as he forced a grin from ear to ear before begging himself into a look of apology and welcome. The Three were not eager to see such an utterly insolent masquerade continue any further. Pleasantries were thrown aside and incinerated in violet flames of bitter annoyance.

'Are the artefacts ready to be transferred to our ships?', Nul'lus commandingly asked succinctly with disdain. Even the relaxed man from Lon'tus had grown weary of his time on M'Gata.

'Yes, Imperator Nul'lus. You can transport them after the treaty is signed'. His words were filled with meekness and anger. For Gn'rys P'rynn knew that the Lis'talla probably had as many as one hundred and thirty three thousand cannons trained on his world right now. Selfishly and obsessively he still itched to tend to his economy but the sheer telepathic presence of the Three caused him to submit himself to his audience with the Trinity of the Imperium Trinity.

'There is another provision that will be agreed to for the H'Raka Imperium', interjected almost impatiently.

H'Renn upheld a cubic ruby neon holo-pad that he folded into the air above the palm of his right hand that contained an addendum to the P'rynn-Imperium contract treaty. 'Lîna had not been made aware of this but she remained in silence to support the comrades she placed so much faith in. 'Iato blew the holo-pad from his hand to that of the bulbous fingers of Gn'rys P'rynn, for him to read one of Y'vis's last commands before he transferred power to 'Iato H'Renn. How the face and facade of Gn'rys P'rynn became fields of lily of the valley.

'I can't agree to this', the leader of the P'rynn begged as he conceded.

But he knew there was no way out. It was 'Iato H'Renn's duty to consider this man the weakest of preys. All it took to defeat the will of Gn'rys P'rynn was for 'Iato to point to the skies over M'Gata. Gn'rys P'rynn knew with but the merest thought command the weapons systems of the Lis'talla could obliterate M'Gata. 'Iato let loose a strike like McManaman and countered with an imprisoning,

"You will."

Gn'rys P'rynn looked into 'Iato H'Renn's ice like eyes for a moment with a hatred bred by jealousy of what the P'rynn were not. Then Gn'rys lowered his head in the realisation like that of losing your soul without even having one to begin with.

He exposed his right wrist as if for it to be cut by the sharpest razor. Nul'lus folded into reality a tourmaline hued palm-sized, self-sealing genetic extraction cube and pressed it against Gn'rys P'rynn's submitting wrist in the ancient tradition of the Imperium in sealing their treaties. 'Lîna turned her eyes to 'Iato H'Renn with a mild perplexed searching expression for what the smug Imperator from

H'Raka was up to but whatever it was it was already done.

Nul'lus took the small cube from Gn'rys P'rynn and gave it to 'Lîna's tender hands who let the cube prick her right index finger for a genetic sample. She gave the cube back to him and he held it out for 'Iato 'H'Renn who pressed the cube with a slap against his right forearm. 'Iato H'Renn did not break the silence that now cast itself down in the cluttered office of Gn'rys P'rynn as he nodded unemotionally to confirm the sealing of the contract treaty.

The Three then turned their backs on a Gn'rys P'rynn who covered his head with his hands as he fell back into his tan leather swivel chair. As the door to the executive office of the M'Gata world systems operator closed behind the Trinity, they could see, telepathically and psionically, after a long pause over what he had consented to, the enormity of it. He returned immediately to his inter-link to try to stabilise the P'rynn economy and tried to hoard what little was left.

Walls were only wind to their eyes, and 'Lîna looked back for a moment for another snapshot of her memories made on the path of war. She watched as Gn'rys kept trying to hook the inter-link into economies that were disappearing and found none to replace their lost markets. She could tell he wanted to kick the inter-link terminals over but opted to pull his own hair out instead from the stress of it all. 'Lîna felt disgusted as she watched him yank out a huge chunk of hair from the side of his head exposing the yellow scale plating of his skull. The path of war would not be easy.

As the honour guard were rejoined by the Three outside their Imperium short-range shuttle, 'Lîna asked 'Iato H'Renn what was contained in the addendum, and what it was all about. He shocked her in his answer to her query; for he was the Hunter.

'Let us just say for now that a decree from a higher power will do for your people what you could never do.'

Then 'Lîna realised what H'Renn had alluded to, and decided it was best to see the matter quietly die. For even she could not make certain choices by who she was. This addendum 'Lîna thought of as a most bitter of fates or the most balance in how trying it would be for those from M'Gata. 'Iato was right, 'Lîna thought, I could never have made such a choice.

When they returned to the Lis'talla, the Three found that the merchandise had been delivered, and their costly supplies were already on their way to the construction grounds. The Three were especially eager to leave this banal world of greed behind them. But war made for strange bedfellows, and there was no turning back on the path of war.

23
The Midnight Garden

The young and perhaps no longer so gentle Imperiatrix of At'Lann was close to creating a psionic gate to the Death of Death. 'Lîna had woven her temporal spindles into a curvaceous trellis like array of soft pink and mezereon. Irises grew throughout the fields of 'Lîna's launching psionic plane. For to fight the Death of Death, it would take a piece of herself. Thick dark greenery spread across a matrix of roman columns with ultra-violet, mauve chiffon covering the landscape with wavy, ethereal trellises. Fate came to exist in as many random temporal points and of one existence that was her very being. The music of Tiësto, on some level, always filled the air.

She could almost see the darkest tunnel to the most vile labyrinth that lay ahead. Whispers of its putrid smell of rotting fowl polluted her psionic realm. The dark finality lay ahead. In response to the immense darkness, the midnight garden began to grow outwards for as far as the soul could see. Even the lilac lit, cloudy nightscape became awash in floral holy infernos.

Flora and faunae abounded Fate's midnight garden. The sky became awash in floral violets, mauves, mezereons, emeralds, dark blues, reds, and whites of the softest of orchid pedals. But even the smell of the most fragrant and most fresh cut of flowers was still not enough to hide the scent that was the dark trail of the enemy and the ultimate domain of evil. Fate had more than upped the ante.

Within her mind, 'Lîna was meditative upon nearly all levels of meditation. Her mind became her homelands. She came to take notice upon all things within her mind. She was being watched. Not just by the psionic eyes of the enemy but also by the eyes of others hidden amongst the ferns. In this realm, she became and desired the path of the crusading anchorite once more.

With the path of war, her path, at times, was difficult to share with others. For the path of war had become her burden. She was being watched by the psionic sensors of the Death of Death and sets of familiar eyes that she could not yet discern. How like fireflies they danced across the waves of foliage within the psionic realm and realms within her mind and soul.

Fate was far from surprised though part of her had to let go of her path alone and she would have other times to be left with her own being. She continued to work the spindles as if there were no foreign eyes inside her mind. For she was 'Lîna and she was Fate. To Fate, these familiar eyes were just as much a part of her as she was of them.

Fate was almost at the final liminal gates she had to open, and the eyes that came to watch her on the path of Fate chanced upon what was fast becoming the unlocking of the dark frontier. She wondered if the familiar eyes that gazed upon her were as afraid as she was of the prospect of unlocking the path to the psionic realm of the Death of Death. She cried out in a soft and subdued echo like that of calling out in the glory of evening,

'I see you have arrived just in time for morning tea. I believe it is almost the At'Lann dawn. Why don't you come out so we can have a sip or two, 'Lus?'

Fate broke herself away from her trellises of temporal spindles and arranged a tea setting for two under a leafy pagoda like canopy. She knew her soul as well as who was inside her. It was an immaculate arbour and made even more so by her eloquently eloquent gentleman who shared her path, and she instantly made the Aristocrat feel at home in her psionic realm.

Fate watched as the Aristocrat poured himself a cup of cosmic, ethereal tea, and watched as he preferred to stand under the violet and mauve moon-glow that made the midnight garden drip with the sweetest dew. It was a perfect setting that even a thespian like Stewart would be envious of and one like Brooks would find challenging. Fate took a cup of At'Lann tea that was a silver glitter of stars with the scent of Earl Grey. Everything seemed to come so easily in the psionic realm without any required thought. For power comes easily in the garden of the soul.

Fate then sat with the Aristocrat who was now convinced to sit and they enjoyed the company of each others mind as they sipped away.

'Surely you have not been at it all night, 'Imiszi?', the Aristocrat asked with pleasant and serene astonishment.

In their minds, Nul'lus and 'Lîna called to each other and their path became one through their soul bond and were affectionate toward one another as their minds swirled. After all, the garden of the soul was an enlightened psionic environment free of most genetic shackles. Souls in this place could swim beyond their programming, and 'Lîna and Nul'lus enjoyed the freedom of all that this psionic realm of Fate had to offer. For Fate, this was no intrusion. In the transual that surrounded them, they linked their thoughts in a way far more peacefully content than their corporeal conversations. Fate always welcomed the Aristocrat into her thoughts. She answered him with the serenity of a shyness cast aside.

'Since the Imperium midnight. I am very close, my friend and companion of the great path.'

Fate's voice was a song of layered joy as she told her friend of her latest progress. Though the glow of other eyes fell back into the shade of the midnight garden, she brought into his mind her latest path. Secrets could not be kept for long inside the Trinity. The Hunter knew and now the Aristocrat came onto the path of Fate. And Fate strived to be the valiant mate of the Aristocrat on the path of war.

'Have we reached M'Goa yet, 'Lus?

'We will arrive in three hours, 'Imiszi.'

'Well no wonder you have had to venture into the psionic realm to drag me away to attend to the affairs at hand. But not before we finish our tea', Fate said with glimmers of a tranquil enthusiasm.

Fate then brought a sunrise to join the moonlight to brighten their shade. It was all quite lovely. The only thing missing was the Pal'ana ocean lavender beaches of 'Mura. Fate was almost going to change the psionic realm to shine with the sun of those days though she chose not to as she thought it would only remind the pair of what they left behind on L'unn.

Fate was, after all, a paradox who always stood guard over her thought while all the while exposing them even in her most fragile of moments. Though the Aristocrat could always see behind closed doors if he chose to, on this day he chose not to. For he knew Fate was kind to her memories. They would savour a few more moments of basking in this place that defined her path, her philosophy of re-evolving, reconfiguring, and refining the place and being of their souls within the universe.

Fate's holy ground became the ways that shaped her and even to some degree the Aristocrat who also walked his own path. B'Dak would have been pleased by what would have been his today. And, perhaps, 'Lîna hoped that a set of those still obscured familiar eyes were his. Still, it was a great moment to relax before the journey that is the gathering on M'Goa.

Approaching the divine, the world of M'Goa was blessedly spared in the first wave by the Army of Two Rings. M'Goa is an evolving world bound by a strict neutrality of peace. Perhaps the Death of Death though their pursuit of efficiency and excess would be their own undoing.

''Lus, you can tell 'Iato that I accept his decision that ninety seven percent of the P'rynn will not be genetically transferred to the Tr'Lann system. I can sacrifice a principle for the sake of the alliance of war.'

For a moment, the psionic sky became a little darker but the Aristocrat was, for the most post, not surprised by how far his once gentle friend was willing to go.

'He was worried you might have such an act weigh upon your conscience when you are needed most. 'Iato has made sacrifices as well before he brought the H'Raka into the Imperium. He broke his covenant with the H'Raka high gods, the 'Hyn, to stand beside you on the path of war. He has your faith except his faith, and as a H'Raka leader that must walk the ancient path and also the path of the At'Lann and their leader.'

Fate had known of this but the psionic reality moved so swiftly now that it seemed like a vague recollection. For indeed the Hunter possessed a worthy soul even if it still remained hidden amongst the vines.

'Well please tell 'Iato to please try and spare me anymore surprises. I am not one for them.'

'You, 'Imiszi? Now that *surprises* me. Will your path not be boring if you know only all that is to come? Your path needs chaos and uncertainty. You must leave complacency behind.'

'You are as wise as you are evolved, my friend. But why do you seek to pry my thoughts at this time and in this place?'

'Let it not bother you. His reasons coincide with a stand to ensure the At'Lann will not be taken advantage of, 'Imiszi.'

'But of course, 'Lus'

She turned to 'Iato.

'Son of H'Raka.'

'Iato bowed out into the psionic realm as she bowed to him.

'Daughter of L'unn'

These were strange days indeed.

'The P'rynn will be a difficult species to mould but it will not be an impossible task for the At'Lann. They will surrender to peace.'

'Well, glad to see you remain a true daughter of L'unn.'

The Aristocrat then reached back in the corporeal world to check the time, and then added, 'So when will you be ready, 'Imiszi?'

Fate pointed to what was woven by her hands and responded, 'This only waits for me to turn the key to enter the dark nether-world. Knowing what will come in the liberation that is the gathering on M'Goa, the second front can wait for a full regenerative day after.' She paused. 'So where are you right now, 'Lus?'

'Outside your door. Its chimes did not wake you.'

'Well there's a first, my friend. I shall awaken now. Hopefully, you did not mind waiting.'

The Aristocrat shook his head in his psionic form. She then asked if he did not mind going from the Lon'tus blend to the House blend of At'Lann in terms of his medical care. The Aristocrat had a hearty laugh before he faded out of the midnight garden of the psionic realm. Though as he left, a part of him was taken aback by the sight of the blooming flowers that abounded for all the soul to see. However, so much of its beauty was watered by her tears of loss.

'Lîna purged her quarters of bio-gel and returned her room to its normal state as she returned to corporeal reality. With her thoughts she opened her door for him. As Nul'lus came into her private domain aboard the Lis'talla, they then decided spontaneously to have a corporeal cup of tea. Though they did not need or require it, the pair simply chose to partake in the tradition.

Nul'lus, dashing as ever, enjoyed the simple pleasure of the morning sunrise conversation with one who knew him so well. Soon, they would arrive on M'Goa. For they knew would be both a duty and a release like no other. And on they pushed on along the path of war.

24

Taking The Last Piece Of Future's Hope On The Great Gathering Along The Path

It was a brave new day. It was a day like no other day that had not come in some time for the Trinity sovereign that still played like aristocrats. This day marked the end of what the Trinity considered an essential trade mission that left each of them drastically empty. Diplomacy on the path of war is a tiring business. All that changed for the Trinity when they arrived on M'Goa.

The azure skies as soothing as those over the Balearic tropical candy skies of M'Goa were a welcome relief and respite from all the misery seen along the way. The final piece of the Imperium omega defence project would be acquired from a beautiful people that chose to go out of existence in style in their mainly photonic sculpted and renaissance styled palaces. For the M'Goa were far beyond the *depeche mode* of how the great finality would be greeted. Only on M'Goa would a situation of Armageddon be a cause to realise celebration and liberation. There was a noble defiance about their peace and the Trinity respected the M'Goa for this reason.

Most of their planetary institutions seemed permanently shut down as their path forever changed. Vessels from lesser species orbited the planet as M'Goa had become the flocking ground for the final gathering, the last dance, where rank would be left at the door. The M'Goa would greet the Death of Death by showing the darkness before all existence that the enjoyment of life can never be destroyed. They had a hard-core faith and perhaps this was what 'Lîna needed. She needed to be blanketed in the faith of others so that it may restore a little of her own, and her fate was to find it amongst those who awaited someone like Azrael to free them. Perhaps, true freedom was already theirs.

In the meantime, the Imperium would trade their entire pharmo-genetic database for that of M'Goa's so that the bio-mechanical systems of the omega defence project could be built, and the M'Goa could have all the hedonism they could buy. 'Iato joined Nul'lus and 'Lîna for their morning briefing. The Imperiatrix also ensured the other supplies requested by the M'Goa were transferred to their world. Though the P'rynn negotiated for them, the Imperium would have given the M'Goa what they asked anyway. The M'Goa were the only exception to Imperium sensibilities as their front-line was that of celebration as their battle. And for having a battle to fight, the M'Goa were a worthy species in the eyes of the Imperium.

The M'Goa had asked for a vast array of items both uplifting and bacchanal from the Imperium: poems, sonnets, ballads, novels, omni-media, plays, as well as visual, musical and literary creations from the entire artistic databases of the Lon'tus, At'Lann, and H'Raka interfaces that composed the Imperium Interface.

Every song, every piece of music from the Imperium was especially valued. From litronica spoken aloud to beats beyond electronic styles of music was the march of the M'Goa. And now the music of the three central powers of the Imperium would also be played on M'Goa to usher in the soon to be coming finality. Taking this positively, 'Lîna admired them for taking both a united and internal path.

Even when the Lis'talla entered the M'Goa home system like in symphonic wave of Van Dyk, 'Lîna could feel the happiness of the M'Goa people soothe her empathic soul with their thought shining so strongly across the soulscape. And by what they had asked for, 'Lîna knew the M'Goa wanted to go down in joy.

It was almost as if the M'Goa would fill their souls with bliss before awaiting release of being rid of the burden of all reality. Erasure would bring a separate peace and final peace to the ecstatic M'Goa. Instead of looking in and looking at the Death of Death as something to be depressed about, the M'Goa had taken this as an opportunity to take a unique path and a unique stride towards a higher state of being. The Trinity found something logical about the approach of this developing culture.

Amidst the girandole rainbow coloured multi-spectral confetti that greeted the arrival of the Lis'talla, 'Lîna could not helping feeling quite motherly towards the M'Goa. For in a way, the M'Goa had already found the freedom the Imperium was fighting for. And for an evolving and developing species, the M'Goa already had the most indulgent of tastes.

The list went on and continued with anti-proton fireworks and sparklers, H'Raka war drums, Lon'tus chemical stimulants, At'Lann cigarettes, H'Raka liquors, aphrodisiacs, Imperium fashion textiles and patterns. Indeed, the M'Goa were to become the last but best symbol of all out revelry as they were accumulating enough supplies for a sustained fifty five years, and even this transaction might not be enough to hold them.

When the Three landed on the planet, they were greeted by the ambient almost ethereal divination that was only the tip of the M'Goa musical spectrum. Like that of Graham of Copeland, of Lashes, of Savage, of Sneak, of Sun, of Sister Bliss, of Tiësto, of Van Dyk, of Villeneuve, of Carter, of Foort, of Keinenberg, of Juarez, of Dan, of Hawtin, of Deep Dish, of Sasha, of Digweed, of Corsten when he came out of the blue, of Oakenfold, of Maas, of Balu, of Heather, of Fontaine, of Moby, of Trevor, of the Chicks with Decks, of Armin, of Onionz, of Fleming, of Mehat, of Jules, of Fergie, of Kai, of Solo, of Warren, all in one and always joins. Everyone's personal essential mix became the only essential mix. Like the flavour of a Djarum, the music of M'Goa invited them to stay the night. In one vibe and beat, many vibes and beats came together to stretch across the azure sky that held the green and silver planet that is M'Goa.

The M'Goa gave the Trinity a planet wide welcome even began playing a song from At'Lann for the highest of their trance beats to enrapture M'Goa. The Three were officially met by their world ambassador, Sy'dosa, and he welcomed the Trinity to his techno-humanized world by having a rotation of selections of music from all three powers cast by the M'Goa music masters for sets the Trinity would not soon forget.

As if with his hands in prayer he graciously invited the Imperium crew of the Lis'talla to join M'Goa in rejoicing in the planetary gathering and all its festivities. It was an invitation made for a night of peace to belong to them all, and one that came knowing that the Lis'talla's crew would soon put their lives on the line on the front against the Army of Two Rings. And it was an invitation extended to the Imperium as a whole for their rest and relaxation until the end of existence. M'Goa would be the paradise in the ring of betrothal Pandora wore after she opened the great darkness.

As the music across M'Goa was as loud as it was silent as it progressed, the Trinity telepathically and joyously accepted Sy'dosa's welcome to his world. In telepathically discussing the night at hand, the Trinity came into agreement that memories for their people of fun and freedom, even if sometimes frivolous, would be something their crew and their peoples would see as another reason to fight that much harder on the path of war. For to know freedom is to fight for freedom, and one can never fight for release if one never experiences it.

The Imperium third fleet had come to patrol the space outside the M'Goa system for their protection and the spirits of the Trinity needed to be brightened after too much of the melancholy of their recent affairs. The Trinity were in full agreement, and Sy'dosa was extremely pleased that the nights of M'Goa would become the Imperium's to enjoy as well. Even evolved beings should have fun when they can, Nul'lus telepathically emphasised this to 'Lîna and 'Iato as this world was once his frequent vacation and commercial destination. He knew their night would be one where the three of them could leave the war at the door. The enemy would be kept at bay and the night would be theirs.

The Three would stay the night for their grateful hosts, the citizens of M'Goa. Safe and secure venues were created for the revelry of the Imperium court. The Trinity sealed the trade contract and treaty and left it to their minor bureaucrats to adopt the finer points of the agreement. It was then agreed that the supply ships carrying one of the most valuable cargoes in the universe would be escorted to the At'Lann system by four H'Raka warships.

The Three felt they had done enough, and 'Lîna knew there were no safer hands for all their precious cargoes. Fate knew the H'Raka would come through and the security task force of the Imperium would protect them in the delicacy of their pleasure and all their moments of fragility. In the time the Trinity had been on M'Goa, nine Lon'tus and nine At'Lann warships also converged on the system to protect the sovereigns. The leisure would be pure, and their leisure would intersect the path of others who have undertaken the path of war.

Among those who would be joining the Trinity during the M'Goa gathering on this night would be 'Xo General 'Ivia who captains the At'Lann warship, 'Garja. Nul'lus especially wanted to meet this exceptional tactician who came from a species that was similar in its genetic configuration to that of the At'Lann. He heard she was one of the best strategists in the fleet. As Sy'dosa began to show the Trinity his world, he also welcomed 'Ivia, the aqua hued, slender muscled soldier, to their night of being a part of the new scene of M'Goa.

If the Three or their compatriots did not want to experience the highest purity of ecstatic delights that lead away and lead to the greatest of decadent states now was the time to reconfigure ones chromosomes to produce geno-trophic hedonic inhibitors, 'Ivia wisely pointed out.

Unsure as to how their enhanced psyogenetic structures would be affected by a night on M'Goa, the Three each activated a minute dose of inhibiting agents within themselves. 'Ivia drank a anti-gene-toxin elixir so that she would remain in an optimal condition in case she was called back to duty during the night to return to the front. Like the Three, a gulping of the taste would be enough for her. For this night, she did not mind as it would be for the Trinity. And at least for now, they were a long way from Tartarus.

The music of the house of M'Goa could now also be heard. As the thumping of the quantum bass grew, the night of pleasures was satisfyingly starting to build. The music was the pump. Fate knew this would be a night they would not soon forget. For the throng of millions, the place was already jumping. The night of mystical sonic adventure was noticeably being appreciated by all. The vibe of M'Goa was already entering the souls of the Three and the sound before them was like skiing through the snows of one like those for a sport of Charles. The Trinity began to enter the loveliest dynamic of this wilderness of the soothing drums of the M'Goa night. For this night, peace and love would be theirs once again.

Sy'dosa teleported the Imperium entourage to his stadia-parlour like area venue of ten thousand M'Goa and their guests including many off-world dignitaries. Everyone was spread across varying gravity platforms allowing for contact on sliding gravity scales with other parties on other platforms that looked like wave gliding steppes moving perpetually within an octagonal stadium. The music was piped in across the planet by sub-spatial sonic fissures in every space of the ether of the wave flowing sealed room that encompassed both massive and small gatherings together.

The music filled every aspect of the room to the point where, the very molecules and the very atmosphere pulsed along to the beat of H'Raka war drums mixed into what had become M'Goa trance. It was the sounds of freedom for all who joined the erotic, tangerine hued M'Goa whose females danced with the sweetest perfection of the purity of faeries and butterflies. And they were butterflies dancing across tiger lily fields in the sun embracing the freedom of the light of existence.

Sy'dosa made the Three and their companion General 'Ivia feel right at home in the libation that was now M'Goa. He lived to be the best of hosts and his private platform was theirs to enjoy. The instant club on a hexagonal platform, was held up by a thicker than usual gravity field, like all others, was illuminated by a smoky field that constantly traversed along with the music across the visual and non-visual spectrum.

Besides a modern and solid triangular table set aglow with azure light that rose out of the dense graviton floor, V-shaped couches of diluted gravitational plush bubbles adorned the right side of the platform which made for plenty of dancing space. This was a strange world. What could one say. Though inside, this was a wide-open space. On the table, there were buckets that had the shimmer of At'Lann poly-quartz, filled with 'Nagashima class, or highest grade, aural activated, meta-neural stimulants recently acquired from the Imperium. Each of the six buckets was filled to the brim with such vials that contained a juniper-coloured liquid.

The excess of M'Goa, whose economy was a thousand times greater than M'Gata's, knew no restraint. Sy'dosa gladly told the Trinity their supply would be continuous for the entire night. The man simply knew how to throw a party the likes of which the universe had not seen before. 'Lîna was amazed to find out this was not even the main course, musically or otherwise. Nul'lus explained the buckets would be filled and emptied the entire night so as to hold as many different varieties of geno-trophic compounds as possible. Nul'lus also told 'Lîna of how the natives drew the massive planetary concept so that all M'Goa parties would be inter-connected and become one through music, vibe, empathy and telepathy.

As a previous visitor to celebration gatherings on M'Goa, Nul'lus told 'Lîna that there was little difference between what would be their night on M'Goa for her and 'Iato H'Renn except for a purer sense of freedom. For the M'Goa existed to experiment with a path of techno-evolved tribal liberation, and this was their tribe. Many worked to bring pleasure together in the end time and all seemed ready to go down blissed out.

With a small armada of the Imperium's elite to protect them, the Three began to enjoy a night of soulful freedom and freedom from restraint. With the loud whispers of one like Myestas thumping the wind of life; it became a happier sirocco for all members of the gathering. And then each of them gently reached into the buckets before clicking off the liquid from the vial as if releasing a ball-point. After the compound was instantaneously transferred to each of their being though their sub-dermal pores, the new gates were opened. Then the vials were thrown casually to the floor, which let the empty vials sink though the graviton platform and fall unto the ground far below. A ground that was stories below the solid and variable graviton platforms.

'Lîna looked to the ground below her and noticed a thin pile of juniper hued glass vials beginning to blanket a once rainbow speckled granite looking floor that in only a few places still peaked through its temporary burial. As 'Lîna pressed the tab, she momentarily felt disconcerted as a subsonic neural signal activated the vapour liquid as it diluted itself across her sub-cells in a dance that became further empowered by what is embraced on M'Goa.

If not for the minutely required inhibitor, the experience of joining the united vibe of M'Goa would be far too jolting for her liking. The music of M'Goa began to sing as part of her being. Don't stop, she peacefully thought. But this was no jagged epiphany. 'Lîna let go of the war. This night would be theirs to savour. Existence became a smooth and balanced symbiotic synthesis with the holy essence of life itself. Truly, M'Goa was a homeland.

Psionic streams waved in the wind of the moon around 'Lîna's being. The effects of the inhibitor began to fall away, yet she was fully in control while experiencing what the M'Goa were experiencing in its full effect. The inhibiting agents within her body reconfigured 'Lîna's neural pathways to input both the psionic and what is reality. Her neural paths diversified into newly created balancing channels. Her mental framework was continuously re-initialising itself to maintain both a conscious state and an altered one. For only an instant was 'Lîna worried that she would keep too many of her inhibitions as her being momentarily psionically fragmented. And then she felt swimming freely in the oceans of Cronos, the oceans of time.

Like a midnight surfer, 'Lîna adapted to ride the psionic and transual waves. The dragon of evil that is war was caught in 'Lîna's grip and contained for what she could feel to be was already a special night. For this night, the evil dragon would be cast asleep.

'Lîna and Nul'lus began to dance away with what felt like the aftertaste of guarana in their mouths. The vibe and music of M'Goa gave them a reason not to hold back. They could see the M'Goa and other species dance on a near countless number of other platforms scattered about the stadia-parlour of Sy'dosa. Even before the Trinity was a few dozen select revellers of M'Goa to create even more atmosphere on the world ambassador's private platform.

Class distinctions disappeared as everyone, even 'Iato H'Renn, who came from a gathering culture all its own, joined in the spirit of M'Goa. And the spirit of transual euphoria wrapped itself about all those across the surface of M'Goa. 'Lîna swam into a united spirit of peace, love and respect. Like swimming in bliss itself.

She looked down as she danced alongside Nul'lus and H'Renn to see the thick ever growing mounds of empty juniper vials beneath their feet. She realised what lay below here was just the discarded remnant of what became another key to spiritual release the At'Lann lived their lives to find. She was converging with the path of Fate. What she felt this night was just as solid and genuine as any glorious feeling that could be held.

The empty vials glittered like diamonds beneath the gathering, and the party intensified above. Sy'dosa explained to the Trinity that the empty vials would be recycled as energy crystals that now acted as M'Goa's primary power source. He told them the M'Goa lived in balance with their world and their celebrations returned their energy to their life-giving world. 'Lîna was especially impressed, for the last time she visited this world when it was more restrained though their people kept many of their world's continents undisturbed for the animals upon them. They were even then becoming a people worthy of inclusion into the Imperium. All that was left was for them to ask. Even the recycled vials acted as an atmospheric cleanser rather than as a polluter. Relaxation became a path all its own.

'Lîna danced to where 'Valis Val'damus was and embraced her affable, steady officer. For they always had been in the mould of electronic children. Tonight he returned to being purely an endearing old friend. She was glad to see he was having a good time in the ethereal excess. Nothing could describe it. The place was jumping and the place was slamming. Everyone was becoming one to the beats of the global house of M'Goa. For this tribe revelled in the wide open underground. M'Goa was simply wondrous. The music seemed to massage 'Lîna's mind as the choral sounds that are those of At'Lann gatherings blended themselves in.

To fully satisfy their Imperium guests, the pure concept of the musical flow of M'Goa was taken to horizons never before ventured. Sound became the beauty of Venus. 'Lîna used her enhanced vision to see the biorhythms of those dancing on M'Goa become synchronous with the pulse of life and a million levels beyond their normal parameters. She realised that the M'Goa were fast approaching an enlightenment all its own.

The M'Goa faced erasure but chose to never feel its coming, for they believed they always remain in happiness no matter the outcome. The continual gathering would keep them free until their last instant of reality. They faced the finality with the bravery of joyous perpetual catharsis. Truly a way of style that was a most beautiful way to face the end.

'Lîna felt the sweet candy of M'Goa was too sweet for her constant tastes while fighting a war but this experience already made her choose M'Goa as her healing destination as well as that of her home. This night was becoming more wondrous by the moment.

On another platform, a circle of M'Goa were joined in an anal and phallic interlock dancing around another ring of nymph like M'Goa women that were joined in a cranial and bilabial slippery tightness of equal measure basking in the glory of the conjoined men. Now 'Lîna had seen everything. For a moment at least. The tangerine hued M'Goa mocked their impending doom with a greatly heightened vigorousness. Such ravenous hedonists, 'Lîna thought gleefully. And then even 'Zaya came to visit Sy'dosa's platform for the crazed festivities.

Nul'lus handed 'Lîna three of his finely tailored cigarettes as there would not be any bio-gel stasis this night. To his surprise, she had a householder pack her a case. 'Lîna did, however, take the three Nul'lus handed her, and in exchange for the Lon'tus doses, three of her own from her obsidian compact case.

'Lîna swayed as she moved so she magically cast herself in the beauty that are the wings of a dove as she let the music of M'Goa massage her body. In the transual saltwater, 'Lîna felt free. She saw Mu'tolma and waved with a touch of redemption at him. He waved back with a weight lifted off his shoulders equal to the restrained emotion in his face that also seemed to lift away. Though not his thing, even he was not about to miss the gathering.

The M'Goa activated their newly acquired At'Lann and Lon'tus pyrotechnics above the stadia-parlour after its domed roof folded into subspace. Ultra-neon rainbows glittered and flowed across the M'Goa nightscape and harmlessly to the platforms and to the walls below.

It was a heavenly beauty unparalleled. Like steams of electronic angels etching across the night side gathering on M'Goa. Bright maraschino and bilberry spotlights waved across the heavens above and below. Her eyes even had little pooling tears by the blessed visual beauty before her. What the M'Goa knew of freedom astonished 'Lîna for the M'Goa only sought its deepest contents. It was for life that made the M'Goa fight so hard in their own way.

They truly were *Hedone extremis.*

'Lîna danced for a longer time than she expected herself to and remained in motion alongside Nul'lus and 'Ivia as H'Renn had decided to have adventures on every other platform. She danced hard until deciding to take a break with those who joined her as Nul'lus wanted to smoke while reclined on one of the couches. She retired with Nul'lus and 'Ivia to admire the gathering from a more relaxed position.

Chilling, 'Lîna smoked the Lon'tus curative, her first of the night. Whatever edge left for the night was worn away. Sy'dosa's platform bobbed along in a gravity flux and thumped mildly with bass. From this distance, 'Lîna gazed upon the majority of the gathering crowd around her. She noticed many S'yana agents secretly placed on many of the neighbouring platforms guarding their sovereigns however unnecessarily. It was easy to pick them out as they seemed attired to up for Wookie, yet were not there for fun but rather duty. They seemed on a different path altogether as they flowed along with the celebrations on M'Goa while remaining in the cover of the mostly tangerine sea of people.

'Lîna commented to 'Ivia that war even in the sanctuary of peace and love still had to remain to some degree. But 'Ivia surprisingly reminded her that such actions were truly necessitous. The foundation of the Imperium could not be left to chance after all. Nul'lus added that the 'Sonann'Nor also watched over them from above and would meet any threat probably before either the Lon'tus or At'Lann forces could react. At last, there was a path of time where the Three would not have to worry until the Lis'talla reached the front.

Nul'lus reminded 'Lîna that it is an aristocratic and sovereign privilege for evolved beings to enjoy themselves too. For even in war, life still has to be lived. 'Ivia then gave her telepathically and psionically linked sovereign companions each a glass of glowing jade, glittering M'Goa 'Qal'latu nectar before taking one for herself. The triad toasted happiness with jarring clinks of their cubic ànd crystal glasses before tossing back the watermelon bubble gum flavoured local liquid delight.

'Ivia was making a strong impression on 'Lîna that night. Her genetic configuration suggested her people came from the Origin Species as did the At'Lann, the H'Raka, and the Lon'tus even if the galaxy her people came from now bordered the edge of the universe. 'Ivia told 'Lîna that the 'Xo were involved in previous wars where the Imperium took up the fight but from unseen fronts on the other side of the universe.

She believed Fate had brought their peoples together at last. But this terrible war had taken a great toll upon her people. 'Ivia confided the Imperium had become their only salvation. War had brought their peoples together. She pledged her life for the Imperium with all her faith that only they could liberate the universe. For this time they could not go it alone.

'Ivia was as beautiful outwardly as the soul, if somewhat askew, that her body held. Like no other before her, her thoughts were as nearly damaged as 'Lîna felt. But the war could not stop her being, that of those who come to know her, to light up with the serenity of a sunset over Mariposa. Like 'Lîna, she was a petal of an iris blowing in the summer wind. Their paths were parallel to one another in terms of what their souls sought and they seemed destined to become friends. Only 'Ivia fought to save and hoped to restore what remained of her people.

While At'Lann was left relatively unscathed in the first wave of the Army of Two Rings, over three quarters of the 'Xo population had been killed from the first hiss of the Death of Death, and what remained of their worlds was barely habitable. Considering the losses the Imperium was now taking, the two races were saviours for each other.

For Fate had brought them together. Genetic kinsman by their commonly aligned matrices, now together they vowed to work with each other to shatter the prison of dwindling stars that the enemy inflicted upon all. 'Lîna clasped her slender hand that was so much like her own and vowed to see her soul through the war as 'Ivia had already done for her.

'Ivia's navy blue and gold highlighted curls blew in the winds of the M'Goa night, and they both felt a sense of home that they seem deprived of. If one could not discern their origins one would think they were cousins. 'Lîna could see psionically into her structure to see their species had also come from the path of the Origin species.

Already, the 'Xo had become a fine addition to the Imperium. Their bond made to one another this night showed how the paths of the souls of their peoples were nearly aligned, and already aligned in finding victory in this war. For theirs was the fashion of understanding existence. It was a beautiful feeling to know that someone like you stands at my side and shares the beautiful meadows of where our paths run, 'Lîna told her with her thoughts. And this was a place where Nul'lus also walks. It was like another trinity in itself that grew out of their paths of commonalties.

She also enjoyed seeing this gathering also gave Nul'lus the time to know what people are into as that was one of his greatest passions. He could distract himself from his burden on a pace that already was for him a path of bliss. ‘Lîna remained on the couch and watched on as Nul'lus and ‘Ivia returned to their allotted dance space that started to return to a denser equilibrium of revellers. Their smiles, as they moved, made ‘Lîna smile with pure delight for the first time since the Trinity truly began to come together.

‘Lîna, for the first time this night, sat alone amidst the throng of party people but was far from lonely. She continued to smoke and as she did she felt an almost familiar presence before her; a presence of similar design. For a moment she thought the inhibitors had worn off as a man who seemed sculptured by *deja vous*, asked her with tender grace if he could join her company.

What struck her almost immediately was that she could not read the thoughts of the mystery man, yet what she could feel his being, and ‘Lîna could see that his place in the gathering was a more than worthy one. The ambience remained calm, yet the flow became a little quizzical, as the tall, clearly evolved man with mauve water colour skin and raven's tightly shorn locks sat next to her on the couch.

‘Lîna then reached into her bucket and handed the man in tight black and teal two handfuls of dispensers before taking another for herself. She could tell the night had moved along as the latest buckets were nearly empty. Though when she looked again, it was full once more, and so was the other. The man told her his name was Kir'rus, and flicked the cap from off a dispenser before thumbing it with a toast of deference to this night and the Imperium, and like her had very good tastes in the colours of his life.

She could feel his heart was without evil and became glad he had joined her. What still puzzled her was that his genetic matrix remained encrypted from her senses that tried in vain to ascertain him. Strangely, when ‘Lîna looked upon him, she could swear she saw a hint of M'Goa blood though she was still unsure as to what to make of this person who came unto her path this night. He seemed both alike and unlike her.

Perhaps he comes from frontier species or one already decimated, she thought. He was unique as ‘Lîna went as far as thinking he might be a lost colonist of Hy'Bor though the night of celebration had made her far too unsure of herself. What she knew for certain is that she had seen him before on a world called ‘Irilis when she glanced over her shoulder before she returned to exploration and space, waving her a farewell for that planet. A world he was definitely not a part of and one that had already fallen to erasure.

He then said he was a fellow traveller from the Us'ka galaxy that neighboured the M'Plura galaxy that was also part of the intergalactic system which the At'Lann made as their home in the universe. She found it almost hard believe Kir'rus came from a galaxy nearly devoid of life and hardly worth noticing but she somehow did since all who existed came from the Origin galaxy. There was something about him.

Perhaps he is the last of his kind or is now. His overt thoughts seemed to say, 'I am like you. I am only so weak because I am so strong.' Fate's interest was piqued. And without hesitation, he told 'Lîna that the path would be jagged but she had it within herself to overcome it all. His cryptic words somehow seemed a soulful truth.

'Lîna was more than taken aback by this prophetic stranger who seemed just as cut with the strives for perfection. But before she could ask any more of him, Kir'rus grasped her shoulder with a most tender, reverent touch that he wished the daughter of At'Lann and 'Mura well. Before she could even say another word or think another thought, Kir'rus had vanished, leaving Fate with only mystery. Even if he had folded away or disappeared into the once again growing crowd, 'Lîna could find no trace of him.

It was as if he became part of the dream of the living dream that was the gathering that became M'Goa. For one that found few mysteries remaining in existence, 'Lîna did not know what to make of this but one thing was for sure, the night would leave with them with no ordinary morning, and the revelry in what seemed an immaculate dream world had only begun.

She wondered how someone could blend into her life for such a brief shining moment only to leave her with only intrigue. 'Lîna fell into a deep introspective of time and thought but M'Goa was far too hypnotic for her. Nul'lus and 'Ivia motioned for her to return to the dance floor oblivious to the brief moment that had captivated 'Lîna.

'Who is he?' she wondered.
'Who is he?'

Φ

'Lîna's thoughts returned to peace and love, and celebration and after a moment of inner meditative transual thought, she returned to the dance floor of the platform. Sy'dosa had swam though the low gravity current to other platforms and then teleported to another party on the other hemisphere of M'Goa to make an appearance after feeling confident that his own was going well, and after promising to return to personally see how the Trinity were enjoying their evening in what was beyond any electronic dream works.

He made sure that his personal staff would continue to see to their needs. After all, he lived to be the best host in existence. For he was the love of the doves in flight in the skies of peace, and the glittering and aglow butterfly of the light of the moon. Words cannot describe the respite into the oceans of ecstasy that souls that long ago let go of their constrictions. This was their time to enjoy Hedon in Eden.

'Lîna could not see or feel 'Iato H'Renn anywhere and wondered how many platforms away the great Hunter of H'Raka was. Yet she could see in his thoughts that the only thing he hunted for tonight was the bliss that is pleasure that is the transcendent uplifting spirit that was M'Goa and its path of hedonism on the path of war. Considering what this early stage of the war had cost him on his path, she thought he more than needed this, and she knew M'Goa had already made its way into his heart. He deserved this just as much as any of the Three and was thick in the bliss that was their night.

She could see Nul'lus and 'Ivia dancing up a storm two platforms away, swirling in the gathering amongst the hard-core M'Goa, the body mass that was the sea of their revelry. The sound of M'Goa progressive trance swished its way through 'Lîna as the happiness of those around the explorer finally felt she could be safe returning to the innocence of her nature. This was a homeland and this would give her the strength to carry on along the path of war. As she danced as M'Goa faerie dancers do, 'Lîna felt she could not ask for more. Like dancing on sunshine. It was wondrous.

Fate chanced to look upon an M'Goa goddess of the dance floor that seemed just as captivated by the Imperium sovereign. Without any hierarchical restrictions, there before her was a young and vibrant M'Goa nymphal maiden. Her name was 'Temisa, and she set her flirtatious sights upon Fate as much as Fate set her sights upon her tight satin smooth tangerine skin, navy and lavender highlighted hair glittering with emerald and diamond like gems along with so many sparkles. Glitter was also a sweat this night. And 'Lîna was especially attracted to the beauty of this goddess of the dance floor's deep mezereon eyes that were so much like her own.

To give her a reason to smile, 'Lîna flash-folded a handful of dispensers into the young maiden's delicate hands that had the softness of white orchids about them. Graciously, she bowed before the daughter of At'Lann and 'Mura, and for her she created a fury of motion on her platform while casting photonic mauve fireworks about. The sensuality of her mind gave herself to a sexual liaison with she who now walked the path of Fate. She was transual.

The soul of her yoni flooded with desire, and 'Temisa felt honoured to give herself to another for the rest of the night. For 'Lîna the explorer, this was one honour that was also hers that she could hardly refuse.

What a bravely beautiful soul, 'Lîna thought to herself. M'Goa may be a neutral, pacifistic world but their people carried in their hearts a fanaticism for life and understand why the Imperium must exist to do what they cannot. For the Imperium made it possible for M'Goa to hold their gathering by protecting their world from enemy attacks, and would continue to do so.

And some like 'Temisa lived to be courtesans for the Imperium Trinity. But as Fate explored her soul, she realised 'Temisa also wanted to experience what love is with an enhanced being like 'Lîna. 'Temisa selflessly offered her body and soul to be fully explored and satisfied by the daughter of L'unn. With such faith and devotion offered by this tropical candy dish, who could refuse. The sensuous daughter of M'Goa who was enlightened enough to be able to begin to give 'Lîna a tantric psionic massage with her tender thoughts. Furhter enhanced the muscle as she danced. 'Lîna folded herself to 'Temisa. How could she not refuse?

Their passion of thoughts intertwined as the daughter of Fate found herself in the arms of 'Temisa. She intertwined herself with 'Temisa as they danced together sharing the enjoyment of the M'Goa vibe. Fate's sexual hunger became their kiss as they swirled in each others arms. To be certain their discovered hunger for one another was taken to another level. The wetness of the sweet nectar of her tongue stroking her body and in rapture with hers was bliss in itself. Her gift would be Fate's heart for her night on M'Goa.

Her glacial hued body was painted in a interlocking ribbon style across her luscious canvas that is the body. 'Temisa's hair was tied back under a hot pink veil and was a buoyant jumble of piano like keys that greatly enticed 'Lîna even more as she ran her fingers through them. Her cherry scented sweat aroused the senses of one on the path of Fate as her eyes feasted upon her shimmering and soaked athletically cut body adorned in what was once considered M'Goa clubbing clothing.

The intertwine of their souls became almost compulsively hypnotic as their humid passions rose. Her clothes clung to her like wet silk, cotton and lycra. The drops of 'Temisa's perfumed sweat also seemed to cling to all in the gathering, awakened 'Lîna's sensual soul. She could smell her essence and arousal everywhere, and few swents are sweeter in all existenceThe kinetic heat was the magical, transcendental result of the revered M'Goa music-mancers. Even Fate dripped with sweat from following the tribe of M'Goa, and that of the cherry wine that dripped from 'Temisa's joyously moving body. It was a welcome rain that only added to the vibe of unity.

Almost seamlessly they began to fit themselves into one another as they danced. The violet fires of their souls began to burn into one flow of flowering flames, and into all the fires of the multitudes of universes. Their waters of thought began to flood warmly into each other's mind. Their winds swirled into one mystical cyclone. From their soils grew vast, lush forest of cedar. Their souls stretched out and into each other. They would become coital in the new thresholds that the other had not known for quite some time.

Having to release the tension, 'Temisa took 'Lîna by the hand and they swam in a low end jade florescent gravity flow to the midpoint of the stadia-parlour high above the other platforms. The house of Sy'dosa seemed to take on ovular curves to its once straight edges. They then flew joined in embrace above the raging dances of peace to its north wall.

A circular aperture opened just enough for them and, while in embrace, they swam through and into the aether and the lofty touch of cashmere that were the private chambers. Chambers for amorous private chilling fit for their Imperium guests became one facet of the place where the gathering came together to strive to find the music of the soul. They floated to its centre softly; stroking and tasting one another all the while. 'Temisa's petite body was positively soaked and was utterly, indulgently delicious to 'Lîna as she lapped up as much of her as she could. It was something to erect a statue over.

'Temisa dripped with the sweet honey of carnality. 'Lîna would let her ravish all the areas of her tight and nimble body. Fate seemed to flow with the fairest dimension of the erotic pulse of her being. They were both soaking and moulding themselves deeper into one another as the juiciness of love began to splurge and squirt everywhere as if it were Aphrodite's fountain of desire unleashed. Definitely a moment worthy of a statue and one building over three storeys in height.

Time moved to be both slower and faster than fast as the seconds became hours and the days became seconds. Time lost all meaning. Climaxes of orgasmic thunder and lightning rumbled across the violet skies of their souls that became a symphony of transual pleasure beyond the bliss that is sensual. Time became frenetic and releasing. Their begging, their pleading for more wrapped itself tighter around the lovers nestled in the musical walls above and below the nightscape. 'Lîna and 'Temisa came to exist as the winds of ecstatic bliss.

For one powerful, indefinable moment of time, the universe was theirs. Like halcyon. The moment they flowed as energy into each other's tantalising orifices let their souls flow into one cosmic energy strand of being. In the blossoms of their souls they existed as one energy, above the friction and lather smoothed mountains of vestal freedom. Their multitudes of pleasure became an infinite rhythm beyond and one that aligned itself with the gathering music of M'Goa. Reality quaked open with the intensity of quarks shattering. Everything was everything else as it all went off.

Their hands reached to pull and clench the walls of the chamber as if they were bed-sheets. Their moans, their orgasmic sensual wails of Eros unbound echoed succulently across their private chamber as the yummy splooge poured and poured out in tsunamis.

They lost themselves in one another before they intertwined into each other some more. Sexual droplets of sweat covered their beautiful bodies like dew before a summer's day. They kissed a kiss of a journey's end with the exhaustion felt by one like Marathon. Exhausted and somehow timeless, their bodies kept on holding on to one another as they fell softly to the plush ground after one last atomic howitzer of sensual release. The light of the heavens seemed to shine and simmer upon them.

'Lîna lit her genomic stabiliser and she telekinetically created a M'Goa twenty one petal cigarette for 'Temisa who graciously fired it up and listened and laughed as everything started going off again. Both relaxed after becoming full from a most carnal buffet.

After finishing, 'Lîna let 'Temisa fall asleep in her arms and let her dream in her soul and of the wonders of their night. The hospitality of M'Goa was indeed legendary. What a night. What an adventure. What an interesting path taken.

They slumbered together for a few hours with 'Temisa knowing 'Lîna would soon have to leave for the front. Though she remained in bliss as she knew Fate had chosen her as her courtesan. They slumbered in a iris hued bayou of deep underwater waves of release. 'Lîna created blankets of tropical waters to wash across them as their silken blankets. Fate was the most equal of opportunists on this night and she was more than assuaged by the afterglow left by the effect of 'Temisa's soothing hands and the passion of her fires.

'Lîna wondered if Nul'lus and 'Iato H'Renn were looking for her but she decided to rest for now in the wondrous sleep that comes after supernovas of love and passionate release. She closed her eyes and decided not to pry, for she knew they would come to her with their stories of the night.

Φ

With the dawn of the M'Goa morning making the chamber of their night passion shine to set alight the opaque graviton welded structure, 'Lîna forced herself to push on back to the path of war once more. 'Temisa passionately kissed her repeatedly to show her gratitude and wish Fate well on the journey and battles ahead. 'Lîna left the goddess of the dance floor beautifully drained and unshackled if only for a night. She left her post-orgasmic slumber with a purr that remained with her spirit as she left. 'Lîna spacially folded her clothes back on and curled back her dishevelled hair that flowed in lilac and mauve like vines past her tiara. She kissed 'Temisa farewell telling her they were now psionically bonded for existence. Fate had to return to the Trinity, and to the war. 'Lîna embraced her one last time promising she would return one day soon.

When 'Lîna returned to Sy'dosa's platform and to those still going in his stadia-parlour, she found the majority asleep from their night of transual movement. What could be said, it is a lot of work to have fun, and the M'Goa more than worked for their pleasure. Hundreds at Sy'dosa's party moved on with the beats and were still going stronger than ever, for being played were their solar serenades. Those asleep rested to return to trance rhythms; conserving energy for the night to once again make the place jump.

The piles of empty dispensers beneath them nearly reached their feet as their systems rested too. The buckets on the table, however, still yielded all the sweet mind-bounty they could want. 'Lîna found Nul'lus and 'Ivia dancing and chatting about astrophysics of all things. Happy to be reunited they both gave each other a haughty looked. Nul'lus had a sly smile stretched across his handsome face as he saw that 'Lîna's cheeks had an innocent violet flush about them. He could tell she had a wild night at the gathering and let her thoughts let him know that it was a wonderful for him to be on M'Goa as well.

As the roof of the stadia-parlour disappeared once again, the freshly squeezed rays of the M'Goa sun poured in and let linger the smoke through its pure light. 'Ivia winked to 'Lîna and she smiled almost embarrassingly back. Then H'Renn jumped down for a higher platform to rejoin his fellow sovereigns on Sy'dosa's personal platform space. And Sy'dosa himself returned to see the Trinity off with delight knowing their night on M'Goa, one of many more to come, he promised, would always be carried in their memories. For they had raised the roof.

Without expectation, 'Iato and 'Lîna high-fived one another after a night of going large. For they had both indulged and found satisfaction on M'Goa in their own way. She also wanted to let him know that she understood his sacrifices in life, and that he understood hers. Though they spent the night apart in tropical canals of bliss, they grew closer in this moment than they ever had so far along the path of war. 'Lîna lit up a smoke for herself and one for the son of H'Raka from her still plentiful householder's pack.

She lit them with a psionic mezereon flame from her right index finger. As she passed it to him, their thoughts linked to say that they would have lots to hang on to on the front-line. Not only their worlds but worlds like M'Goa would be carried in the memories of their souls so that they may truly survive this war. As 'Iato H'Renn took a drag, 'Lîna blew out her still sparkle flaming finger with the satisfaction she felt from her night on M'Goa. They all savoured these last few drops of concentrated peace and freedom.

The Three had indeed enjoyed their one last night of peace on M'Goa as they decided to remain in the morning light for one more round of enjoyment. Sy'dosa shook each of their hands to give them his prayers that they would defeat the Army of Two Rings in what was no secret to anyone, in what would soon come to be the biggest offensive of the war thus far. 'Ivia embraced the Trinity with the warmest of gratitude for them as she folded back to her ship saying she would eagerly await their orders on the battlefield. As the Trinity remained in the vibrant sun of M'Goa, they took their last looks of the place that freed them for a night from Tartarus's chains. But the time soon came to leave the magic of this world behind.

Those of the Imperium returned to the Lis'talla and their ships. 'Lîna had such a beautiful time there that she needed little persuading of her allies to agree to having M'Goa relocated spacially to the At'Lann home system of Tr'Lann. The dreams sought in this place could not die an empty death. The P'rynn may have bought their genetic security but the butterfly beauty of M'Goa and the drive of their spirit alone ensured that they would remain for as long as the Imperium would fight.

None of the Trinity wanted M'Goa to be degenified by the enemy. 'M'Goa should always remain in our safer hands,' declared the Aristocrat. Even the H'Raka desired this gathering place to be the jewel that shined on, and would further become the enlightened spa for the collective soul of the Imperium. And for that, 'Lîna had one last reason to smile as she headed back to the dark frontier of war. The path of war awaited the Trinity once again. It was time to go into another kind of night.

25
The Front

The Three had arrived at the final barren steppes of space, to the sobering promised land of battle with their hearts still pounding to the rhythms of M'Goa but where the drums of war now also thundered loudly. As the Lis'talla left the stars behind at the edge of the U'kra galactic system, the only lights ahead were those of the Imperium armada. Yet beyond that lay the immense darkness, the end of all they hold dear. It went beyond unnerving.

It seemed to fill the Trinity with a bitter calm as they saw before them their warships and fighters. M'Goa seemed a reality away as they reawakened to the grim reality of the battle ahead. The crew was as well rested as could be hoped and as battle ready as could be. Their motivation had been fuelled by what was now a rare breath of freedom both sensual and encompassing. They were more than ready to go. 'Lîna was especially gladdened to know the 'Xo, like those who joined them on M'Goa, also found the same drive once again in order for the full potential of those who stand on the side of the Imperium can be released.

For regardless of gender, the At'Lann possessed a genetic stream of a near maternal drive to protect species of life but to especially protect species which were close to being worthy of integration into the At'Lann race. Like the goddess of sparrow waters, this drive would enable them to bring souls to unite in oneness as they feel about L'unn and existence. And like the H'Raka on their psionic realms, would find the ultimate truth of freedom in the phoenix blessed fields of *sosna.* 'Lîna had taken an eye to seeing to the 'Xo surviving as much as she would for her own. 'Ivia, like her kind, shared the path of war, and for Fate there was no other way.

The hull of the Lis'talla had been reinforced with the strength of Atlas and carried the crew directly into the heart of their armada of hundreds of thousands of ships that gathered in what was once U'kra galactic sector nine five three. The Lon'tus once again had the chance to be inspired in their continued mastery of artistic flows. Nul'lus was chosen quite obviously to remind his people of what noble creeds to follow as their model for the pan-aristocracy to avoid decadent self-destruction. Fate knew he had been chosen due to his refined soul. For he was close to perfection but like the Fate and the Hunter chose to strive and survive in its path and pursuit.

The Three had strong thoughts to cherish before they would be left to a battle, and though Fate hated to admit it, probably the first of many. All the joy from M'Goa seemed to be exhausted as she prepared herself for what lay ahead. She even wondered if there would even be an after period. She shuddered to think about any of it at all.

Her thoughts turned to her parents as 'Lîna thought of how Mother and Father would disapprove of the night that was before taking on such a challenge on the path of war. 'Lîna always regretted that they could never understand her logic. But she knew she now lived in times of war that At'Lann had never before known and she was their Imperiatrix.

And the At'Lann stood beside the H'Raka, the Lon'tus, as well as all other species of the Imperium. Like making your way through the snow blanketed branches and trees of the black winter forests of war, the Imperium hegemony had found itself in a place where the light drew darker. This would not be an easy day.

Val'damus spun around from his interface station to face his Imperiatrix and his Imperators that sat on their command thrones in the central area of the Lis'talla's bridge. With 'Lîna at the head of the triumvirate aboard her ship, she looked to her officer seeming to know what he was about to say. The At'Lann flag-ship had been performing well thus far, and had reconfigured itself smoothly for the paths of the Imperium Trinity on the path of battle. The Lis'talla extended itself out perfectly for them as her cannons were adapted to tear into the enemy.

Val'damus smiled to all the Imperium founders as if with a sense of calm before a great maelstrom with an assurance that all that had been done was done.

'H'Raka upgrades to ship defences, sensors, and weapons, all on-line and at optimal.'

'Excellent', Lîna answered a glib stone face of stoicism which all warriors paint unto themselves in battle.

'Iato H'Renn, you may order the fleet to fire when ready.'

'Lîna dropped her lace glove from her right hand. Her words were in the tone to remind everyone on the Lis'talla's that for every second the enemy exists, the path to a place like Volhynia continues. The three linked themselves in a shallow psionic field with the interface data stream to facilitate fleet communications. They dove deep into the core Imperium Interface data-stream. The rewards of their biotechnology soon brought them also to a place like Roma's road works as the psionic became part of their enhanced strategy. The faces of the Three were painted in readiness as their souls became congruous on the path of war.

'Lîna's eyes became surrounded with mauve as if she had found the cosmetic artistry of Cleopatra Jones. Below 'Iato H'Renn's was the grey of the vicious silence of a hungry wolf and the angry bolts of red through his eyes. Beneath Nul'lus were the most fashionable turquoise southern crosses which were a more tribal symbol of the Lon'tus. And even he enhanced and tranced the paint of war across his face.

The Three were set to direct the battle for the Imperium. Their minds became both synchronous and independent of each one another. They were as ready as they could be. The path of battle became wide open.

The Lis'talla converted its outer hull into its armour block mode with her Bofors like guns splicing the dense armour like a growth of turrets set in a grid pattern as if quills growing out to protect them across every plate of their shell. Their weapons stood ready to smash through the omnipresent skeleton that shackles their reality and awaited to hopefully smash the enemy with their fiery bolts into ashen bits. Fate was especially eager, as much as any in the Imperium Trinity, to have justice served.

'Lîna had addressed the At'Lann Imperium in her morning broadcast, and she did not want to repeat herself with any out it now but she did want to convey to Val'damus and her crew, the spiritual meaning of this moment.

'Today the enemy will burn from fires that seek to only bring death. But we must not fear fire for even in hell we fight as the angels of our very existence. Though we fight upon its cursed earth, know that we always find a way to fly above it. Remember that the fires of your soul burns through you to always crush that which seeks to destroy you. Have faith in yourselves this day. Whatever steps we take, the Imperium walk only to victory.'

As Val'damus proudly nodded, she turned to 'Iato H'Renn and smiled with a serious sharp-edged beauty all its own. 'Lîna looked to Nul'lus as well. And with her thoughts told 'Iato that he was born to be wild but the fires of war would tame him into balance. She told both 'Iato H'Renn and Nul'lus with the slight nudge of her mind that the three of them would find balance in one another, and most surprisingly of all that they would find Fate in one another.'

'FIRE!'

'Fire.' 'Iato H'Renn spoke with a zealous calm.

'Fire.' Nul'lus said with a zesty aristocratic and sovereign patriotism.

'Fire.' 'Lîna said with a bitter soft uppercut that were the first steps in taking revenge for the dead.

Toward the empty wall that lay ahead and toward the dead coil that imprisoned them, their fatal fury was let loose. Fate could smell their rotting stench in her mind. She could feel the vastness of emptiness and what is like the thirst of vampires ahead. Every cannon, every gun, every lethal energy wave became the opening salvo that shattered the fortress of Hell. The gates of war were flung open with a heavy kick that ripped opened the bone-yard of torturous ruin, and they were flung to the sullen crisp earth of the underworld. Cannon fire came to deadly life with the brutality of a hale storm that could shatter black holes.

Every energy shell shot was off into the heaven's of the universe's precipice with the light of the fireworks of Guy Fawkes. All shots went heading off into the body of the most vile constrictor to shatter its scales in a colourful loveliness that is an energy of existence.

The first ring, the zombie army, the scourge of locusts that elliptically orbited reality in its slither that had drawn itself across ten thousand galaxies, was hit like what would be shovel plunging into the head of a serpent. Fate was unsure if they could cut off the head. The entrails from the scaly ring became shredded by explosions at the midpoint of the macro-vessel link; precisely hitting the enemy targets.

For a moment, the fleet thought they had punched a hole through the now smouldering crater that stretched across a thousand galaxies that was the now burnt scales of the enemy skin. As the smoke cleared after the flurry of all the Imperium could throw at the enemy in sledgehammers on photons flung at warp shot into the scaly flesh of the macro-vessel links of the Army of Two Rings, the terrible truth lay exposed. Every citizen soldier saw the depressing spectre of the Second Ring, the sinister viciousness that is the purity of nothingness.

The darkness of reality shaving itself away into erasure lay exposed by the advance of the Imperium armada beneath the constriction of the first ring. Nothing described nothing, and nothingness was unsettling to those who looked upon it this day. Fate could feel the utter absence of life before her. She was already frightened but had to stay strong. This was the apocalypse, and the finality must be escaped and fought to the death.

Then with a sounded scanning warning, the counter-fire and counter-attack and defence came. The vipers hissed into them. As Fenris's throat lay slit, the once empty sky became littered with crossfire. Subspace quakes shattered the last of the battle peace and the last of the calm in the hearts of the Trinity.

The venom seared the fleet as the fangs of the ultimate deluge flew into the Imperium warships in energy pulses that could easily tear through planets. The scales of the dark coil shot out as the warships of the enemy were launched towards the crusaders. Blood was already spilling like that once draped itself over Guadalcanal. Theirs was the despair of Scott at his journey's end. The Vistuta already seemed polluted from the dark storm from the east. There was little time to react to what was hurtling towards them.

'All hands brace for impact.'

The enemy bombardment hit the Lis'talla and the fleet without mercy in joyless explosions of fire. Imperium ship after Imperium ship exploded and many ships in the fleet splintered apart from the collisions and impacts. Like hale pounding into rose petals. Small fires erupted on the bridge of the Lis'talla. Lu'va was flung out of her chair and lay unconscious on the floor.

In space, bodies, countless bodies, were sucked into the vacuum of the frosty steppes of the last reaches of space and were pulled through the wound the Imperium inflicted unto Dante's serpent of hell, into erasure where they could never be saved. The latest breed of Apollonians were already falling in this battle against the Army of Two Rings. The other sword of the Death of Death was already infecting the Imperium with the plague that had become their killing fields on the path of war. The voices of the Trinity became the chorus of the fleet riding into the valley of Death.

'Launch fighter wings 6199 through 8527.'

''Valis reallocate emergency power to the weapons systems.'

'Move the Lon'tus heavy bombers to grid 010.'

'Wings 427 and 853 have been decimated.'

'Enemy fighters closing in on the J'vok. Have the 'Ilann fortify her shields.'

'Quantum fissure torpedoes away.'

And on and on it went as the Three became the gift of Kosciuszko upon the new dominions. They walked as Caesar and walked as all crusaders do when in the thick of the cold yet scalding cauldron of combat. They were under siege as cannon shot, fire, destruction and doom seemed to surround them as the great horror of the wall of erasure edged ever closer like a dank shadow over the misery of fireworks below. All things considered, this was a bold deep blue gambit.

H'Raka squadrons swam like sharks but even they were not immune to the swarm that outnumbered their armada.

'H'Raka squadron 4 through 98 reinforce At'Lann squadron 303. They are taking heavy casualties but are pushing through to secure another firing position.'

The dark Zeus speared them with his bolts as the Lis'talla collided with several enemy fighters. The bridge shook but their minds were only on the battle.

'Move the 'Xo warships to cover the H'Raka flank.'

' Fleet Admiral M'on of the Lon'tus flagship is dead.'

'Enemy fighters are continuing to ram our vessels. We've already lost a fifth of our fleet. Fortify our shield amplifying satellites.'

'Fire at the wound again. Maximum firepower.'

The crater grew but as quickly as they pierced through the scales, the constriction was now almost instantaneously restored.

'Take twenty two hundred H'Raka systems killers into the path of the enemy sorties in grid 929.'

Another enemy warship then broke through the lines and rammed the Lis'talla only this time tearing a third of the ship asunder like Hela's fury in the twilight. The main bridge was, for the most part, engulfed in flames, and support struts collapsed through the ceiling in crackling explosions luckily avoiding the Three who paid no heed to the falling ruin about them. They were massively outnumbered. The Fleet had now lost a third of its strength. Something had to be done. The Trinity dove deeper in the vastness that is the interface data stream which co-ordinated their efforts against the apocalyptic wall of emptiness whose soldiers began to leave them as skewered martyrs.

'Zaya came to the bridge and took over a tactical station and gently pushed aside the dead male bridge officer and used her own telekinetic might to reinforce the Lis'talla nearly exhausted shields. Their path of war was falling apart.

Val'damus, one of the few bridge officers not struck down at their posts, returned to his feet before getting back in position, and though battered and bloodied, kept the guns smoking in the carnage the Imperium found itself in. For the Trinity found themselves on shores like those of Dieppe, and in quick span of time had to protect the worthy remains of their offensive force while pressing on into what now became a vain hope that they would somehow succeed.

'Lîna looked proudly to Val'damus and 'Zaya for a moment amidst the strife before returning to the depths of the data-stream. The Three decided to diversify their structure. H'Renn folded himself like the strike of a white wolf and took direct command of the H'Raka flagship. Nul'lus flash-folded himself to the Lon'tus flagship, the K'meria, to take direct control over his forces taking the place of the dead Admiral M'on.

The bridge of the Lis'talla was attempting to repair itself and even managed to reconfigure itself for 'Lîna's sole physical presence. A young, excited lieutenant named L'krk, like a young lad too excited to remember his shoes on the way out to meet a car load of beautiful women, shouted not to 'Zaya, or Val'damus, but to 'Lîna directly. 'Imperiatrix, half our guns began to fire on a new target on our port-side. It's a temporal incursion.'

'What!' 'Lîna said with a tone of surprise and lack of forewarning in shades of James Earl. Impressed by the urgency of his words, 'Lîna brought part of herself out of the data-stream, and for a moment 'Lîna blinked, the guns of the Lis'talla fell silent. For a blink of an eye, At'Lann's offensive enjoyed silence and fell silent. Thankfully, the enemy could not take advantage of it with 'Zaya mentally reinforcing the shields.

The interface brought up on the main holo-screen, a scan of a sub-temporal region the enemy was tunnelling through outside of their ring of constriction. The enemy was now deeper into the universe than what they faced before, and their trajectory placed them directly through the path of the Imperium fleet. Four enemy vessels, each twice the size of Imperium flagships were pushing on in the subspace of their reality. Fate could feel their presence working their way through reality. At any cost, Fate knew they had to be stopped.

One enemy vessels flash-folded from inter-reality to reality and began firing, creating a pincer like thrust in perfect tandem with the revolving descent of the first ring. Nul'lus shifted the deployment of the Lon'tus ships to compensate for this deadly new player as did 'Iato H'Renn.

The storm of battle was growing darker in spite of the growing intensity of fire being exchanged in lightning like thrashes across space. The Imperium fleet were barely holding the front, if at all. Though the H'Raka were continuing to pound the enemy with quantum bind bombs, and systems killers set on auto-pilot for delivery to the scaly surface of the first ring, their efforts were meeting with little success.

The war between fighters was fast determining the outcome. Outnumbered and overwhelmed, there were simply too many for the Imperium fighters to contain. With the enemy dreadnought entering the battlefield, to cut the fleet off from space, this only made matters worse. The struggle in the sky between dogs rabid and dogs nobly vicious was continuing across the dark lit expanse of the empty steppes on the path of war. And as valiant and as brave as they were, this day was the enemy's.

Enemy fighters were still able to clear a path for their dreadnought that had tunnelled its way in from the first ring, and which now had a clear shot of the Lis'talla. A systems wide plasma blade cut its way through the Lis'talla's port-side. Though partly shattered, the Lis'talla fought on; burning in space, still armed and operational.

'Lîna lost consciousness for a moment as the data-stream began to drown her. With a great gasp of breath, 'Lîna returned reality to herself. 'Containment fields holding, Princess 'Zaya. Repair crews already on it' as Val'damus assured and reported. 'Thank you, Commander,' 'Zaya said with distraction laced courtesy as she fed tactical strategies into her interface station. Even she already knew the battle was not going well.

A status one report came up on the main holo-screen. Over half the Imperium fleet was destroyed and their fighters were outnumbered a thousand to one and rising. Even their high number of kills was not enough to continue to protect the fleet from being wiped out. The safety of the At'Lann flagship came into jeopardy as Imperium warships could no longer protect her. Thousands of enemy fighters poured in and the Lis'talla found itself in constant small bombardments. Her armour was being penetrated as the Lis'talla depleted her shields and 'Zaya began to burn out. Fate decided it was time to change the pursuit and focus.

The battle continued with the wreckage of shot to pieces fighters, warships, drones, and satellites cluttering and spinning out of control. The fleet was in disarray before the siege. Energy blasts and explosions continued across all one could see save the constriction and the erasure of the Death of Death. For this was the foaming of waves of the red tide over the dry dusty dirt of a land of battle like the Somme.

The spears of all the Valkyrie could not twist and plunge deep enough into the ring of the great snake to destabilise its structure. Its most critically vulnerable point, though accurately hit, was not hit with enough strength to slay the dirtiest of beasts. The misery would continue and still nothing could be done about the nothingness that loomed ever closer. The Three, from their various vantage points, saw their ships adrift and passing through the macro-ship infrastructure or though the holes their blades had managed to make. And they watched as they saw life washed away into nothingness. They could only watch as life was consumed by the last scavengers of existence.

Though a difficult choice, the Trinity decided to fold heavy mines unto their fallen ships in the hope that it might inflict greater damage upon the enemy. They succeeded in only inflicting superficial damage upon the dark locusts ahead.

Though the Imperium database filled to the brim with strategic data on the enemy, this was not their day, and the armies of the Death of Death were far too strong for the Imperium to prevail this day. And even with the spirit of their 303 squadron surging through the dark storm more than most would fear to, it was not enough force to hold the enemy back. Their lines were continuing to crumble and the locusts of the horde continued to prey upon Imperium juggernauts, destroyers, frigates, and fighters. The Imperium in spite of the gallantry of her soldiers and pilots, they were all starting to weaken in the face of the swarm.

The Army of Two Rings, was being continually reinforced using their inter-dimensional gate of invasion that lay along the spine of the body of the dark serpent. The enemy continued to surge in and now outnumbered the Imperium ships, fourteen thousand to one. 'Lîna fired the main gun of the Lis'talla and enhanced the blast's power with her own and obliterated the enemy dreadnought and as many ships as she could target in closing the temporal conduit in a symphony of rapid fire pulses. The Imperium was still faster and the enemy incursion beyond the ring seemed curtailed for the moment, and 'Lîna did not bother worrying once their tracking signatures disappeared from the interface holo-display. The Imperium pilots had let the dark horde know they would resist until the end. The symphony of the fires of war burned and a siren call out in a thunder across this corner of reality.

'Zaya, in a torn uniform that matched the look of most of the bridge crew, including their Imperiatrix, looked on, continuing to input tactical patterns into the interface. Her white gold brocade of the house of 'Mura was scorched and covered in drying blood, yet still clung to her. A piece of console shrapnel had grazed her temple. She could no longer reinforce the shields as the Lis'talla's auxiliary shield power kicked in.

Val'damus looked to 'Lîna who was rapidly drowning in the swiftness that became the data-stream once more. She was manoeuvring the fleet as quickly as her mind possibly could to still give the fleet a fighting chance. Val'damus and L'krk watched on as she moved so quickly in the movements of her mind that she slipped intermittently in and out of phase. The dark demonic strength of the enemy continued to heavily outnumber the fleet just as the dead continue to outnumber the living in linear time.

The Imperium fleet was slipping ever closer to the scales of the constriction of the first ring and the second that lurked with the dark hunger of erasure. The enormity of the first ring finally dawned on the Imperium. While they were fighting, the enemy managed to tear away from existence another thousand galaxies. The fleet almost seemed to fall into an abyss by the futility of it all. What was for sure was that could not hang on much longer. The battle could not endure.

' 'Lîna, get us out of here!'

'Zaya had said it and thought it to bear notice in her sister's nearly overwhelmed mind. 'Lîna knew this was a losing effort but could no longer keep trying in vain to make something happen to turn the tide. Her mind could barely remained linked with Nul'lus and 'Iato's to guide the fleet and their course. Things had gone so badly that it was time to warrant a retreat from the battlefield to fight another day. 'Zaya's hurried insistence of how the dire the need was to extricate themselves from the clutches of death was enough to shift the path of their fate this day.

Retreat became the only option. At the very least, there was solace in knowing more of the enemy so that they may learn to defeat them before the omega project psionic generators would be constructed and save themselves a lot of time in the struggle. But somehow everyone knew there would be no easy way out. The Imperium fleet began to evacuate and fold away still firing away at the most vile of enemies. There had to be a way to ease the suffering of reality but it was not to be found this day. The Imperium sought to find it as they stood on the path as those on the path for the last salvation for reality. They found solace in keeping the faith that as long as they existed, they could re-ignite the reality of existence once again.

'Lîna linked with Nul'lus and 'Iato to combine their minds to fold what remained of their fleet on the battlefield back to their own space before the fleet would slip any further off the precipice. In one last vestige of strength, the Trinity, in the blink of their eyes, brought what was left and what could be salvaged, and folded them back to their central galactic system and to other areas of the Imperium. Bitterly, and for now, it was over.

Φ

On board the battle ravaged Lis'talla, 'Lîna sat back alone amidst the still smouldering bridge. The experience had taken its toll upon her. Her skin and body fluttered in and out of proper phase variance almost continuously for a few seconds. Enough time for those left on their feet to watch their Imperiatrix in the pain of genetic instability, exposing the exhaustion of directing the At'Lann fleet. She was far too weak to be embarrassed by pride. Her nose and eyes began to bleed as her body returned to a proper state of genetic cohesion. Her dark violet blood dripped unto the floor about her throne in growing pools as she brought herself to stand after looking as if she had vomited, and surveyed the fleet through the holo-screen.

What she saw as she stood in the debris of her damaged main bridge was that the spirit of their people though tattered and torn had survived their first real push against the enemy. The H'Raka had lain their lives on the line defending her fleet and had with done so to the greatest of their ability. Without them, their losses might have been far too great to survive against the vast numbers of the horde. Their fighters left their mark upon the enemy with massive bombardments that kept their retreat removed from that of the search for the sea at Dunkirk.

Though she saw her tattered fleet, one worn down by the flames of hell, she saw inside her thoughts so many that were lost for no other reason other than that an offensive had to be launched against the enemy. 'An enemy that continues to enslave us', she thought. She felt her fist shoot out in failure to smash into her interface console. It was if it were an involuntary action as the pain of the battle overcame her after the sound of the crackling collision. 'Lîna felt so weak and seemed ready to fall to the floor. Since there was nothing good to say, no one uttered a word.

'Zaya and the bridge crew collectively feigned ignorance of their glimpse of 'Lîna's condition and how serious it had become as she quietly excused herself from the bridge. The Imperiatrix of At'Lann fourth-walled back to her private sovereign quarters. Regardless of whether she remembered that her state was weakened and exhausted, she began to let loose the fury once held tightly in her heart during the course of the battle that had been a waking nightmare of an undertaking. She back-handed a bulkhead with her fist with such a velocity and ferocity that the entire ship shook from her display of diluted power. For this was a moment of misery.

If not for the expectation of it, after all the suffering, the crew would have thought it another enemy attack but they were tied into Fate's soul and knew her suffering. The thorns of the hunting grounds of Diana dug deep into the flesh of her mind. It was over for now but far from over on the path of war. She felt so useless, and 'Lîna also found a terrible form of release as she collapsed to the ground in a pool of her own blood.

26
In The Temporal Currents

The Fate of tomorrow had remembered this day and its lessons well as she looked back to see the enemy ships flee the temporal stream where they once swan like the plague to intercept their temporal ship. Though she was one who had swam the front-lines in so many yesterdays, Fate was still all she remembered herself to be. The reunited Trinity was on their way to make their final stand. The Fate, the Hunter, and the Aristocrat were on board the advanced At'Lann prototype ship that zoomed past the sight of one of their more tragic days on the battlefield deep as they trekked on in the currents of the temporal oceans. The Trinity were on course towards the end of their path taken.

In truth, it was a dangerous quest as they were but drops in the vastness of the temporal currents. A single temporal collision would act like a defensive mechanism that removed pollutants from the time stream as quickly as infinity. There was little to comprehend in the chaos of this dimension. It was both stable and entirely unstable. And no one knew if erasure would overtake them at any moment.

Reality took on little meaning for the reunited Trinity, and their minds tried to compensate by sheltering the reality of their flight to focus on their mission through time. Their path continued as they pushed ahead in their temporal ship in a trip that seemed to have an aristocratic distinction about it by their adherence to appearance that became their image upon the course. And, sometimes, even in the worst of times, image was still everything.

The Fate looked out the Polonian styled windows of the ship to watch the psychedelic scenery about them in the temporal flows. She thought of how that day of the battle seemed to stretch itself upon her once more as what she felt then as her worst days of existence was felt again. Her sullen feelings even seemed to stretch into days in her mind as she remembered the time after the failed offensive. What an awful time to be reminded of, Fate thought.

She remembered 'Zaya pulling up her blood soaked head from the floor of her quarters, opening her eyes to her sister frantically shaking her, screaming in what seemed like silence for her to awaken. Black violet blood seemed to spray and drip everywhere in 'Lîna's private sanctum. How the floor, how the walls were stained by their drenching. Fate remembered awakening to her younger sister's pleading face, and 'Lîna breathed once again to escape the victory sought by the Death of Death. On board the temporal ship, the deeper the aether breathed into Fate, the more their winds blew her into a closer genetic lock.

Back then, the gene drift had almost pulled her apart. Fate knew then that her greatest enemy was not the hand of the Death of Death or the Army of Two Rings but that of herself. Being a creature of possibility that had become and yet remained an explorer of war, Fate had few fond memories other than M'Goa in the year of hell that followed the events of the battle.

The Fate went from one memory to the next as she wore her driving faces. The Aristocrat and the Hunter recalled with almost despondent gaiety all the memories from a time that seemed on a course for oblivion before time became the oblivion overtaken. Even though they seemed the one solution to reuniting the universe once again, the Trinity did try to follow other paths. Make no mistake, whether in vain or not, the Trinity decided to take the fight to the enemy. Taking risks was a sign of an evolved people, and though returned in the past to their home space all but torn apart, the battle had to this day left its scars and fortitude attained from this day of the past for the trinity of souls looking for tomorrow.

Miracles were not performed on what many considered to be a draw though the Trinity considered it all a defeat. The Imperium was still there, yet any shred of innocence remaining in the Trinity was now gone. The trip to M'Goa had only served for the Three to yearn for better days. The battle simply showed how far the Three would have to go on the path of war, and perhaps in striving to be worthy of victory, found that there could be no quick way around it. So much had changed after the battle.

After three trillion and three years, the events of the battle still left an indelible mark upon the Trinity. The Hunter turned from the epic he was composing, and created by what seemed the inspiration of Moroccan shores. The Aristocrat also shut off a play he was watching on a holo-screen called the Lon'tus Shrew of all things. As Fate looked to those who shared her path, their thoughts merged into one in the style of psionic pottery being shaped. They remembered the battle through different eyes as Fate watched in the waters of the soul.

She watched young Nul'lus through the temporal windows, aboard his flagship, as he took the Lon'tus wing deep into the ooze of enemy fighters pouring into them with a calm and cocky swagger. 'Lîna had warned him against this while in the command link but he would hear none of it as he knew the Lon'tus were brave and wanted to give the Army of Two Rings a proper thrashing as only they can deliver. 'Lîna tried her best to cover the Lon'tus flank by giving even giving her squadron 303 and other elite squadrons to engage the enemy alongside the Lon'tus attack fighters.

When the enemy became too numerous for them to push ahead, and the Lon'tus fighters began falling from the skies into the erasure, Nul'lus brought his ships to fall back, and he did so by having the Lon'tus warship fire off the last of their explosives. He even did so from the K'meria, which he had taken command of, to honour the integrity of the spirit of the Lon'tus flag by leaving the winds of Trafalgar upon their sails. It was a message that the Lon'tus would return for a victory befitting of Sir Alf Ramsay.

Nul'lus swam like a dolphin-shark through the data-stream of the command link, and manoeuvred the fighters like Jubei stationed in play. He fired as many inter-fold disruption mines as could be shot, and did his best to make the enemy pay with remembrance of why the Lon'tus flag flies with such exalted esteem. But the exerting ordeal had already cost the young aristocrat his noble vigour. When the battle ended and they returned to Imperium space, he returned to his stateroom on board the K'meria to his place that was both home and away from home that Churchill would feel unworthy in.

The effects of the phase shift were further exacerbated in a far more lethal fashion by the cost of the battle. But Nul'lus, who was bloodied and scorched, stood on as his faith was that one disastrous defeat would lead to one thousand Lon'tus victories, even though he was left to wonder if the Imperium's day would come.

As the aristocratic spirit glided into it latest path beneath his veneer, the romantic optimism for the future still lay strong, and perhaps that may have explained the way his enhanced form moved in and out of genetic phase with a flutter of more and less subtlety than either 'Lîna or 'Iato. Though he knew the Trinity walked away from the battlefield even more forged in the fires of the path of war.

Purely constructed water beaded and dripped from him like he had walked through the steam of Myestas's boiling silver cauldron, and overturned its contents. He vomited water as if he were the source of a brook. How he shook and flooded his latest inner sanctum and fell to sleep on his bed in the position of his collapse. Someone had thought ahead to upgrade the K'meria and his quarters automatically filled with curative bio-gel. He slept as the Trinity did for six weeks after the battle drifting in and out of reality.

In the moments that he returned to reality, Nul'lus instructed the Imperium Interface to give command of the Lon'tus fleet to 'Ivia during his respite. Thanks to the latest strategy undertaken by the Imperium to reinforce their hold on existence using cross-lateral spatial mine detonations, Nul'lus, like the Trinity, and the Imperium fleet had time to recoup.

Φ

Everything had gone wrong, yet everything had gone right. In the temporal currents, the three souls looked back to remember what was. Though the Imperium fleet was close to decimation, their interface had gathered enough intelligence on the enemy to level the playing field with their numbers and technology in the next times that they would meet. This was not over yet. And Fate, pledging to do whatever it takes to win the war still had their faith and grew it all into something stronger. Her belief in those at her side kept them striving on.

So strong was her faith in the Lon'tus and the H'Raka that as she healed 'Lîna gave the Imperium everything she had. She insured the At'Lann chose strategies that brought their fleet up to operational strength in only a month's time. Though the bodies of the Trinity were being repaired from the latest battle they had to endure, their minds reached out through the interface to oversee all they must do. Fate remembered that she linked minds often with Nul'lus and 'Iato during this time, and if she was too weak to, she prayed for their souls and all those of the Imperium that the salvation found in the galactic museum would rule their day.

'Ivia embraced the task of restoring the Lon'tus fleet, and the chosen military woman went about her work with devout charity. She represented the 'Xo well and her good will was freely given to the path of the Imperium. The daughter of 'Xo also found a new genetic affinity and aspiration in the fold of the At'Lann. The only exception to Imperium integration was the autonomous H'Raka Imperium which was far more selective. Only a select few At'Lann and Lon'tus served in the H'Raka military aside from the segregated Rz'hro who were taken in by the warrior state. 'Iato H'Renn would have none of the charity of other Imperia as their only way, sometimes, was the pursuit of strength.

In the battle, the H'Raka fleet had fought long and hard and gave more in ships and lives to protect the Imperium Trinity, once again gave the lives of the greatest of hunters a purpose. Ironically, the earliest of wars were between the H'Raka and the At'Lann though few cared to remember. But through their wars, each people came to understand that together they were part of the balance of creation and could come to work miracles. It was said the At'Lann warriors of those conflicts exchanged souls with the great H'Raka hunters so that both could understand peace, and so that the H'Raka could learn to mesh such concepts into their soul and social culture.

In the short times of peace which the At'Lann and H'Raka shared, art was painted, written, heard, felt, and tempered into the H'Raka, and though the great hunters once tried to conquer those of L'unn but could not, had always cherished the beauties of At'Lann. Not surprisingly, 'Iato remembered history well. He remembered the ancient tales of how their wars ended, not with guns but with the will of souls filled with ideas and ideals that created respect amongst the souls of the two species. If only there were more from that time, 'Iato once mused. Perhaps that was why 'Iato H'Renn fought so hard for the greatest conflict his people faced were against the At'Lann, and strangely a species not suited for being warriors at all.

As 'Iato fought beside 'Lîna, he found her spirit as unbreakable as her people. These warriors of virtuous ideals found worthiness with the H'Raka in the battle. Though their day was lost, the one who would become the Hunter knew his allies in the Imperium would have the strength to fight on. Almost reluctantly he had found a kinship with this people never before known by his kind. But there could be no other way as he possessed the soul of a poet that sometimes found solace on the path of war. He was blessed with the hands of a powerful scribe and that of the hands of a swordsmen.

The Hunter's path had always been one of difficult choices though he had found little difficulty in founding the Imperium with his other allies. After the first real offensive, 'Iato almost felt assured that they would learn to do what must be done and those at his side were worthy of the support of the warriors of H'Raka.

Still, 'Iato had obligations to maintaining the genetic hegemony of his empire and in maintaining the naturally selective rule of the H'Raka state. It was the heritage that the H'Raka set themselves apart and if they changed their imperial chemistry too much they would soften and fall from the power of their place in the universe. For theirs was to strive to be the benchmark of strong, and that only the strong would prevail. 'Ivia did not take any other this personally for the feelings of her people. The H'Raka way was their burden, and few could survive their path.

After the battle, 'Iato's experience in the field evolved him crackling with fiercest bole of Ares unto the path Y'vis desired for him, the path left for the strong select, the finest few. The many who were few, who would sacrifice the balance of their souls in the filth of war, for the sake of the cause. As he became more and more the Hunter, he became far more edged by the winds of war. The battle had been a costly one but it made him realise how far they had to go on the path of war. The Hunter, in the temporal stream, now wondered if it was all worth it.

The At'Lann even in their expected loss to the enemy came to a better understanding of the enemy and unified them even more into the Imperium Trinity. As their armies were being rebuilt, 'Iato H'Renn could not help but be impressed. For they faced the war with the same strength that 'Lîna has, that of striving to live, to sacrifice, and to continue with whatever must be done for the sake of victory. After the battle, 'Iato H'Renn came to think of them all in a different light. The Hunter remembered it all with a wrenching fondness.

The Hunter recalled with stoic tragedy of how that single battle changed the flow of the war, and how it changed the entire course of their path. Fate also remembered it well and was impressed by the Hunter's enlightened sight for temporal paths. Though victory seemed so assured, in the great combustion of many of their forces, it seemed so far, far away. 'Iato H'Renn wondered how Y'vis would have fared in the war on the front lines with death and erasure. He could feel within him an ethereal gaze watching him, judging him, and protecting him. Somehow, the Hunter even then knew the answer. Even during the battle, 'Iato could feel his presence that lay so deep in the shadows.

The Hunter recalled that during the battle he arrived on board the H'Raka flagship, the 'Brulak, to find its bridge crew dead. He bound himself into the interface of the ship, and swam the data stream like a wolf bounding through snow, to constantly reposition his fleet. He had his fighters take on the locusts and his dreadnoughts the storm. Though the controls are far more cramped than the Lon'tus or At'Lann fighters, the H'Raka war fighters were laden with the heaviest firepower known to the Imperium. Like the saliva and blood, flesh dripping grip of the Fenris, 'Iato chose well where to burn and blow away as many of the dark beings as shots would allow.

Still, it felt to the Hunter as if it were one wolf against the permanent midnight spread forth from the most terrible of winter's cold. And the cold of the steppes of Tartarus had blown too wildly into his soul.

On many occasions, the enemy was able to penetrate the H'Raka lines, and 'Iato H'Renn could do little but watch as the bulge into the enemy territory burst. Fighter after enemy fighter acting in the way of the *morituri,* flew into H'Raka ships, and that of the raccoon paw shaped configuration of the 'Brulak, time and again and one more time than needed. With a heavy shred and explosion, one enemy fighter pierced itself unto the bridge, and exploded directly in front of the lone seated 'Iato.

He knew the enemy sensed which were the patriotic hands and those who rose to enchant and lead the fight against them. Before the command inter-link was severed by the force of the enemy craft exploding, 'Iato managed to redirect a few H'Raka wings to bolster the defences of Nul'lus and 'Lîna's command vessels. 'Iato's H'Renn's enhanced structure easily allowed him to shield himself from the raging flames of the enemy fighter exploding, and from the hurling shrapnel of deck and hull plating that flew everywhere. 'Iato H'Renn then wrestled back into the command inter-link by attaching his thoughts to another interface console surprisingly undamaged on the bridge.

He once again dove into the data-stream as the fires of exploding plasma fires continued about him. The 'Brulak was spinning out of control but H'Renn worked quickly to cast a quick, tight telekinetic ally enforced force-field across the section of the bridge gashed open and exposed to space. He was more than able to re-route power. He reconfigured his throne and had the ship also repair the command link console.

As he neared finishing repairs to those critical systems, he realised the damage inflicted by the enemy left him open to spatial and warp crumbling as the ship had drifted closer than most ships in the fleet to the scales of the deadliest of constrictions. Space at this point lost cohesion as it entered the first steps into erasure. Space at this point only served to wreck havoc with his genetic cohesion.

As the battle raged on, 'Iato began to realise how much it had begun to tax him. His genetic structure had come to lose cohesion in many areas of his body. His cellular walls were especially hit hard causing many of his inner organs to shred apart. Fate knew first-hand as did the Aristocrat that this was not particularly pleasant. The bones of his right knee were shattered like an iron bat coming down upon a ball of chalk at warp. The silent explosion of bone and blood dust shattered out from his knee, the left side of his ribs, his shoulder, and left ankle. Globules of his blood flew into the force-field barriers before they were shot through into both space and erasure. The environmental containment fields were porous from the haste of their construction, and his blood, for one terrible moment, floated freely into the vacuum of decaying space that lay before the void of nothingness.

'Iato H'Renn used his telekinetic prowess to reinforce the barrier over the exposed bridge and that of his link with his ship as he bit down on the pain. He fired a brutal, continuous blast of photonic torpedoes at the enemy target ahead of his flagship. The hunt grew and grew, and battle became the wretched in the madness that is all out war. Though feeling almost invincible in pain and power, the Hunter could have fought on until dead but as the word was given to fall back, the great hunt was not to be concluded that day.

The Imperator of the H'Raka was furious with having to withdraw. He hardly noticed the pain creeping over him as he cried havoc as the Imperium forces began to withdraw. He laughed at the exhilaration and misery of it all. Stalingrad was a pale shadow of this battle. But he did feel the pain as it drowned him with its embrace. With such extreme damage to his form, he slumped over as his blood gushed as freely as the waters of a Manitoba flood down his side and that of his warrior's throne. With his will of triumph being cast to cinders like those who made a bitter return to the Rhine, the one who would become the Hunter did his best to stare away from futility.

Even in his unconsciousness, the work of war set him free as he pushed the data-stream of the interface to restore open grazes and gashes that covered the armour of the 'Brulak. He reawakened as quickly as he went out, and though nearly spent, he did not want to appear weak in front of the H'Raka warriors who came to take the place of the fallen bridge crew. He gave command of his fleet and vessel to Gr'dak, the most senior officer left alive on board. Then ceremoniously, and without another word, he slash-folded himself to his quarters where he let himself collapse to writhe in pain.

And even with the bio-gel invigorating the automatic healing process, it still took over a dozen hours for his body to close all the wounds inflicted upon his form. His only thoughts during that time was of how his blood needed to run with even more iron. He let joy come from the pain of his genetic core re-stabilising itself. To honour Y'vis, his blood of iron would cast him into an even more devastating sword of truth.

During his rest and longer rest that followed, his thoughts turned to 'Lîna who seemed to knock recklessly on Death's door. She had to be protected at all costs for she has a fate to play, he thought. The daughter of 'Mura proved herself to him once more in the battle that could not be won whether she knew it or not. He expected no less from Nul'lus, who by his effort on the battlefield made him proud once again of his aristocratic friend.

And most strangely and strongly, even in the strangle of pain, hope did not leave H'Renn. The path of the war was simply changing directions and the hunt had just begun. After the surprisingly short time it took to rebuild the fleet thanks in large part to species who volunteered their time to factory and assembly work, 'Iato Hrenn linked his thoughts with 'Lîna to find that her condition had worsened. 'Zaya contacted him that she had found a new solution though one that would change a face of the war. Drastic days were ahead, and 'Iato H'Renn even then could feel their coming.

Φ

The Fate, the Hunter, and the Aristocrat were closing in on their final objective. Their circle of war across time was drawing to a close. Their path streamed by so many memories of days that were so dark and incomplete, and yet so wonderful and happy when it came to M'Goa and the bond that grew within the Trinity. The warm embers of those days and ivory sepulchre had emerged from the glimmering emerald forests of the past. Soon all would be complete. Fate fondly remembered the days when no one noticed how the pieces would fall into place. The peace of Polonia was seen as at hand in the same blurry haze that it was envisioned in their younger days.

Fate looked back to the temporal stream behind their ship, and wondered if there would be no more surprises along the way of this long journey. She had a paranoid thought that enemy fighters still pursued them. The Aristocrat patted his friend on the shoulder, and to make her feel better, reached his mind into the interface for their vessel and launched a temporal mine to relax her thoughts.

The Hunter turned as if to display there was nothing to worry about. And then the three all caught sight of the explosion as three cloaked vessels exploded as they were ripped apart in collisions with multiple time streams. The Aristocrat smiled and said, 'See nothing to worry about, 'Imiszi.' The Trinity then resumed their watch for the end of their path. Soon would be the time of the convergence.

27
An Awaiting Long Slumber of Restlessness

Time seemed to move at a slow pace, and all at once time bolted through reality again to herald the changing face of the Imperium. The young Imperiatrix returned to At'Lann feeling hardly a hero but as the crowds of At'Lann greeted her with mauve neon photonic ticker tape, they demonstrated to her that hers was still their path, and that they had not abandoned the cause of victory as 'Lîna had not either.

During the time 'Lîna had been away, Za'szu had completed the utterly magnificent restoration of the cities of At'Lann and 'Mura. So beautifully were they redone that many speculated that their perfection had been improved upon thanks to the Za'szu's detail orientated path. All palaces of the houses of 'Mura, At'Lann, of 'Mura'Lann, were also enhanced with a touch of what one may call modern neo-baroque adornments and furnishings.

Though she did not like to admit it, 'Lîna was beautifully impressed. After every place the path of war took the Fate, on this day At'Lann had never appeared as wondrous as it did for her return, and, in fact, it did look better than it had before the dark hours of the war began. 'Lîna was in heaven to return home to 'Mura. And thanks to 'Zaya's efforts, 'Lunn's ecosystem was restored and modified to be instantly savable to the interface.

Even the face of the Tr'Lann system had changed as thousands of Imperium warships and defence drones were deployed in a grid across the entire system. The face of Tr'Lann also changed by the asteroidal like debris from the melted hulls of the enemy vessels and At'Lann vessels destroyed in the first wave of the Death of Death. The central system orbit of the debris and graveyard became mockingly and prophetically known as the 'Third Ring'. Outside this hammered ring was hull of the largest enemy vessel which came to become the closest body to the At'Lann sun.

It all amazed 'Lîna how much had changed in only a minute blink of time, and how much more was to come. She felt ashamed that her health was failing her so, and worried that her path neared those set aside for invalids. Yet 'Lîna did not get too carried away with herself as she still had a few tricks up her silken sleeves.

After the Imperium Trinity were safe once again and after looking in on 'Lîna during the time she was still on board the Lis'talla, 'Iato H'Renn did not follow her to At'Lann as Nul'lus had. The K'or and Imperator returned directly to H'Raka to further stem the latest paths of enemy incursions. H'Renn set about having more and more mines deployed along the ever falling front in order to slow the advance. He was also at work on a new super-weapon for the Imperium. A strange way to heal was to build a bigger gun, thought a puzzled and still weakened 'Lîna. He would have to tell her one day of what he had cooked up.

Nul'lus returned to At'Lann as was the way of his courtesy and chivalry to his long time and forever friend. But he too soon had to leave as he had return to the seat of Lon'tus's throne for his official coronation and take the crown given to him in Lon'tus's time of need. He also had to take care of greater affairs of state that he needed to attend to, such as the growing illegal refugee influx taking place on his Imperium's furthest frontiers. That particular problem escalated daily as neutral worlds evacuated their worlds in search of safe harbours from the erasure.

Initially, the Lon'tus were able to take in those seeking whatever sanctuary remained but overpopulation and crowding of Imperium supply lines forced his government to rescind such benevolence solely to more evolved species. Those who missed their opportunity the first time around were lucky before laws of the Lon'tus Imperium were changed. Of the species let in, those who were not conscripted into the Imperium forces were made to work in the Imperium war factories.

The steady flow had already become a steady nuisance to the Imperium ships on their way to the front as their displacement of space delayed their faster than light travel. Convoy vessels were disrupted by the sheer number of mostly rusty and dilapidated migrant ships clogging their vital shipping routes and supply-lines. Action became necessary.

As their own defensive technology and enemy dampening fields made spatial-folding a much more difficult and power draining concern, spatial fissure jump routes were becoming more and more heavily relied upon and made the problem even worse as the transport points stretched like a web across to the front and the refugee fleets. Some of the H'Raka and 'Xo captains were already forced to fire on migrant vessels to clear a path for their warships.

Though 'Lîna disapproved, she lived by her word that this war would have to be won at any cost, and did not question the actions of numerous members of their forces. Though H'Renn and 'Ivia had attempted to curtail such practices amongst their troops, they found this procedure had also begun being used by ships in the Lon'tus and even the At'Lann fleets. By the time she heard about all this through the interface, she had little to say anymore to protest the matter as the delays to their fleet started to interfere more and more with the war effort. A solution had to be found soon, and one the Trinity hoped they could live with.

Though 'Lîna had little time to concern herself with such affairs during her homecoming, she saw this as losing only another piece of herself in order to find victory. She once only thought of living in peace, and now her thoughts were of making peace with her beloved sister Za'szu before she would go into long term stasis to restore her genetic cohesion.

'Lîna returned to the seclusion of her home, her lilac pyramid and sovereign throne over the 'Mura'Lann cities. Though Za'szu ran the government from the traditional palace, 'Lîna never did take a liking to the throne in the other capital on the main continent. As much as she had loved her parents and their memory, her vibe was simply not there, and she had always been like Clotho on 'Mura as it was there that she always bonded and became one with her world, and blessed her on the path that explores. Besides, Za'szu had always taken a fancy to the Imperium residence in At'Lann.

Za'szu and an honour guard composed of S'yana and Sz'yana greeted 'Lîna and Nul'lus as they returned to the surface from the still heavily damaged Lis'talla but only under the facade that is some functions of state. Their feelings remained icy and buried under the emotional tundra while the celebrations gathered around the daughter of 'Mura returning home from the front. Though few expected a quick victory, all were gladdened that she was still alive and had been valiant in her pursuit of victory.

After a few simple and sombre speeches to the At'Lann clerisy, the sole class of the At'Lann that gave the gift and path of leadership to their sovereigns, 'Lîna found one last chance to relax in her lilac pyramid, and settled all that she could before her health must be attended to. On the large aerie balcony atop the slightly behemoth structure, 'Lîna found a small measure of freedom once again amidst the tide of reflection and quiet realisations. All that was left was to see Za'szu and restore what was always there, and set the balance right.

The damage of the war, to her genetic structure, to her way, to what she sacrificed for existence, already seemed far too harsh a noble penance. 'Lîna took what seemed a long look around to her home that had returned to and the beauty that it was before existence came to have a death sentence over it. She felt abandoned by joy itself. Everything ray in the sun, and every breeze in the relaxing skies seemed so fleeting knowing how much of herself had already been abandoned in order to protect it.

'What am I doing?' she thought. But she knew she had to strive on. For if there was to be a tomorrow, Fate had to choose cruel and twisting paths. That was why there was no debate by any between the relationship, the duality, between the Imperium and M'Goa, and why time still changed the reality between the two sisters in their understanding of one another.

As Za'szu joined 'Lîna on the deck, all that was repressed and all that wanted to be felt came forth in their long awaited embrace as they held each other in a true return home. Their rivalry, their differences, were forgotten with the swiftness and benevolence of Hermes. Their holocaust seemed their time apart. Their sibling conflicts were thrown aside, their love that begins with blood flowed though each of them and bound them tightly together once more. Sisters like these should never be apart in the dark times of war.

'I have missed you as much as I have yearned for us to set our differences aside.'

The thought seemed to flow through both of them. If was as if their differences seemed to become their commonality.

'Thanks to 'Zaya, we are brought together once more. She has kept me alive as much as she is the fulcrum like Nul'lus is for our Imperium. I love you, Za'szu.

Let us fight no more, 'Lîna said with a long awaited devotion that lay in her heavy heart.

Za'szu began to have tears of joy flow from her soft cheeks from the sweetness of 'Lîna's candour. They both lay their hands upon the black hand-railing on the platform of the lilac pyramid of 'Mura and looked out to their world before they folded inside to sit and talk.

The Regent of L'unn brought up the holo-interface display as they sat back together on a plush couch in the Imperiatrix's inner sanctum. Though neither was as yet interested in strategic discussions, 'Lîna saw ,displayed before her, data on a new drive technology Za'szu helped develop as well as that of the latest enemy design. The panacea smoke grew as Za'szu lit a smoke for 'Lîna which became cut by the sun of At'Lann that poured in as their embrace of thoughts continued as they came to hold one another.

'Zaya sobbed, almost pleasantly, 'You were worthy all along. I was foolish to think that you could not stand so strongly on your own. 'Imiszi, your devotion is to your path. I understand now. You have protected me, you have protected so many of us from the path of war, and you strive to protect us all. Your selflessness really is one of your paths. At least today, the war between us ends. My fate will remain in your hands without any hint of discord from now on.'

'Lîna's tearful smile was filled with pride. Za'szu had always been one of the most logical and intelligent daughters of At'Lann but lately her logic had been given little her shelter by the far away evil that spawned winds of war. She realised 'Lîna had never cast her bond with her away, and kept her love for her in the deepest region of her heart throughout the campaign as she did for all she cared for.

As they further relaxed themselves and distracted themselves with the constant flow of the data-stream which 'Lîna continued to be mentally linked to, and as she perused the interface, 'Lîna lit another cigarette. The light kept on piercing through the Djarum like smoke which reached to engulf itself across the room. Za'szu lit a milder *triketracel* hydro-filtered concoction of 'Zaya's for herself. 'Lîna was not the only one to make sacrifices for the sake of the At'Lann. 'Lîna who was paying a far heavier price but only because she was further ahead on the path of souls.

'You do not look well, 'Imiszi. It can only mean that this was the right time for you to return.'

'After defeat?'

'You and I both know that this war will not be won in such a fashion. Stop punishing yourself, 'Imiszi. Let yourself heal.'

After a pause, 'Lîna had a laugh laced in lament, 'I am not sure if I can. I am a lost place. I have lost so much of my innocence. Perhaps you were right. Perhaps I am not strong enough to survive.'

'Lîna seemed to end her words with sullen dread but Za'szu immediately shook her head in her ursine way and immediately said,

'You will. You will, 'Imiszi. For peace is a song of the phoenix. Your soul fires will always burn. You will always light the fire.'

Far be it for 'Lîna to disagree, and as her confidence seemed almost restored, she smiled a happily painful smile. Her form fluttered with a lavender and lilac glow of luminescence. Their reunion time was drawing to a close. They spent the rest of their time listening to music, and let their thoughts of eternal togetherness enrapture each other. They savoured their new peace and felt at ease around each other that they had never before known.

Their minds and souls linked and saw the future and knew they would be apart until a month before the final battle would take place. Yet they would never be apart. Fate reminded her that there were still paths she had not yet seen for Fate rules nothing out. But they let their thoughts flow into one another in soothing seas made as it were their last chance before the path of last hope remained. The sisters decided to enjoy the time left to them by returning some of their favourite childhood pastimes.

'Lîna flash-folded a hand-held music creation station player into her slightly trembling slim hands that had been out there and back. Like a small, unbridled tray size, black, satin metallic sketch etching pad cast itself and spread itself across 'Lîna's neatly crossed legs. It was an At'Lann child's toy that allowed the user to paint, spin, and curve music across the air and aether. Not to miss out, Za'szu had the interface trans-locate a diamond needle shaped teal hued prism flute-keyboard used by At'Lann children to create psionic mathematically and logically derived rainbows of colours cast and glowing geometric photonic forms.

'Lîna played as if she were Sasha spinning, and felt the vibe of Charlton as she found passion on the pitch, and Za'szu moved her mind to the songs of 'Mura and At'Lann. As 'Lîna mover her hands in the chaotic flow that is the wave of glow stick waving during a night of M'Goa, the music made the colours of the light become far more bright than that of their setting sun. The beauty of their transual song spun out across L'unn like violet butterflies on a spring morning filled with an amber sun over fields of wildflowers. Their song reached to 'Zaya at the main laboratory of the Imperium ministry of psyogenetics, and she too joined her sisters by folding herself over to 'Lîna's sanctum.

'Zaya had the interface bring forth her old silver low band psionic scissors-streamers casting wand that she moved as if she were creating the wisps of a dragon's tail. Her streamers and lime photonic neon danced and moved their way through the music and sculptures of logic. The realm of the electronic moved as life does for the music of their living planet.

The dimensional enhancing and genetically activated brush of 'Zaya's kind hands completed the beautiful art of that which is the canvas and spiritual landscape of the daughters trinity of 'Mura. The scissors-streamers snipped away in a trance nation at the photonic landscape that grew like a midnight garden all around them where one like Armin would be merry. Like the art of Lachesis, Clotho, and Atropos, theirs was a canvas that is the intertwine of life. The superstrings of life were hers for the playing.

The music of pure thought danced through the waters of their souls and around their being as their minds linked in the trinity of their sisterhood. They flowed like a glimmering white nebula light across the souls of the Imperium to almost say don't give up. From afar, Nul'lus had a gladdened smile for his aristocratically becoming comrade. From their song, he smiled one the most beautiful smiles for them. He was touched and his fondness for them comforted him. Then out of the blue, and like being hit by a bolt of blue, he was invited into their psionic transual symphony.

When he was a boy, he also played what 'Lîna had as it was he that led her to embrace the station player, for it was he who gave it to her. He linked his mind to them and his station player to 'Lîna's. He had never forgotten how she had embraced a more Lon'tus style of play, and how together, the music of their childhood nights would warms their hearts. Though he had rarely played with all the sisters at once in his youth, he felt ecstasy to make music with them today after so many dreary days.

His friendship with 'Lîna was bolstered by the many commonalties of their souls. So similar were their songs that they usually bound into each other to become one. His flow easily gelled into that cast out passionately by the daughters of 'Mura and added an even more refined edging to their music and photonic sculpture. On another part of existence, 'Iato H'Renn had the beauty of their song bring their savoury light into his being, and though not as hard and driven as H'Raka's music style could sometimes be, a tear of bliss rolled down the lion-wolf's war torn cheek. He let himself be wrapped in its beauty for what seemed like a very long moment.

As with 'Iato H'Renn, the song became introspectively cathartic for many of the souls of the Imperium. Battles would be won for things such as this; for art. Art was worth fighting for and worth saving. If life imitated art and art imitated life then it became only logical to assume this symbiosis should continue for eternity.

Sometimes the enlightened songs of children create the drives needed to protect them and to save them at any cost. Their art left them and their people awe-struck amidst the wonder that still remains across the succulent universes of the soul. It served as a reminder to all that art could and would save them. For many evolved beings, it drives them to take the steps on their paths for completeness of purpose. Something the P'rynn, their soon to be orbital neighbours had all but forgotten and needed to be re-taught in their materialistic, lethargic response to erasure. And now Fate left many paths to transcend above into a more complete path of existence. Victory was sought for those who value life and art.

For the Imperium would not forget the simple pleasures of existence that creates cradles for complexity. Art could always save them and catch their fall. The music of 'Mura seemed to play on until their dawn. And then a wind of change seemed to blow across the morning sky. The time came for ‘Lîna to enter healing stasis, and their song faded into their hearts.

Φ

Surrounded by her sisters, those of her noble clan, her S’yana, Sz’yana, Nul’lus and the inner clerisy of Mura’Lann, ‘Lîna lay herself into bio-gel solidifying interlock stasis chamber shaped like an onyx hexagonal looking coffin. She wore a mauve cere that was seamlessly and precisely cut. She hugged ‘Zaya and ‘Za’szu with her usual style of petting hugs and clenching of hands. She embraced Nul’lus with equal and mutual measure. After one last look, she lay her self down in the plush photonic lilac petals of pillows and sealed herself shut with a thought as the words of an At’Lann holy man, ‘Perna who reminded one of Korzeniowski. They were the last words heard. Sadly, there was little time to hear the rest of the blessing which sounded more like a dirge.

As the bio-gel solidified about her, ‘Lîna gave her thoughts to the Lon’tus Imperator. She told him she would see him soon, and how much she had joined the addition of his oceans of sound to the songs of L’unn. She promised him she would see him again in three days. After a brief meditation before once again taking the chrysalis path, she would come to exist in temporal multitude within reality. For she had found a way, both on the psionic realm and on the path of war, to the Death of Death. And she had found another way, and she would not rest in stasis if she could not continue on the path of war.

‘Lîna conveyed and confided in a secrecy that would be only so long before the same fate lay ahead for each of their trinity as each of them continued to psyo-genetically evolve. Nul’lus was happily and cautiously taken aback as he let shine his pride in her by how far she journeyed on her path. As their minds linked, he kissed her as the brother she had come to know. ‘Lîna then began to fall into the trance of the ether sleep as she bid him farewell as she slipped out of consciousness as her body went into stasis.

The onyx chamber then in a swirl of violet shimmering energy folded itself into the core of J’Poko, the under construction At’Lann component of the phase generator array, part of the omega project, that orbited in the distance past L’unn shining brighter perpetually as it neared completion. ‘Lîna would await in a restless sleep for her time to properly return to the path of war. But even for the next three days she would continue to pursue the enemy. On the psionic plane, she had woven herself a more enhanced psyogenetic structure and reality for herself. For she could get no sleep, and would remain awake outside her healing but still frail body.

‘Lîna would continue to stand on the front in her mind as she delved deeper into the enemy mind. She was Za‘Lîna ‘Imiszi ‘Mura’Lann, and she was Fate. Like her midnight garden, she grew herself into existence once again as if into the core of the At'Lann sun where there still burned the fires of hopeful dreams. Fate became her own creation as this was her path. Fate would be and would do what 'Lîna even with all she sacrificed, could never do. Fate is a tireless worker of paradox. And as she was born into reality as a dream warrior, she knew on the path of Fate that she would not stand alone.

28
Fate Unbound

She was all that and more. Fate's imagineered psyogenetic matrices were the ultimate prototypes known to Imperium science. She was now the living and walking dream split apart from herself. She had engineered herself to extract genetically derived loyalty in her subjects and had redesigned herself to better channel even more psionic energy through her being. Though if she decided to make her presence known, she would need little coaxing to inspire others; for she walked an enlightened path for her people.

The time would soon come where the people of At'Lann would still come to call her 'Lîna, the ghost reborn of Fate. She would retake her place as holder of the tiara crown, the faith of the At'Lann, by wearing her own as she returned to being the Imperiatrix through her other path of existence.

Fate would take a more reclusive profile to stifle the efforts of enemy monitoring to detect her, and as not to encumber herself with too many official duties while on the path of war. Her mauve skin visage lay under a cowl of many sheer layers. Unceremoniously, church and state on At'Lann became one as the Imperium of her home walked the path to amalgamation as 'Mura'Lann. Now Fate had everything about her to induce obedience from her people and their allies. She made herself a worthy heir to absolute power, and as Fate she could call on what she wished for the missions ahead.

Her fleet would be taken care of by 'Ivia who was transferred to the At'Lann Imperium as the Lon'tus was returned to their direct control. During her time away, 'Valis Val'damus was given the captaincy of a new At'Lann Tr'Lann-class warship, the Kam'manu. A promotion well deserved for his grace under pressure during the battle with the Army of Two Rings. The pieces were falling further and further into place.

As Fate, and though existing as an incomplete mist of a being, she felt and flowed with more knowledge, power, enlightenment, and far less innocence. Fate survived the vivisection of the first crusade upon the path of war. She was taught and became experienced by the lessons of the battle zone. She began to know where to cut the heads of the hydra that are the enemy. For Fate, her path was her mission as the daughter of 'Mura remained asleep though quite awake.

She flash-folded herself through a spatial gate cast in mezereon glimmers, to her rooftop of her lilac pyramid, and marvelled at her own evolution. She became the fires, the dark passions of war. Fate gazed upon the ever so slight fingers of her hands. They were as precise as the blade of So. She looked at herself as she looked through what remained of the universe in amazement of her creative genetic artistry and that of the tireless work of 'Zaya and Za'szu.

She felt she had become a perfect vessel, a true path of bold and dangerous virtue. She felt fierce, and she felt the rush of her power. She laughed a sweetly haughty laugh, and Fate felt a freedom apart from the pain of sacrifice of certain ethics to preserve the greater good. This was the exciting insanity of Fate's first true steps.

Fate's sporadically infectious laughter seemed laced with cries of dark sorrows of war thinking of how pathetic it all was. And these were the easy horrors. Whatever is to come, she wondered. Victory was already tasting as bitter as defeat. She longed to keep her conscience contained. Whatever was to come, in any way, it would be dreadful. But Fate kept in mind that it was worth it. All she had done and all she strived to do, the path Fate walked was for existence.

Since old habits die hard, she lit herself one of her old cigarettes as she looked out to her world continuing about without any sight of her. She smiled as her fingers twirled her violet nebulous dusting of her hair tangled about her soft shoulders, and breathed in what was now a panacea of no effect. Though only once a habit, it did not matter anymore.

'Zaya had done what she could and thanks to her selflessness, and with the enemy invasion, it had come down to this. Fate no longer felt ashamed, and the flexible glaze of her light mauve skin seemed to soften into something far more beautiful than the way she once was. For, she seemed composed of empathy as she seemed to find release amongst the souls of her people. And she felt so far beyond herself. She was her own reality and she had found purpose.

Fate would fight holding nothing back to preserve the great path of life so that souls may continue to journey to where the beginning exists with the end. She cast the pain of the losses that cut deeply into her heart. If she was Fate, she would be the alpha and the omega and all in between. And if she was Fate, she would bring herself to exist as eternity itself as all is determined and all is unwritten. In order to realise the future, Fate first had to find it. She knew where to start, and knew the Trinity would soon be reunited on the path. Soon the Trinity would be once again complete.

By any means necessary would they walk the path, and they would come to exist as, perhaps, something more. Fate no longer wondered what she was. Now and forever, she was Fate, and she was the sermon and the coy temptress of the path for those who pursue destiny. She was the living memory and the forever memory. Fate walked further down her path. Somewhere, temporal ship continued on.

A beautiful soul both lay asleep and continues to walk the path of war. The end would soon be the beginning once again.

Φ

Fate vowed that the enemy would garner far more dread from her, and would require a little bit of duty from those of the Imperium. She was the theistic core of her people after her awakening. The more things changed, the more things stayed the same. Even with the universe collapsing, what was to be always was. Fate was the empress of whispers and shadows, an iris in Y'vis's nightscape, and Fate had taken the bold and perilous path. For, she knew how far she had to go. Fate was now unbound, and the victory she now lived for was all that remained.

In inter-reality, a tie-dye of mint and azure energies, Fate stroked her fingers along the side of her dark violet cowl, and folded herself onto the ship that would take her to her destination in the galactic museum. Without notice, Fate boarded, the N'Lurr, an At'Lann destroyer, commanded by none other than Captain Mu'tolma who had improved his position through accepting it.

Originally, Mu'tolma was the third officer of this class of ships which were less than half the size of the Lis'talla. He had redeemed himself to the At'Lann and Imperium command by also discovering several improved target areas on enemy vessels through his own metallurgical scans no less. 'Lîna also thought she was a little too harsh with him as well, and decided to give him a little redemption.

As the Imperium Interface continued to grow in oceans of data, the At'Lann Imperiatrix had decided, in one of her commands across the data-stream, to give him a ship patrolling a vital defensive position well behind enemy lines. In spite of his prior ways, he was still a good officer, and was grateful to Fate for giving him what his soul wanted during this stretch of the path of war.

Mu'tolma simply wanted none of the madness, the chaos of volleying thunder that the war entailed. He was not ready for it in his heart. Fate realised this, and let him heal in this patrol route until the time he would be called upon. His soul found salvation in the Spartan simplicity of his new quiet existence. His first officer, An'sze, was a third cousin of 'Lîna's who shared Mu'tolma's creed.

Captain Mu'tolma and his First Officer, greeted their once and before Imperiatrix, and in some way, was still their cousin. It was plain to see that so much had changed and that any rapport they might have had was all but gone. Still, Fate was cordial as were her officers that walked the path of the new ecclesiastical order. They were souls apart but all were enlightened enough to know a true understanding of the path each took. Mu'tolma certainly did not envy or covet Fate's power, for hers was a most perilous absolute freedom. For Fate was a prisoner of freedom.

She almost frightened Mu'tolma and An'sze in the ready room of N'Lurr's command section as she almost unexpectedly folded her way in. Fate kept her distance as she came into existence at the other end of the room from her blood relations in silence, her form draped and cowled. Fate had cloaked her form to spare her cousins from the burden that could be seen in her eyes of walking unto the unconstrained dark places of the soul but she could see in them that they knew all too well, and they seemed to hasten to conceal their shudder from the enormity of the reality she walked. Fate still surprised them.

Under her lavender glaze, she was still 'Lîna but she was 'Lîna no longer. Fate was kindly more severe. For, she was the inherent spirit of the At'Lann to win this war. 'Lîna walked the path of war to the point where all she was, was Fate, and as she became herself, there had been little looking back. In truth, this had always awaited her. And indeed, this was a strange reunion along the path.

An'sze greeted her with her usually gilded way of affection said, 'Why cousin, you look so cheerful today. After all these years, you have not changed a bit. 'Good to see you too', Fate said groaning with a smile and a slow swiftness. It was a curt reply to the tempered excitement of seeing her strong spirited third cousin once again. She had changed little either, from her auburn curls, to her husky yet slender frame. An'sze was near 'Lîna's age but seemed to have a gruff wisdom all her own.

Fate then took Mu'tolma's hand and shook it with only a drop of grudgingly tart water. Fate no longer cared about their trivial discords from the past, and she smiled genuinely at her cousin.

'The ship is yours, my Imperiatrix', Mu'tolma proudly told her.

Fate smiled. 'As it should be, Captain. Set a course for L'Ja Prime, and have us there in one hour', Fate said in her incontestable voice of command confidence that came with the expectation that she would not be disappointed. And without considering his own thoughts, Captain Mu'tolma said with the most sincere and proud commitment as he bowed to her, 'It shall be done, my Imperiatrix'. Fate then folded herself to the inner temple of the ship after waving farewell with her hand in a shamanistic way.

Anti-gravity spectrum crossing photonic emitters were anchored to every wall. There was no fourth wall as the chosen families of 'Mura and At'Lann would not have it any other way. The photonic floating lava danced across the room. Like an Inca temple, this place was made for those who walked the path of Fate. Lily-of-the-valley and blueberry was the scent of the quiet air of this place. The temple was a stone plating of dark copper flames. Fate clasped together her hands as if she were in prayer. Like a buddha of last resort, Fate set her time aside to transcend, and entered a state of oneness within existence constrained, a virtual Lubijanka over what remained.

Fate gracefully leaned her head back and breathed in unity and angry despair. She found balance in a brief moment of clarity. As she stood with her legs semi-apart, her hands held up high, Fate fully leaned herself back for as far as she flexibly could, and touched the sky with her eyes. Her vision was the path of Fate. She became one with existence for what seemed the blink of an eye. Fate then lowered her head and raised it to see her symbol, the mauve and violet sliver crescent of L'unn.

The photonic dance circled and hovered about Fate as if like the devoted before a glimmering show about her symbol, and her covenant with existence. She activated the holo-interface within the temple. The reflection of the data-stream glow shined like moonlight upon her exposed face. Fate entered a command data pathway. She was Fate and she could do anything.

She set out, in complement to the decrees from her path of sleep, new orders, directives, and strategies into the interface. The data-stream flowed across the Imperium in a perfection that would have saved Paddington Station a terrible tragedy as what Fate desired became part of her new order. The data displayed on the interface signalled that her orders were already being carried out. It was a new day to be bold.

Fate casually keyed another sequence into the interface as one like Devi would. She was calmly filled with guilt by another morality being sacrificed. She smiled with a slight blush about her. She smiled as she felt like a god now. She was not sure. She had a smile that was the mask of a hard,imperial trance. Soon the shell would become even more hers. Fate said a blessing for her people and those she found worthy, and then left the shrine, almost unsure of how much time had passed.

She entered and folded away into an adjoining office held with the inner temple in the hidden subspace architecture of all Imperium vessels. Fate sat back on a L'unn heron's delphinium feather chaise and routed the interface data-stream before a simple diamond shaped table of onyx. Fate saw a new path of information drift across the data-stream that verified what she already knew in her mind. Fate had her bombers swoop down on the P'rynn and had them drop a gene-lock quantum field module onto the surface of M'Gata, and placed the entire P'rynn population into genetic storage. Their population was reduced to quantum field patterns on At'Lann macro-quartz data crystals the size of small scented candles.

Fate watched as a barley hued crystal was flash-folded onto the precisely polished onyx surface before her. She was anxious before she seductively laughed. She gently grabbed the data crystal and playfully threw it up into the air before catching its quiet fall. Fate held the crystal in her hands and she then spoke to it without hiding her empathic heart. But her words were sensuously curt.

'Your pursuit of selfish wealth will not deliver your souls this day. Most evolved species stand ready to accept sacrifice. Yours shall be thrust upon you. Though you shall remain genetically held in storage, you shall remember all that we do to save even your kind.'

The daughter of Mura almost let slip a near audacious, indulgent laugh at beings that had been reduced to nothing more than frozen accounts. She placed the gene-storage crystal back onto the table, and shook her head at the desperation of such a people that craved such limited treasures. They had bought their way in without ever paying for any of it. Fate made sure even the P'rynn would pay their tab. The vaults of the At'Lann seemed so much richer with the potential of what could be. Fate watched the face of Gn'rys P'rynn flush with a zephyr of fury frozen in a data sequence. He must have wondered if he could have made a better deal with the Devil. Fate thought it a pity that this soul had so far to go.

She was then interrupted from her musings as the N'Lurr jarringly slowed to drop out of its subspace sliding corridor. She casually moved away from the edge of the table and had the M'Gata crystal folded to their sorting station on Nu'Ata before they would be taken to At'Lann. She uncrossed her legs and stood feeling a little of the madness. Fate then flash-folded herself in a monsoon of photonic rays and colours to the main bridge of the N'Lurr without another thought.

Φ

With a veiling stream of psionic glitter, Fate made her way onto the bridge. Captain Mu'tolma gave the Imperiatrix command and appraised her of the situation. An'sze stood at Fate's side looking quite bored and accepting of it all. So much had changed and so much remained the same. Mu'tolma looked at his cousin and saw he had no longer a need to worry for he could trust her with their fate. Fate reclined as luxuriously as a soldier could in her carbon tanned leather centre throne couch. In a most stoically glamorous way and transual fashion, Fate sat back as the holo-screen displayed the space ahead. She had a decision and a judgement to make.

The impediment ahead was a degradation of subspace caused by the power distribution networks of a conjoined fleet of refugee vessels from the H'Bdkas galaxy which had fallen to erasure. Twelve million antiquated and unregistered vessels composed the conjoined fleet strewn like seaweed across a galactic spindle.

Though limited in the skills they could provide to the At'Lann war, they refused as a whole to contribute themselves to the war effort and had moved illegally into Imperium space without their consent. Fate did not like that someone had sneaked in, and immediately modified the Imperium Interface to reinforce their security, and to make sure the enemy would not take advantage of this. Somehow the H'Bdkas had folded their way in. Their bile grey ancient turtle shaped vessels, each half the size of the N'Lurr, covered the space ahead.

Even with their co-operation, considering the rough shape of their vessels, it would take days for the H'Bdkas to evacuate their ships out of a region of unstable space which their pollutant, antiquated power sources had created. It was not just their power distribution networks that degraded subspace, it was the aggregate of their patchwork vessel technology. Truly, a people not prepared. The H'Bdkas had trespassed themselves into a region of space which they made into a North West passage to overcome. Fate was not pleased by what choices she had to make.

Fate folded her left leg tenderly across her knee with the hushed sound of a satin drive-by. She watched to see who watched her. The crew knew who she was, and Fate did not mind. Perhaps the Imperium will see more of me, she thought. She lit herself a cigarette that she folded into reality, and felt sympathetic during her judgement in finding a solution seemingly to be only found by viciousness and exactness. She puffed away and in a lamenting assured voice said as she turned to Mu'tolma,

'You know cousin, I find the best way to overcome an obstacle is to eliminate the obstacle.'

Mu'tolma nodded as to how to proceed, and to acknowledge his crew would do what it would take to win the war by whatever orders their Imperiatrix wished to be carried out.

'Commander An'sze. Reconfigure and align the N'Lurr for Imperium Protocol 'Mura'Lann attack pattern 'Anu seven.

Fate, it seems, had made a few changes to the Imperium Interface. As the N'Lurr stood in space, the weapons banks rose swiftly out of the patrol ship's armour. Ironically, the ship would not have this new technology without having capturing it from the enemy. Technologies created from analysis of enemy warships from the debris left in Tr'Lann to scans taken during the battle on the front. Mu'tolma stood on silently observing it all.

'Have the ship generate a meta-phasic tri-genomic (trionic) field pulse fire before firing the main weapons banks at maximum firepower for a sector field. These actions are to be forever classified. These events will remain secret and will never become part of our recorded history. Understood.' Fate said as she looked around the bridge to see she would be obeyed by all. Her words seemed to flow with a stark solitude about them and coercive caresses. Saying them sadly seemed that similar orders would have be be taken from time to time.

Captain Mu'tolma bowed quietly and would see that what Fate asked for would be carried out. Fate now seemed to have sanction to dismiss ethics and moralities that seemed less suited for her but she did not want to be remembered by her people for necessitous, desperate acts of war-time. All media and recording equipment of any technology was jammed by the N'Lurr, and rendered useless. The crew of the all-At'Lann warship would live forever abiding by their oath of silence for such matters.

The interface displayed that the captured weapons enhancements were on-line with maximum payload energy standing by and waiting for Fate to choose a path. How they waited to be fired. Fate inhaled and exhaled the latest 'Mura'Lann Agent 27 smoothly and slowly. She looked at An'sze and Mu'tolma to let them know that this burden was hers, their souls were to become encumbered only by what they were about to witness.

Fate then turned her attention back to the galactic expanse ahead to where she would direct existence. She activated a communications channel and directed a message to the conjoined fleet ahead. She spoke through her thoughts as she sent her message out.

'I am the path of your souls, and I am the war for existence. A choice has been made today that your species has no choice about. What you give today shall not be forgotten. You shall not be forgotten, and you shall be given tribute for this day…farewell.'

Fate then hit a neon mauve coloured key on her personal interface console. Though this action was everything she was not, Fate had to do whatever it would take to win the war. The L'tca corridor was vital to the war effort. She had done it. The protocol became reality. 'What have I done?' she might have wondered but there was no time now to ponder her actions.

The weapons of the N'Lurr came alive as the moment came to pour cannon shot upon the H'Bdkas. Pincer like platforms, the size of spires over the heart of Europe, protruded from the hull and in a symphony and by the beating of tribal drums of war, shot in unison towards their target. The N'Lurr's cannons subatomic shear pulses flew out into the fear strewn space ahead. The pulses rained into the H'Bdkas ships like stain-glass shards raining down to shatter the tainted peace of this region of space.

With the resolute stillness of a wandering gaze, a change swept across the universe. Trionic lightning danced almost menacingly around the utterly terrified aboard the conjoined fleet. As the bridge crew of the N'Lurr looked out into the galactic expanse, the ships were silently gone. Not one of H'Bdkas ships remained in the eerily quiet space ahead of them. It seemed a pasture of solitude once more. Fate remained under her cowl letting no one see her eyes as she watched the dreadful moment where silence was plundered as the guns finally lay silent. The interface promptly erased the events of the day. Fate was not impressed with herself.

To maintain the arrival time for L'Ja Prime, Fate chose to be cruel in her decision to impose erasure upon the H'Bdkas species. Fate can always be wrong but she made her choice the day her reality fell apart and darkness descended upon everything. Looking out into the beyond before her, she could feel within herself the loss of the species of life from existence as she did of all life that fell to the erasure of the Death of Death. It was what tore away at her before, and today Fate only added to her wounds. The time the Trinity would unite on the path once again was still slightly ahead in the future. She could have had the species stored in gene-storage data crystals preserved in particle reduction stasis until the war is won but Fate chose not to this day.

Fate, the empath on the path of war who could feel extinction and death everywhere, found the madness of it all far too consuming of her drowning soul. Her path was perilous, there could be no mistake about it, and she was willing to show, even to herself, how far she would go for the sake of victory. How it consumed her at times. Fate then sequenced into her interface that the Imperium fleet was now authorised to forcefully remove non-aligned vessels by way of gene-storage data crystal extraction.

As well, the At'Lann fleet were now authorised to destroy non-aligned vessels who obstructed actions of war. Surprisingly, Fate chose the future actions be recorded for access via a public data stream. But this day would be Fate's burden to bear.

Fate could have psionically re-weaved the memories of the entire crew of the N'Lurr but she chose not to. She had their faith and their word, and in the sad reality of their times, a little fear. But Fate believed by choosing this path she would save reality. Fate buried the pain of her soul under her silent lavender shell. There was no turning back on the path of war, and Fate unleashed and unbound what little remained of her innocence and filled herself with the ice-blood of the coldest warriors even though Fate hated the discontent of the cold. And now, her soul seemed far below the dark winter snowdrifts.

Fate rose from her centre throne, and released the end of her cigarette onto the ground with a well executed toss. She looked to see An'sze and Mu'tolma with their faces aghast by what they had seen. She was no longer seemed to be anything at all like the one they knew.

'Maintain course and speed, Captain. The bridge is yours. Inform me when we reach L'Ja Prime. By my calculation we should arrive in thirty minutes.'

'Yes my Imperiatrix. It shall be done.'

Fate said no more as she left the bridge, to let the souls aboard ponder the events of the day. She could forgive disappointment but not inefficiency. The crew of the N'Lurr would continue to give her their best. Like the blink of time that they passed through, Fate flash-folded back to her temple without the skip of a beat from the way of her grace. Her only satisfaction being that she could do now what she could not before. Fate had lost herself to war. How she longed to exceed the limits of M'Goa as many on the gathering world already did.

Whatever the case, the Imperium knew she was back, and had already enacted many of her directives. As M'Gata took its place in the Tr'Lann system, the Imperium commandeered the world and modified its technology to serve as a medical facility for Imperium soldiers injured on the front. Fate hoped the nectar of the healed, through her actions, would bring a sense of peace to an otherwise gloomy first day of returning to the battlefield.

Fate knew what lay ahead, and though the firth was silent now, it would not remain so forever. She had to muster all her strength to continue on her path. As she let her thoughts fall into balance, Fate knew L'Ja Prime would become a turning point whatever the outcome. The thorns below her feet on the path Fate walked felt like sharp and shattered cobblestone. The path ran with a river of violet blood. Innocence was forever lost.

29
The Once and Future Wasteland

The surface of L'Ja was akin to what was the east of Tunisia. The land before her reminded Fate of her days of youth and her times with her legendary uncle T'Koris. She had always been fond of his retelling of tales of his travels to worlds like this. In fact, it was he who told her of his visits to L'Ja when there was still a small trading post there in the days before the galactic museum was sealed to most visitors.

All back in the days when T'Koris was a King of 'Mura, and back when At'Lann was governed using a dual monarchy system. All long before the next generations would govern differently. The daughter of L'unn created her model of governance upon many of her uncle's principles, for he was a man of civility and noble destiny that even the Lon'tus would approve of. Governess of the Imperium, Za'szu, who shared most beliefs as 'Lîna did when it came to sovereign rule, continued and maintained the returned traditional rule that 'Lîna had embraced. However, much had changed since T'Koris's reign.

Hyper-accelerated psyogenetic enhancement, sibling fighting, absolute rule, sapphist lusts fulfilled, extermination of species; Fate wondered what Uncle T'Koris would have thought of it all. But like Fate, T'Koris was an explorer, a Kosciuszko, a Peary, a Putaski, a Korzeniowski, a Scott left unscathed, and an Amundsen without the canine stigma. And he too came to find balance on the path to L'Ja as Fate came. All that was left to do was to wait before the others would come.

In actuality, Fate remembered being here before. In fact, this was her third visit to L'Ja. As a child it was one of the first worlds she could visit as it was within acceptable spatial fold distance limits from her home system. She returned to gaze upon the serenity of the wasteland before her. Fate remembered T'Koris who seemed with her as if showing her, for the first time, a silent ancient world. And now, Fate had returned.

Uncle T'Koris once found the same peace of the desert planet's sirocco massaging itself across such a holy wasteland. 'Such possibilities. Such paths.' he always used to say in the way one as noble as Cincinnatus would. He was a man of a different time from the age of high volume inter-system trade. Fate hoped T'Koris was smiling upon her on the day she arrived on L'Ja. A day that was long past her arrival time. One half hour that became an extra day as a random enemy sensor sweep had to be evaded. Fate seemed only a little unfazed as she knew she could be wrong and excessive wishes cannot always be met.

Fate left the N'Lurr after holding private holo-meetings with Za'szu and 'Ivia before having a holo-conference with her favoured cousins from T'Koris's great house and clan, the house of Ta'al. With unconditional support her cousins greeted Fate, photonically on a portable floating triangular holo-interface, to do whatever more she asked of them in order to aid the cause. They folded the requested weapons and technology to Fate's Imperium scout shuttle.

After polite and not as distant farewells as before to Mu'tolma and An'sze, she disembarked. They had brought Fate to L'Ja. Fate now telekinetically and psionically carried a hockey bag size grey violet metallic rectangular case which her cousins promptly folded to her and now which she had brought out of her landing ship. Fate made a decree that only the Trinity would now walk the white gold sands of this world for the duration of the war. Captain Mu'tolma had the N'Lurr returned to its former course as if nothing at all had happened. In barely visible meringue swirls did the winds and sand blow about her.

Fate stretched out her hand to shield her eyes beneath the cowl from the brilliance of the sun that was so strong that it even took her psyogenetically constructed eyes a moment to adjust. She thought of the resonant hold the desert already had on her as she stared out into the wasteland of L'Ja that already haunted her mind as it did in her youth. This was the place her thoughts brought her to. She could feel the immensity of the life that once resided on this world, before the Origin species decided to walk the heavens, in each grain of sand that blew past her.

A long whisper whip of her dark violet cowl blew in the wind, almost dancing to its trance swirling twists, about the crusader. It now seemed sheer enough by the light of the desert sun to make out the details of her tiara which Fate had folded back onto her slender head above her sad yet tenderly silent face. Like Artemis she stood preparing her thoughts for the path ahead in the desert sea that had the lines of Baikal. Like Virgil's day and that of Remus and Romulus, Fate stood on an outcrop of stone that once held up a great edifice which more then likely rivalled any in the Imperium. She was way out west. Fate would have no choice but to wait for the others before the great task ahead. She sent her thoughts into her enhanced meditations. This would be her time alone before the others would soon be at her side.

Even the legendary endurance of the Lon'tus and H'Raka genetic structures could not hold out much longer and were falling even now to the burden and the strain. Like the sun over the Atacama, the red giant shining upon L'Ja radiated across Fate's dark mauve and amethyst eyes. Her eyes held the reflection of the dry serenity that would have made for an ideal Burning Man.

Her thoughts became transual as time no longer mattered. She awoke her thoughts once more to reality to find the path envisioned about to become the path taken. It was time. She could feel winds change direction about her. Then the humble march of the enduring Lon'tus seemed to fill the skies as Fate reconfigured her cowl into something like a *kaffiyeh* that trailed off in the wind above what seemed like the same coloured At'Lann *dishdasha*. Then her thoughts were awakened to a presence. He was here at last.

With an Edwardian lined walking cane in hand and in fitting attire for an aristocratically sovereign leader for a stroll through the Sahara of their hearts, he came to her side a day after she arrived, after she let both her mind and body wander across the surface of the desert planet. The Aristocrat came to her side and theirs souls found the ocean of unity this world would give them. Their bond had remained unbroken.

The paths of the Fate and the Aristocrat had once again converged. Now the Fate only awaited the arrival of the other dynamic soul of the Trinity. The desert of L'Ja was their rendezvous point before they would begin the path ahead in what would be the objective below. Fate watched as he walked from a great distance across the sands towards her as his thoughts came to dance around her. The horizon was wondrous as it lit the desert in pastel fires for the gazes of the pair that had been out there and back, and now, back again.

The Aristocrat walked with his usual dapper prestige through the ruins of the gods that came before. Now and again, he would tap the tip of his cane to the hallowed ground with the eloquence that elite souls should carry themselves with. He looked as if he were a warrior of Anfield out upon a safari. He was impressive. He was very impressive. He walked like a son of Wessex through the sands through the desert estate of the Imperium. So here he was after all this time.

The Aristocrat bowed and took Fate's hand which she freely gave to him. Fate wrapped her hands around his triceps and looked at him in the bliss of his return. 'A divinity amongst all divinities,' Fate thought as she looked deeply into him. The short span of time made the pair seem so different, so beyond one another, and yet exactly the same. And though starkly different from what they had been before, their psyogenetic bodies, all but their immaculate eyes, seemed impervious to all that had changed them. But when one looked into their eyes, one knew that they had been forged in the fires of war and the bliss of peace.

The Aristocrat's hair had become long and tied back in a perfectly edged Lon'tus style that is the fashion one takes before conquering lions as they used to in their ancient days. He was the hearty patriotism, the greatest masterpiece of a superman upon the genetic canvasses. The enemy seemed almost an antithesis of the Aristocrat. With his arrival, the Death of Death seemed all the more the feculent absence of culture. She could feel the enemy here. And she felt within herself the spirit of her bond with the Aristocrat and both sadly and sardonically with the Death of Death.

Fate and the Aristocrat could feel the enemy nearby, and it seemed so clear to the Fate that the enemy had, unbeknownst to them, allowed the H'Bdkas to enter so deeply into their space. How the dark one must have laughed as the few paths left were ones of dark choices. Fate could see the effect on Nul'lus's soul as the covenant of existence seemed to shatter. So much was already lost. The art, the music, the splendours that are love and duty, the things the Aristocrat and the Fate appreciated almost seemed forever gone.

Their reunion was both joyously subdued and the continuance of what is endured on the path of war. The Aristocrat maintained his vow to stop the Death of Death for the flag of Lon'tus that always has to be flown with victorious distinctions and always must fly above defeat. For the path of civility must always be worshipped while in combat and with comrades. It was a noble path to choose that now had become as it was with Fate. And now the path ahead on L'Ja waited to be taken.

The Aristocrat and the Fate briefly linked minds. He saw the Fate had been eviscerated as the last of her innocence had been torn away with her soul desperately trying to hold onto the last few shreds dangling in the precipice of erasure, and of what she was before the enemy invasion that brought the raping plunder of it all upon them. She had remade herself into the serenity of the path of zealous slaughter. Fate almost hated herself but kept her optimism alive as she would do whatever was necessary to gain victory. Her path had never wavered. The Aristocrat found his return to reality sliding back into balance as the Fate was there to share the path.

The path of souls returned to its ever flowing unity as the Fate and the Aristocrat embraced once again, and embraced as warriors and comrades. Childhood's end was found in both their eyes from this miserable war that had all but killed them. It was etched deeply into them as they did their best to remain positive.

Imperator Nul'lus lay in stasis within the core of the Lon'tus macro-phase generator, Sol'linko, after degradation to his genetic cohesion became too much to hold together corporeal and stasis became imperative. Their paths were now one once more. They hugged and laughed telepathically as Fate told him he was a day late. Perhaps if their path was to culminate in glory, this world might once more flow with tranquil waters like those of the oceans of L'unn like those from the days of their youth, and it was a youth that seemed all but gone.

Their thoughts reached out once more and became one. The Aristocrat's soul was filled with flair and strategies of graceful conduct. And as his thoughts came into her, Fate's calm and hidden tenderness surfaced for a moment as she half-jokingly told him she did not foresee their deaths in the next few days at least. Soon the Hunter would come to unify the Trinity as he would sink his fangs deeper into the wretched necks of the vermin that tore away existence from all life. They would await him as the pair would not seek destiny before him but awaited him knowing destiny was possible upon this path. They wondered if they truly were the last remnants of infinity. All that was left was for the Hunter to join the hunt once more.

The pair awaited him while they traversed the desert and walked past many flecked obsidian outcroppings protruding defiantly from the while gold sands lost to time. They ventured deeper into the wasteland of the bone-dry sands of a beyond ancient ocean bed and shores of even more ancient lands. They thought that perhaps the Hunter was already stalking their position and was amongst them even now. But it was still not to be.

The terrain became more like that of the Gobi as the pair pressed on as their souls healed, readied and adapted for the great task ahead amidst the enemy being felt everywhere they surveyed. The peace of the desert thankfully lulled their psyches as they looked out to the horizon of white gold dunes, and after walking for so long that they had almost forgotten when they began.

The distance ahead seemed the same wind worn sand of dead snow that in the absence of maintenance had become planetary granular corrosion. They were close to where the path below would begin and could feel the Iblis like a shadow stench infesting its way up into the atmosphere from below the surface.

The pair could sense the enemy presence intensify as if there were a cancer growing beneath the relatively still world. They traversed through the enormous salt beds of a once deep ocean with hills of salt being twice that of the size of 'Mura. The salt crystallised itself to their militaristically soled boots and left a tinge to them as they kept on. The desert of L'Ja seemed a tomb fit for the pondering of a silent sunshine as the pair trekked on. The Fate and the Aristocrat could feel the winds drenched in a certain current temporal wisdom of what was to come by what had happened before. Fate wondered if even the transcendent had fallen to erasure as well.

After a day of walking through such sameness, the Fate and the Aristocrat thought their minds were playing tricks on them as something emerged from the dissipated stillness. For, there could only be two answers as to who or what it could be. Fate could feel an energy charge build. She could hear the sand savannah have its calm shattered as a weapon system armed itself with a healthy hush and strangled desperation. Neither the Fate or the Aristocrat were sure if it was their comrade or their enemy as the *vrreeeeee* sound of weapons charging intensified around them.

With a lightning strike of one like Silvinho after some mystical dribbling, reality came almost full circle. All at once the Hunter de-cloaked holding a modified sawed-off length nova-pulse anti-personnel rifle as if he were Figo ready for battle. He held it to where the Fate's jugular might have been if she were still human. Fate could feel the power surging with the weapon that shattered what seemed the silence of the dead. She did not turn to see him but recognised the evolved lines of the prototype weapon that 'Iato H'Renn had designed during his inventing times, and which the Hunter had built himself. For, there could be no other way. Whatever his intent, he was a Macgyver of futures past.

Moreover, it was quite obvious that he had stalked the pair as prey since their arrival on L'Ja. Fate could see he used a doppelganger to conceal his steps on the next aspect of their psyogenetic transformations in the same sense in which the Trinity now walked. As Fate looked to him, she came to see a living statue carved from the essence of Gibraltar and that of the Harz; cut like a Mark V in trim black dragon leather. The Hunter in his lightning strike was a powerful invasion.

'Go ahead and pull the trigger if you stand with those who pillaged Hy'Bor and all reality. Even if you do not, pull the trigger. The Aristocrat would be most pleasantly surprised,' Fate said in a tone reserved for reunions with kinsmen.

She could see in her mind the weapon was set for maximum pulse charge. Fate smiled at him provocatively before turning away from the Hunter. The Aristocrat was calmly aghast by what was afoot. Somehow he knew, this was merely a good showing of what was returned to them.

'No need to be nasty, 'Imiszi.', the Hunter said almost playfully.

But then the rifle went off. The Hunter's eyes became the union of the hawk and the jaguar as the trigger was pulled. The nova-pulse energy shredded out of it like Cerberus tearing away at the dank but burning reality of Hades. The blast sailed through Fate's body in a blaze of high order energy disruption. She did not move or flinch as the blast passed harmlessly through her and into an adjacent dune that was rendered into a jagged heap of oozing glass from the blast. Fate returned her gaze to the Hunter with a peaceful smile. Their combined technology remained harmless to any of the Trinity.

'Welcome back from the dead, 'Iato. Did you miss me?'

'Of course.'

The Hunter turned to the Aristocrat as well.

"Lus. You look well, old friend. What do you think of the adaptations I made using Origin species technology?'

'Impressive, old friend.'

The Aristocrat marvelled at the extent of their war drive innovations. The Hunter even had two additional nova-pulse rifles for his companions. Since Imperium technology was based upon what is beneath the surface, the various weapons components continued to gel together with a synergy that only the enemy would find to be a threat. It also made combat a little easier as one could fire through their comrades in order to hit enemy targets. The Three were now complete and ready to face the infestation of this place as well as the impediments left behind that kept the planetary core safe from intrusion.

The thoughts of the Trinity became one as the plan, for their path became clear. The Aristocrat was an expert of the technology buried beneath L'Ja and could tap into the central core's systems. A vision from Y'vis's oracle gave each mind of the Trinity a map to the central core of L'Ja. But traversing the technology of the planet was a far more difficult path than it would first appear. The Hunter would battle alongside his companions and would take on the task of sniffing out any enemy incursions, deployments along the way and would eliminate them as the others of the Trinity would also do.

Like the great Fenris, or she who watched over Romulus and Remus, the Hunter holstered his rifle as Fate held his elbows with her tender hands. He had the enhanced frame of a Colossus, and he was more than ready for the path ahead. Fate welcomed his returned existence. He bowed before the pair and placed his hands upon the shoulders of the Aristocrat. The Hunter's soul flowed with how glad and happy he was for his comrades to see him.

His presence completed the Fate and the Aristocrat. And now truly they were the Trinity of the wind, the water, and the moon. The Trinity then began to walk deeper into the wasteland of L'Ja which always seemed to stretch ahead, and even Eliot would have found far too encompassing. The place seemed burned with visions to come but the Trinity had to press on through the horizon of dried out lands. The Trinity seemed to walk endlessly together in their thoughts as they would soon begin their descent in the underworld of L'Ja.

Hours seemed to pass until they reached an equally uneventful place in which to stand in the salt encrusted sand. The Aristocrat then etched a line in the sands below and parted them in a way Moses would think had great style and circumstance about it. Salt and sand blew away from desert sands until the shell of L'Ja was revealed. The sands blew away to reveal a large rectangular hatch in the same dark plum hue as the advanced metal of the ghostly shell of this world beneath its dunes. The hatch was roughly the size of a typical At'Lann dwelling, and it was the only portal into the wettest of Tesla's dreams that lay beneath them. A path through the silicone labyrinth of thorns awaited.

The ancient technology was already starting to have the effect of dampening the enhanced abilities of the Trinity, and the Three understood, the further they would go, the more gruelling it would become. Legends said that all sense of direction can be lost in L'Ja's heart and they would have to be on guard against this. In all Fate's visits to this world, she somehow always feared descending into it. Now, she understood why, and ironically, it was her job to navigate the Trinity.

As their thoughts joined to open the armoured flesh of L'Ja to open the door to its ultra-mechanised heart, Fate felt as if she were about to descend beneath the soil of Katyn, of Volhynia, and into what now seemed the dark void that is the walking slaughter that is the Death of Death. In both reality and on the psionic plane, Fate began to open the gate into the dark realm that is the enemy. This was to be a walk into the underground valley of Death. This was just another way to lay her sword into the absent heart of the sketchiest of beasts.

The Trinity would descend into a world of micro-particle ultra-conductors and the frozen once molten core of supposedly divine and restricted technology. The planet was sealed by the 'Ri'Muria'Lann court of At'Lann's third generation after uncle T'Koris retired to his own pursuits. It remained a museum until this day when it became a battleground, and a mausoleum. L'Ja became an inanimate sponge of poly-aligned, equi-molecular icons of sacred steel beneath a desiccated and once living skin.

Fate prayed with her hands held open towards the direction of her world as the Trinity set forth on their descent into what had become another cancer of darkness upon existence, and the deeper they descend, the more the darkness would drown out their psionic abilities.

She hoped they would be enough to complete their mission for themselves and the Imperium. Power would have to be conserved as a countermeasure to the dampening effect of the enemy and the ancient technology. The plague beneath L'Ja had to be dealt with before the enemy could use their very worlds to defeat them. They had to complete their mission.

The Trinity were here especially to stop the enemy from stealing and using their coveted technology. Fate knew they had a chance to turn erasure back upon the enemy. But in order to do that, the enemy had to be stopped from acquiring what was a virtual Rosetta stone for At'Lann, H'Raka, and Lon'tus technologies. The Trinity were ready to do whatever was necessary to win this day. Fate used her psionic sight to scan the dark silent corridors for the enemy whose intentions she had intercepted through the insight of her temporal spindles. This was clear to her as her mind shifted into an enlightened focus. For the explorer Fate was a dark beauty found as her kind had never been inside L'Ja before. And she knew there were other things to decipher, and something to be found only on L'Ja.

The Aristocrat remarked with whispered astonishment that what lay beneath the planetary sheath remained, for the most part, untouched by the hand of time. The Hunter stowed a harpoon like sword of the knights of H'Raka and even he could feel the pulse of L'Ja's technology still active and that of what crawled through her subterranean mechanical reefs of splendour. The prey before him would quench his blood thirst until he would give his might to the omega project phase generators in what he wanted to be the final battle with the Death of Death. If the Hunter could kill the evil one here, all the better he thought.

Fate did not quiver in her composure as she stood at the edge of what was a hatch ramp. This would begin the reckoning. She embraced the power of her will that was the spirit felt by those who climbed out of the underground after night after night of the Blitz to stand once again in defence of freedom. Fate craved such a redemptive baptism like that of Highbury's fire. Fate would let slip the guns of war. The parasites of desecration that heralded the finality of erasure waited below. Locked and loaded the Trinity stood before the gate into the black plague with the enemy drenching every corridor beneath L'Ja with its stench. The Three walked the path and were on a crusade to be L'Ja's liberators.

Fate placed their provisions in a sub-dimensional pouch that could sustain itself to the very core of L'Ja and could be accessed by any one of the Trinity at any time during this cavernous crusade, and she flash-folded her new nova-pulse rifle to her hands. The rest of the arms her cousins had diligently packed for her and remained safely stowed away for the Trinity's needs. The Aristocrat then flash-folded a nova-pulse rifle into his waiting hands as he outthought an L'Ja encryption sequence and unlocked the final lock of the gate to the bunker that was L'Ja. The Hunter steadied his rifle.

The techno-tomb hissed open desolately with a rush of dust particles exposed to the desert air and gases like those of Bhopal that vapoured into flight from the planetary sarcophagus like freed prisoners of time into the hotter than Moroccan heat of the aether of the desert wasteland. Billows of coffee bean stained dust like particles ejaculated away only to blow away from what seemed a sunken mirage. The ramp door whirred itself open to serve as a rampart to what was below. The Hunter tightened his grip on his killing instrument and stalked his way covertly into L'Ja ahead of the others.

The Fate and the Aristocrat covered his flank as best they could as they followed the Hunter in. They would let him have one rampage inside the planets to begin their foray inside.

An enemy drone satellite was the lone guard snared for the Hunter's first feast of his firepower. The blast from the nova-pulse rifle shot loose as if it were burning napalm shot forth from the eye of a black hole. The blast detonated every molecule in the lone sentry that wiped away another zombie terror from existence. Nothing remained save for the stub of the drone's finger as the Hunter had programmed into his weapon such a desire before setting it off like the boot of a Bergkamp volley across the face.

The linear whalebone corridors of L'Ja's interior of technology, both greasy and humming, remained impervious to the blast as it continued to rage brightly down one of the dimly lit corridors for what seemed like forever before finally disappearing from sight. For an instant everything came to be stopped as only one like Di Canio would do. The dark corridor no longer danced in light with the macabre energy pulses unleashed by the Hunter, and returned to their once undisturbed dark silence. The tar mustard and slightly rusting sea foam green walls were barley aglow with large tracts of lighting placed at the intersection of where the walls met the floor.

The Trinity walked below to the centre of an arena sized chamber and shut the ramp hatch behind them. The ancient machinery whirred to shut itself with a piercing clank that went unwarranted by the attentions of the Trinity. The Trinity shut the Erebus like gate as they moved below and walked luridly deeper into the nightmare. For, there was no escape and no turning back. How messianic it sadly was.

Fate looked to the Hunter as he reset his weapon to auto-exact the charge to maximise his kill-to-reload ratio. He was still the equinox of the lion's heart. He enjoyed his little indulgence as he simply wanted to showcase the latest additions to their arsenals. 'Imperators and their toys,' Fate thought.

The Aristocrat appreciated the craftsmanship of the same toy given to him by the Hunter, and knew they would be a part of their success against the enemy. The H'Raka gift was more than on par with the creations of the gunsmiths of Lon'tus, and the Aristocrat commented to the Hunter on his prowess. He smiled to his proud friend that helped bring unity and balance back to the Trinity with a little friendly banter. The Three still had not forgotten who they were inside their blossoming souls. And in a way, Three became One.

They moved so synchronously beside one another across the darkened arena space. This was a nightmare where their strength all but waited to be abated. Their first steps into L'Ja came easily but every step taken would be harder to take than the last. The Three would have to hold their own and hold hard to their unity. Corridor after corridor intersected one another at the furthest reach of the chamber where the Trinity now stood.

The Three were before a descending labyrinth of seemingly eerily humoured sepulchre of grease dripping conduction coils. The mechanical tunnels became a little darker as the Trinity moved on, deeper into the interior of L'Ja.

The Fate could feel the enemy surrounding their location, and her thoughts were relayed to her comrades. Without waiting for the other side to fire, the Three shot first with hand and handled arsenals of freedom. Their psionic hands pulled the triggers to unleash an energy mayhem of nova-pulse bolts. The Three shot in every direction in their triangular defensive stance, and in every direction shot, a target was eliminated with perfect accuracy.

So hyper-realised was their killing efficiency that the enemy had very little time to react and were only able to fire their cannons sparingly at the Trinity before being mowed down by the briefly perpetual hale storm of energy fire. Energy fire of royal purple, blue, and red shot out, and for a trance like passing moment, their gunplay fully illuminated the corridor the Trinity entered.

Fate brought the Trinity to the appropriate corridor for their descending path to the core, and the Three hopped briskly over the fallen hell spawns of blunted and blood pooling dead that only seconds before stood in the way of their holy path. The path of war was resurrected as the Trinity moved on.

After criss-crossing through several corridor junctions, the Three found their way to an anti-gravity lift platform that took them to a lower level thousands of leagues in the sea of technology below their starting point. The lift worked silently to lower them down a shaft with a Navaho like derivative layout of wall gratings that whooshed past the Three as they delved ever deeper towards the core of L'Ja. How the duo-trionic energy singed behind the gratings which seemed grafted to the skeletal structure of every wall of Hadrian within L'Ja. The metallic grating beneath their feet vibrated slightly as the lift came to a stop and another pneumatically sealed door awaited the Three.

The Aristocrat held the thoughts of the Hunter, causing him to not open the latest door of L'Ja right away as his caution to flowed out instinctively. The dampening field generation of L'Ja's core by their progress from this point on would appreciably affect their powers. The traps of both the Origin Species and the enemy would become far deadlier. They would have to conserve as much ammunition as they would their own energies.

The Three each reached into the dimensional pouch to grab an additional rifle, only this time, of standard Imperium issue for themselves. The Three would heed the call of the war drums with two guns to be shot in the heated style of McCoist charging at the net. The Trinity were infused with too much of Kanu's work ethic for what could be a room full of enemy troops awaiting them in their task at hand. Yet, they were still not afraid.

After slinging her rifles over her shoulders, Fate delved into introspection for the sake of the mission. She had a power up her sleeve, one which she used only in rare circumstances. Fate brought her hands together as if she were in prayer and tightly pressed her hands together and began to open another facet of her own arsenal of freedom.

Fate flowed in the song of her psionic reality. The aged lavender waters smashed themselves violently against the indomitable cliffs of Dover within the bliss of Fate's once innocent mind that somehow remained in balance even if the enemy did its best those same cliffs into a soiled powder. She opened her eyes and reached her mind into the controls systems buried in the geometric marrow of the walls about them to open the door.

As Fate reached to press a neon green holo-glyph that lit up before her to unlock the door ahead of them, she could feel the entire level was filled with the horrid and hissing hideousness of rattlers being burned alive. One of her psionic thoughts shot out through the enemy soldiers to slice them down. Though the enemy is necrotic in nature and Fate abhorred any choice that takes away life, she hated this action as much as she hated her actions throughout the entire war. Fate watched her thoughts flow into the sharpest of efficiencies. A war that had already left her little choice in terms of what one must do for victory. The Dead of the Dead should be no more, she reassured herself. Yet, she was a little beyond what she used to be also and savoured taking the lives of the wretched vermin that lived to end their existence.

Fate started to doubt herself and almost stopped herself but she knew what was at stake and she finished delivering the killing blow in a joyless silence. Her psyogenetics adapted itself and enhanced her darker armour that protected the fragility of what little possibly remained of her blessed purity. Fate looked down at her boots and watched the enemy blood pool at their feet as the door slowly began to open. It seemed as wondrously disgusting as moments of Nero's reign where moral feculence ruled the day. Fate pressed the shattered stick pattern holo-glyph and the door began to open fully to what lay ahead.

The door cranked open and the bodies of the enemy dead lay scattered in a demonic Jonestown throughout a dark hall before the Three. The better preserved lighting tracts made this hall a little more visible than the last but the rotting dead before the Trinity hardly made it a better sight. On the contrary, little seemed different than the last corridor other than the dead, and more sacrifices were made to further along what now seemed something akin to Persephone's rescue.

The Fate turned to the Hunter as they hopped over more of the dead. To ease the tension, Fate telepathically said, in a comfortingly sardonic and darkly optimistic tone, 'Do not worry, my friend. You are still ahead on points.' The Hunter, though amused, was hardly mollified as he believed it to be always his burden. This was the battlefield where war dreams were becoming reality, and there was no other way on the path of war.

The Hunter somehow was not yet feeling the glory of the battle progressing with every step into the occupied hinterland of the Death of Death. For the Hunter, this was not the essence of pursuit, the K'mja, as the H'Raka call it that was once their sport with the creatures of E'de. How reality had digressed, the Hunter thought. At least Fate had entertained them with her inventive attack of altering the genetic makeup of the enemy soldiers by ripping out a few essential chromosomes here and there, causing their neural paths to overload with spectacular haemorrhaging results.

Indeed, the stench of the enemy blood made its way into the Hunter who began to stand at his best for this tour of duty. He was the king that would quench his thirst with country; a country of the slaughter of the enemy who stood against them. If not for the challenge of the dampening fields, there would be no chance for glory. With their powers reduced, this would become the drudgery of the Somme for the Hunter and all the Trinity. But the Hunter, deep within himself was delighted to press on deeper into the bedlam that had become L'Ja.

As Fate walked on she somehow began to feel a coldness that is the captivity of where the path of war had brought them and she felt frigid to her very bones. She could feel the infestation everywhere and all around the Trinity. This place was dank and humid but now felt far above the climactic distinction of Ulan Bator for the Fate. Considering this level had even more geothermal conduits than the last, Fate's chilled heart seemed to be entirely lost. She saw the dead laying about her in every direction as she kept the Trinity on the route to the core.

The Trinity pressed on through what now became seemingly endless rusting and greasy corridors before coming to a set of stairs that was just as dingy as most of the core thus far. This place was already beginning to wear Fate down. The Three were covered in sweat and coolant gases condensed upon them in this messy place. Viscous drops greasily dripped down from Fate's tangled hair as she continued walking on through the electronic subterranean jungle. The hair of the Hunter was similarly drenched into long follicles that now draped down like the talons of a raven. And the Aristocrat's hair looked like he had spent a hard-core night of clubbing. The Aristocrat's body was dripping in just as many oceans of sweat as did his comrades.

They knew the silent stairs before them would have to taken below. The chill of this place seemed to grow as Fate moved deeper into the hellish field of fire, and such cold fires they were. The Trinity moved on below to continue to risk it all for the sake of freedom.

Φ

Something was bound to go wrong in such a weakened state of being. After zig-zagging, blind corner fire fights with enemy platoons, and after descending the stairs of what felt like a thousand CN towers, the ordeal that is the path of war was bound to land the Trinity finding themselves in a trap. Their battle senses adapted to be so heightened that the Three ignored the obvious.

In a small corridor, a pressure plate was activated by the presence overhead of the Trinity. Moloko's time was now. Splintered particle chains flew like javelin tossed teal hued neon train rails hard tackling their way across the walls of what had become a miserable place. One hit the Aristocrat on the left side of his rib cage, one particle rail shattered the side of Fate's right knee, and one cracked apart the right shin of the Hunter.

A door swept open. Fifteen enemy soldiers oozed out from it firing. Fate and the Aristocrat fell to the ground writhing in pain from the cloaked enemy trap. Fate chided herself for not being more vigilant as she lay beside the Aristocrat in agony. The Hunter somehow stayed on his feet returning fire, as if he were an American fighting the Cong, until all the enemy puppet drones before the Trinity were all dead or he was. He held his nova-pulse rifle and blew away the smoke that rushed out of its thick barrel. His pain was so excruciating that he was laughing at it.

Fate clenched her latest At'Lann equivalent pulse-rifle that fell with her to the grating of the ground as the Hunter helped her to her feet before doing the same for the Aristocrat. The Hunter looked to her consolingly as she was braver than most but Fate should not expect to be everything. The equally stunned Aristocrat brushed himself off and pulled out some Lon'tus cigarettes from his personal platinum case for the Three. Fate felt eased of her pain just by the offering. The blast had left her with a slight limp. Her healing factor, as it was with the rest of the Trinity, was all but off-line. She lacked the strength to heal herself of her minor wounds no matter her psionic repairs. The pain remained and Fate was glad to enjoy a Lon'tus cigarette.

The pain almost consumed Fate as she took in a drag, and she felt ashamedly jubilant by it. The Fate laughed, as if in fever, as the sweat continued to drip down her face and body. The Hunter and the Aristocrat hardly seemed better off and were hardly amused in their battle aches. Their bodies were cut open and battered from multiple enemy hits from energy bullets to the latest trap. Their condition would slow their progress of what had become something beyond a pilgrimage. The Three continued to rest for a moment knowing they had to push on. Their fate depended upon it. The Trinity continued on the dark descent of the path of war deep in L'Ja's wired heart.

Φ

The Three were able to make it to a position two levels below where they had been battered by the particle rails. They found a ventilation shaft to secure for another moment of rest. The Trinity were still en route to the core. Their current location seemed far removed from the path of days before their steps upon the surface sands. The Trinity sat back against the dusty and greasy walls with a final cigarette before the last leg of their journey into L'Ja.

The Aristocrat was injured to an extreme that he wore his suffering wearily. The son of Lon'tus still had enough strength within him to push on and take up their watch. The Hunter, ever the perfectionist, was fully engaged in bandaging his battlefield wounds thinking of all that lay ahead. He knew this path of war for the H'Raka would be one of their most gruelling yet. The Fate, getting to the point where she was nearly overcome by all the pain inflicted upon her tried to psionically exhale it away with her smoke. Her bones, after the last engagement, were all but shattered, and held in place by the tightness of her slender musculature as well as a telekinetic endo-skeletal integrity field-emitter.

The device was a mauve amethyst like crystal triangle the size of a cameo which Fate slapped unto her tank top above the Imperium crest after pulling it out of the medical-kit from her dimensional pouch. She kept herself awake out of fear that her dreams would only continue her horror.

The Three Crusaders had the feel of soldiers left behind in the Demyansk Kessel as their cold seemed to grow amidst the rising heat, and left them almost wondering if their cold carcasses would be left to be eaten and defiled. The Trinity had to believe they were close to their goal as they were already paying a heavy physical penance for what became their ground war. Though outgunned, the Three had made it deeper into the mechanical sepulchre of L'Ja's heart than any of their kind had since the more ancient times.

Seeing the enemy consume their own dead to retain their strength against the Trinity showed Fate how far she had gone. Pleasant musings of reality all but seemed lost. Reality was far more difficult to liberate in their own domain. This place had become yet another dark lair of the enemy that even encroached into the trans-psionic. Fate was worn down by the pain and the frigid wasteland of suffering felt in her soul. She knew she had her own prophecies to fulfil. The Trinity had to win at any costs, by any means necessary they would have to overcome this stretch of the path of war.

Blessedly, the Three found a chance to think of the salvation of hope once again in their moments before pushing ahead. The cramped confines of the dingy ventilation shaft brought their bond with one another to a whole new transcendence and enlightenment. The Trinity did not utter a word to one another but spoke deeply with their usual eloquence to one another through their telepathic link. During their latest rest, the Three went through a variety of topics before the time came to move on with the mission.

Fate revealed to the Hunter and the Aristocrat that she would find her soul mate of love on a path far removed from this one. Waiting for it was another sacrifice for the sake of the war she told them. She confessed her grief of At'Lann's losses had struck her so violently that vengeance was all that kept her going. 'I am a ghost,' she sobbed in her thoughts. She became a little more of what she was and lightened things back up by suggesting a vacation to M'Goa at the end of this latest round with the dark forces of the Death of Death.

The Hunter confided he no longer felt a pressure to succeed rather a pressure to survive. He said they were making their way through the sludge of madness that was the infestations but defeat always seemed imminent. Together, he still thought, they could make it to the core. The Hunter still carried less and more selflessness to the Trinity as part of him still existed to earn Y'vis's praise and to be found worthy of his legacy. The length of the war had begun to humble him and he too felt his pain pressure-cooking and cauterising the tragedies that inflicted themselves upon his beautiful soul. He almost felt betrayed by his soul of scribe quill and sword. The war seemed to rob him of his callings, and felt his soul could never again touch the sky like the first steps of Remus and Romulus.

The Aristocrat lamented the vacancy of culture even more than any in the Trinity. Deep down, the Aristocrat hated war and one that already had stripped away the destinies of great peoples across existence including their own. This place for him truly seemed as great a precipice as was felt by those left behind at Dunkirk. With so much invested in them it was all but expected that the battle would be theirs. But expectations on this world, like those of war do, not come easily.

The Hunter and the Fate nodded in consensus with their faithful comrade, who always aspired to the grace of living, that that they had to push on for the sake of life. Existence itself depended upon it, and the Aristocrat was the cherished eloquence and refinement that kept the momentum going for the evolution of the Trinity. For the Aristocrat was the great motivator. The Hunter patted him on the back before leading the pack along in their weakened, lumbering state.

Fate communicated the path to the Hunter while she took on the watch of their flank as they once again continued to descend even lower. The humid plaque stained ventilation shaft became the latest route to the core of L'Ja. In their current state, the Trinity walked as mortals. They vowed to continue pressing on to the core or die along the way. And no one, even bludgeoned and battered in the Trinity, wanted to die by being buried alive in the technological sarcophagus that is the underground of L'Ja.

Φ

Days turned weeks and weeks to months, and soon it was no longer pleasant or inspiring to think of how long the Trinity had been fighting their way through the hot, humid gunk all the way through to the core of L'Ja. Ooze like that left behind by the liquefaction of fire-ants was inches thick on every floor and on the walls of every corridor. The deeper the Trinity went into the maze of geothermal conduits and bio-gel circuitry, the enclosing only seemed to grow thicker. However, the Three made it far enough to know they where they were and to know they were close. In this latest boiler room type sub-level, a more critical defensive posture was held by an enemy encampment the Trinity spied upon.

The Trinity were down to their last few rifles, explosives, and munitions as well as being down to the wire in terms of how much more of this they could take. If this was not the moment to break one of the last of the latest enemy lines, they no longer knew when it would be. And if they would not break free, the Three would be left with only their fists to pound into hopeless exhaustion of being buried alive and waiting to be purged from reality.

At the end of yet another ancient hall, an enemy unit protected a position using a regenerative force-field pill-box configuration. The Three each began to take turns firing away at it before retreating behind the protection of a corner provided by a pewter hued corrugated bio-gel conduit filled with luminous green biochemical components. The cleaner passage itself, if not for the fire-fight, was lit by a dim mulberry hinted glow that ran through the ceiling of the story high passage.

Fate could see clearly that the pillbox was defending a tremendous source of power. This could only mean that the Trinity had arrived at the core. Out from the pillbox volleyed away plasma charges with the speed of a viper and the thunderous permafrost shattering power expelled from the main gun of an ancient T-72. Worst of all, the weapons of the Trinity were all but ineffective against that which stood between them and a large dark lime hued marble steel looking door that would be the last before the core. They sat once again for what became another countless time behind a defensive wall, only to listen and watch the enemy fire fly by.

The brutal strength of the enemy artillery was comparable to that of quantum pulse energy, and the Fate heard the blasts ricochet off a row of adjacent conduction coil tanks in a plundered regatta of explosive consequences. The Hunter squeezed off a few remaining rounds of his nova-pulse rifle before ducking back around the corner with the cliché of enemy rounds ripping, shredding, and puncturing into the bio-gel conduit corner as he returned to the safety of their defensive position. Fourteen enemy soldier drones were encamped inside the rather large pillbox that could still call upon reinforcements from other sections of the L'Ja interior.

Fate could see in her mind how the Death of Death had imbued them with only the desire to destroy life. She could see it within the vapid empty shells of the enemy which fired away at them viciously from their so far impenetrable pillbox.

Fate wondered if she killed them how many it would bring the total to of all the enemy she had killed by her own hand on this path. Many thousands? Many tens of thousands? Many million? Many trillions fighting back? She had lost track. Death was everywhere and time no longer seemed to matter. Fate had let herself be denigrated into a position where survival and success had become a seemingly never ending quest.

As she sat back in the muck she thought, 'Is this my essence?' Fate no longer knew what she was except she had every sanction to be a merciless soldier against the evil the Trinity continued to face. Ghosts of enlightened purity were the relics of her soul. Fate constantly judged herself far too harshly, and even with the misery of war, Fate was still the wrath of all that was left behind.

The Aristocrat was equally as weary. He was still the dashing Imperator of the Lon'tus though he sat so grimly for one of the few who did so much. He perished a terrifying thought that reality had been torn away in his absence and he was all that remained of the Lon'tus. As he took his shots he feared the enemy trap was to imprison them in a false path on L'Ja while Lon'tus falls to disunity and erasure. A multitude of senses and abilities seemed hardly enough to know what to do. He wanted out of this nightmare just as much as Fate and even the Hunter to some degree. The Aristocrat kept himself going with thoughts of Rimisz'tii and of Lon'tus, and of their seas and shores. He was, after all, the pace of the Trinity.

The Hunter had the glazed, post-orgasmic eyes of a GI that had cut the ears off the decapitated heads of Cong to complete a trophy necklace. Everything seemed utterly tragic and reckless in all the chaos. He tossed his depleted rifle to the metallic floor, and reached into the dimensional pouch to grab a genetic de-cloaking and intensifying module. It appeared as a rectangular onyx stone that folded onto his belt buckle.

The Hunter had noticed this hallway was of the same configuration as the last they had bludgeoned their way through. Since they could not yet activate the main systems, the Hunter decided it was time to overload them into activation so that L'Ja's defences could finish the enemy for them. He would hold on to hope that he would survive and that the enemy would not.

The Hunter explained his plan of directly accessing L'Ja's systems and its probable outcomes. Even at their peak levels the idea had been discouraged as too dangerous but the Hunter convinced his comrades that the access juncture for the L'Ja data-stream was fully integrated at this level for the entire planetary core.

As he would dive into the L'Ja data-stream, the Hunter would be met by the same particles chains that would hit the pillbox and would hopefully destroy it. It would go off like a neutron bomb so the Hunter explained to his comrades to be ready by doing what they could to stabilise their psyogenetic structures. The Hunter folded additional units onto his comrades and explained they would automatically activate when he made contact. There would only be one chance for success and even the Fate had her misgivings.

'Do not take this path. Even I do not know what this will do to change your existence,' Fate pleaded.

'My honour would forsake me if I did not become one with the legendary weapons of L'Ja. This is my place in the Trinity to choose. You especially should not demand to take upon yourself every burden. You and 'Lus have done almost all you can. I will do this. If I survive, I will remain true', the Hunter said assuredly with his thoughts.

Without any further hesitation the Hunter nodded to Fate and she nodded back with her eyes. He wave saluted to the Aristocrat, and the Hunter walked casually into the hallway that continued to be a field of fire. He pressed the onyx cloak once to deactivate it as the Hunter viciously and methodically plunged his fist in a lightning strike like that of Thor's through the metallic floor into a bio-gel data conduit that flowed through all of L'Ja's interface system.

In one mountain shattering strike, the path of war changed. The defensive mechanisms of the hallway automatically registered the Hunter as a threat as it did with the Fate and the Aristocrat who held onto one another around the corner. The hall became a killing field as L'Ja's defensive systems unleashed a girandole shower of countless faster than light particle chains across the core.

The enemy pillbox and its enemy soldiers were instantly vaporised in the shower and waves of fuchsia flames. The Aristocrat and the Fate left the cover of their taxed psionic cast shelters, all but worn into a refuse pile, into the now bright and smoky hallway with weapons raised and with guarded stances. The Hunter had somehow done it. They rushed to where the Hunter lay sprawled char-broiled, bleeding, and broken on the ground. Through their link they had felt the Hunter momentarily gain access to L'Ja's systems as his psyogenetic structure locked, allowing for him to survive his plunge into the sea of ancient thorns.

The exposed conduit began to automatically reconstruct itself around the fuchsia hued data energy stream, and only a trace of bio-gel remained on the Hunter's fist which had all of its knuckles broken. He was lucky to have survived his contact with a soul-stream like Tesla's. The regenerative shields of the enemy were no match for the falling axe of L'Ja's traps. Fate estimated that almost half of the enemy occupation force had succumbed to similar fates across the core, and smiled in her pain as she could feel the momentum shifting.

The Hunter's blood dripped, burned, and smouldered as much as his usually impervious skin had been inflicted with the torment of particle fire. Fate knew of no other being who had ever survived such a massive bombardment before. 'He truly walks the path of the Trinity,' the Fate and the Aristocrat thought together in mutual astonishment.

'You are a mess, my friend. Remove your mind from worry. You will heal quickly,' Fate said with shocked casualness.'

Fate flash-folded the last of their medicine, a psyogenic renewing mist of trans-psionic particles over his battered form. She spread the malachite fog telekinetically over the Hunter with a revitalising sweep of her hand. He was barely conscious as the Aristocrat placed in his hands a fully charged At'Lann rifle which just had to do. The Fate and the Aristocrat then dragged the Hunter to a sniper's position before the coveted door and signalled with a wink as he awakened that he could fire at will.

The Fate phased her hand into and through the wall beside the door before them. Her out of phase hand disrupted the L'Ja interface locking mechanism with a gentler stroke to begin to finish what the Hunter had started. Fate only dipped her feet into its data-stream, and she could see it could now be theirs. The Trinity could make things happen. The oak thick door whirred up and out of sight.

Their weapons were set by the Hunter for full tracking mode. No matter where an enemy would flee a Hiroshima damaging bullet would follow. There would be no need for any backtracking and it would never have to be done again. The last of their arms would have to suffice. Out of breath and more comatose than cognisant, the Hunter began to fire away into the inner central chamber. After only a brief moment, he collapsed as his body could not heal quickly enough to carry on. Fate and the Aristocrat let loose their battle cry and stormed the final inner chamber.

At last. Their goal had been reached. And now everything was on the line. The pair found themselves in a inner chamber with a different dimensional configuration as the wall became the floor. The blue fluorescent glow seemed to give the room a chilled feel to it. At its centre was a great glowing sphere, nearly the size of a typical At'Lann scout-ship, which was the source of the forget-me-not hued seemingly ever expanding glow. There were three, story high, aquamarine nave banners of luminescent *dixeritium* plating hanging, slicing the compressed cylindrical chamber into thirds around the central glowing sphere, the true core of L'Ja.

The Fate and the Aristocrat made the last of the necrotic enemy soldiers that guarded the central chamber say hello to the firepower of their little friends as they blasted away. The Fate found it all deceivingly climactic as her rifle went off with a *Pum Pum Pum Fump Pum.* With the chamber secure with the last enemy falling to the Trinity, the Fate and the Aristocrat dragged in the Hunter, and locked the only door in and out, like sealing the lid of a coffin before a dirt as dry as L'Ja's desert would fall upon it.

'Time to alter the interface of this ancient world to our needs', the Fate said to the Aristocrat implying also that their time was running out and a little alchemy would be required.

She could feel what remained of the infestation converging on their location. Her rifle could no longer charge. She reached into her pouch and there were no weapons or munitions left. Fate could barely stand, her brow was covered with sweat and violet blood. She tossed away her arms and took hold of one of the Hunter's which could still squeeze off a few rounds. The Hunter lay hunched against the wall inactive and not moving. The Aristocrat had about as many rounds left as the Fate, and he knew he would have to make every shot count. Fate could feel the enemy would soon break through.

The Aristocrat tapped his mind, as did the Fate, and each dove into the immense data-stream of the L'Ja interface that was strangled in the assimilating modifications that the enemy had built into it. It was like diving into Mooney's Bay after a heavy summer rain. Fate kissed his cheek. 'Work quickly,' she whispered to him with her thoughts. She had a right to be paranoid as enemy forces seemed on the brink of breaking through.

Decrypting enemy lockouts and defensive systems in the data-stream loomed as a even more daunting challenge. They had to swim faster than they ever had before. For in their weakened states, the Trinity would make for quick prey.

The Aristocrat's mind reconfigured itself to operate as if everything was under control. He immersed his mind like a gliding dive off the peak of Gibraltar and plunged deeper into the data-streams than he ever had before. Like the caressing dive of a polar bear gently into the ice, Fate dove into the murky interface waters.

The Hunter would have to hold out until the pair could inject a decryption sequence directly into the data-bed at the deepest depth of a energy churning sea of dark orange and bone white firestorms.

The legacy before Sin and the dark temper of Fate seemed all but exhausted as she let off her mauve trans-psionic shot to the data ocean floor through the temple of her now sinking head. She began to sink to the bottom of the dark Gatanica like waters. The Gatan, of course, being a spirit, a sub-consciousness of any data stream. A flow often unappreciated, yet a great paradigm of the universe, and one of the Imperium's catalysts for change.

Fate could no longer remain in the L'Ja data-stream and had to make her way back to reality before she would drown. It would have to be up to the Aristocrat as she could do no more. Fate flash-folded back into reality. Fate found that thanks to her improved psyogenetic structure, she was still able to modify her natural psionic energy to telekinetically open psionic disruptions through small swirling fold-gates. Her mauve energy ripped out into reality like throwing stars cast towards the darkest storm. She fired a few trans-phase micro-quantum pulses through the wall to the eventual storming of the inverted Bastille.

She was able to shoot off six before being reduced once again to a more mortal existence. She picked up the Hunter's storm-knocker that still had a precious few rounds remaining. She steadied the weapon and aimed at the onyx door.

' 'Lus, please hurry,' Fate pleaded while trying to contain the lava flows of her anxiousness.

She could feel the weight of the sinister grow around her. Fear grew around her as every successive and concussive pounding on that lonely door heralded the flood of vermin before another gate to the onslaught of Hell's fury. Then a split-second seemed to fall into hours as Cronos seemed to stumble into a silent snow and bleed as the Hunter did. A stream of his blood abundantly began to flow to the centre of the chamber.

The Hunter started to convulse in silent and time stretched shudders. Somehow, the Hunter brought himself to his hulk-a-sized feet. The door exploded in a spattering of both ancient and sizzling dust. The Hunter reborn in his second wind cocked his rifle and fired away at the enemy, who surged like a mob mass through the door, with what nova-pulse rounds remained. Fate steadied her weapon once more before firing at the dark penetrating invaders. How she savoured the moment that could just as easily be that of their final stand.

Deep in the data-stream, the Aristocrat found an epiphany, a solution, to their perilous enigma. Three became one as revelation became computation. The Aristocrat split his world casting hand into three and discovered the desired access inter-link. He swam through the access stream. His mind became the bridge to a unity of technologies. The L'Ja interface was brought on-line and reconfigured by the Aristocrat to Imperium standards. The momentum shifted once again over.

A shunt was spread across as many elliptically, nearing spherical, trans-temporal junctions by the immense and ancient interface. The combined L'Ja and psyogenetic technology inter-link transformed itself into maximum output which, like a wounded falcon surrounded by prey taking flight, removed the dampening field. The Trinity were restored to their proper balance. Their enhanced psyogenetic powers were fully restored in the same moment the Aristocrat set the L'Ja's central core for automatic destructive overload. Fate hoped her cousins remembered to enact the command they would need to rely upon.

The Fate, Hunter, and Aristocrat fired like quicksilver the last few psionic pulses at their repulsive targets. The Fate blew a both seductive and vindictive kiss of death to the enemy who still poured in. The Trinity felt their strength restored as they saw a way out of this buried distortion of the path of war. Fate looked calmly to those who stood at her side knowing how they had all been robbed of so much. The Trinity flash-folded out of the existence of L'Ja; as the world exploded like the death of Vega. The amber hued gravimetric shock-wave ruptured through the entire L'Ja system. And L'Ja was destroyed.

The Trinity were able to flash-fold themselves onto a nearby Lon'tus dreadnought, the 'Tainja, the ship which was Nul'lus's father's captaincy in the days before the ambassador to At'Lann. 'Lîna's cousins had come through for the Trinity. From the greasy and infected ancient marrow, the Trinity came to collapse flash-folding onto grey and burgundy St. Anthony's like cross adorned couches. The 'Tainja, located a sector away from L'Ja, could only watch as the planet of L'Ja became galactic debris for the galactic museum.

The Trinity found themselves in the parlour reserved for the Lon'tus Imperator. His private interface terminal popped up and zipped across its holo-display a plethora of new data.

The first ring of conjoined ships of the enemy had crackled apart like a platinum bracelet of thorns dipped in psionic liquid nitrogen. By using the technology of L'Ja to alter the flow of reality, the enemy's corporeal stranglehold over what remained was, for now, at an end by doing to them what the enemy would have done to them. Except the Trinity did it first. The Aristocrat was able to alter the resonance flow of reality.

Realising the enemy would continue to use L'Ja as a way out of their realm, and would stop at nothing to once again obtain this far too valuable technology, the Aristocrat destroyed the mechanical world.

The Aristocrat had solved the enigma machines of L'Ja before the enemy, and with the result being Imperium space was further reinforced from enemy incursions. And with the enemy fleet cracked in more manageable morsels, the Imperium fleet was able to move in and make quick work of the decapitated heads of the Hydra. The Imperium forces launched an automatic offensive that reduced the enemy forces into minute fractional remnants of their previous strength though its remains were still a threat along with the dreaded and horrific erasure that still awaited. Their hell spawned reinforcements would still come from a realm the Trinity had yet to access other than on the psionic plane.

The Three looked at each other with long awaited relief as a continent or two fell away from Atlas's shoulders. Their bodies were covered in sweat, dirt, dried blood, deep gashes, cuts, abrasions, and even a little disenchantment as they realised their victory in the battle and felt everything change. Their wounds from being hit in the field of fire were countless. The nightmare had ebbed for now.

The Trinity tried to relax as they reclined and let the burning of their wounds heal. How a shower became so prized even with the ability for psionic bathing. It was as if they had become the dignified rubble and shambles of Dresden. Their well earned rest came with an extremely intense restlessness. From this point on, the momentum of the war shifted so dramatically to the cause of the Imperium that it seemed both false and surreal, even superficial. It was the uncertainty ahead that plagued the Three.

Except for facing the Death of Death in the shadows of the mind, the Trinity of the wind, water, and moon had yet to directly face the living embodiment of viciously imposed nothingness and erasure. The burnt skies they flew away from still loomed with the spectre of final erasure that affected everything remaining in existence. Would the Three prevail? Fate looked upon their wrecked forms and then with mild shock as she read for the first time the date on the interface. The Trinity had been in the tomb of L'Ja for four of their years. Their sacrifice had never to dawned on them until now. Time, even though running out, seemed to have taken on less meaning during the intensity of the battle inside L'Ja.

Fate stared out to a giant rhombus shaped, thick plated window to a space where many of the candles of its cathedral had been snuffed out. Reality had changed for the better and for the worse. The view seemed a pale reflection of what it had been. She stared blankly and sombrely. Fate said with a shell-shocked and tattered crispness,

'At what cost came with this day?'

No one knew.

30
Languishing in Restlessness

It was an uneasy voyage home for the Trinity. The Imperium they returned to was as psychologically and as temporally worn as they were. The flow of life hardened itself to expect the worse. Everyone seemed to wonder where it all had gone. The Trinity could feel there had been a mass paranoia that the Trinity had been lost to erasure, and that the doom of final defeat had become even more impending than it already was. The Imperium culture had become far more mistrusting and selfishly fearful.

The forces of the Imperium, even with the return of the Trinity, had lost their morale, and were exhausted from their efforts even at peak strength. What was considered their cause became one of little hope even with the victory over the First Ring on L'Ja. With the return of the Three, the hopes and happiness could bloom once again in a field like Flanders torn far more asunder than when they had left. Even as their people found their cause to be one to be joyous about once again, for the first time in years at that, the winds of Hebe seemed withered in the hearts of the Three.

The Trinity had spent years in the dank, dark cellar of Tartarus, as if surrounded by the submerged dead of the *Kursk*. And even after all they had been through on the path of war, none of them considered that they had earned any sort of victory. For only in the nightmares of Fate had they fought the true face of the enemy, the ever-changing face of evil. They were an immortal, yet very mortal, infantry that had strived to have the strength like that of an undying six hundred and seven still trapped in the Crimean.

The Fate and the Hunter transferred to the Lis'talla, which came alongside the 'Tainja, as the Aristocrat, who remained on board had to return to Lon'tus as he was on time to give his blessing to the players of Lon'tus telekinetic football for their world cup championship match on the Lon'tus home-world.

He had often joked that the bulk of his support came from his decision not to cancel the tournaments during the course of the war, and from what Fate knew of the Lon'tus people, he may have been right. Eager to see the match, to return home, and to forget about the war until he would have to step back upon their fields once again, the Aristocrat bade his mates farewell as the 'Tainja warped home. In a way, everyone needed time to heal.

The Fate would have went to the Lon'tus home-world as well to enjoy the match but the call of her home compelled her to return to a place the years, at times, became one that was all but forgotten. As they watched the 'Tainja warp-stream away, the Hunter and the Fate, who returned to the Lis'talla, were greeted by a familiar face who the Fate had left so much for her care. 'Ivia fourth-walled in from the main hanger where she had given medals and greeted their victorious pilots. She was now in the gathering space of 'Lîna's quarters which remained untouched until the Trinity returned.

'Imperiatrix, I return to you what has always been yours. The crew of the Lis'talla standby awaiting your orders', said an overjoyed 'Ivia

'Thank you, Fleet Admiral', Fate said with a wink to her official greeting.

'Very well then. Set a course for home with a detour to Kul'mir along the way.'

'I will see to it at once. The bridge is yours any time you wish.'

Fate saw that this soul from 'Xo had never for a moment lost her faith in her. Her well placed covenant remained with her. 'Ivia had maintained her ship and the fleet with a most diligently and most precious care. With the enemy fleet reduced to something akin to being treats for piranha, the vastly expanded Imperium fleet could now maximise its efforts in deploying spatial shunts to slow the rate of erasure.

Advances in their Imperium technology even led to relatively fewer enemy incursion into the ever shrinking reach of Imperium space. And now, due to erasure and deployment, the Imperium reached across all that remained of existence. What was left of the universe was theirs in a sadness like that of Midas's grasp. Still, Fate was quite pleased with the effort of one like her.

'Ivia had just as much of a sense of order as that of Za'szu's and 'Zaya's. Later that day, Fate bestowed the ethnarchy of her people as 'Ivia's new crown. She was worthy enough, in the eyes of Fate, to have sovereignty thrust upon her as her peoples voice within the Imperium. Her home world was set to join the Tr'Lann system as it was Fate's choice to bestow safe harbours upon models of virtue. 'Ivia would not disappoint as she kissed Fate's hand graciously and humbly before fourth-walling back to the bridge. The Hunter looked to the Fate with a persuading smile as he brought up a interface holo-display.

The course for Kul'mir had been plotted and engaged with the efficiency of 'Ivia and with a professionalism above her usual high standards. The Hunter had convinced the Fate to go with him to the planet of H'Renn's macro-villa on one of H'Raka's royal retreat planets set aside for the K'or. Already they missed the Aristocrat after their claustrophobic tour of duty. After modifying their clothes and style to the latest trends of the Imperium, the Fate and the Hunter went to the bridge to watch the few stars that remained glide by on the main holo-screen.

As if Fate had only been gone a day, she sat once again in her favourite centre seat as the Hunter stood quietly at her side watching the stars that remained stream by on the screen. The crew went about their duties as if nothing had changed. For the first time in a long time, Fate felt as close as she could to being complete. It was a new day again. As she sat back, Fate wondered what Za'szu and 'Zaya would think of her now.

Φ

The watery crimson sky was stretching itself into a wondrous peculiarity of sunshine splashing down on sands like those seen along the east coast of Ionia. The jagged, ashen mountains seemed a world away in the distance as the Fate and the Hunter strolled down a beach of inviting heat of waters that had the temperature of half that of boiling water. It was a welcome change from an L'Ja that, at times, had been both bone-chilling and confining. Though somehow less of the heat could be felt by them through their tactile senses, it was still a welcome feeling.

The Lis'talla stood by orbiting Kul'mir along with twenty H'Raka super-dreadnoughts over a world owned by H'Renn since his first days in the H'Raka Imperial Military Academy. Both the Fate and the Hunter walked quietly in the sun toward a rock vista of bone, mint hued coral. The two shared their thoughts to one another on what had been the necessity of desecrating a section of the galactic museum.

Even as psyogenetic beings, there were many beings above them, and their actions would be noticed whether those higher beings took the path of war or not. Such was the path of life. And though those above them seemed to pay no heed to the call of war, and seemed to all but crave the descent into erasure, they could still be ethereally sentimental about what they once were.

But as they walked in their here and now, the pair felt a small measure of exhilaration that their methods were seemingly beginning to pay off and their rule as split corporeal vessels was not opposed other than by the enemy. Their place and theirs alone would chart the history of their peoples as they saw fit.

The Trinity had made itself absolute, and enough so for the Fate to indulge her more hedonistic side, and told the Hunter she would take in a retreat of her own as she enjoyed the sunshine of a world like H'Raka. However, the Hunter told her he came to Kul'mir not for its beauty specifically but to train for what lay ahead. On a faraway temporal stream, Fate was the first to return to what seemed only like another day that made for a beautiful memory.

'So you are off to M'Goa before you return to At'Lann?' the Hunter queried the Fate with a friendly, almost excited expression.

'Only for a week. Besides, like the M'Goa continue to teach us, to fight for freedom is to experience freedom. And I will continue to do both. After L'Ja, we all need a vacation and that is where I choose to go,' said the Fate admitting her desire for a guilty pleasure taken before returning home to her people.

Fate preferred to remain blind to her own deification and remain true to her old reclusive and individual path alone which she had always walked. Her family did its best to put up with her free-spirited nature that also would have to be understood by the Trinity as her way. She looked away from the shimmering ruby waters full of notable aquatic predators, and looked to H'Renn's macro-villa. It was like looking to ancient Roma, and she felt the same uncertainty in her decadent silence before it was overrun by another horde.

In the temporal stream, a future Fate wondered if Roma would ever again rise from the ashes of Hy'Bor. Of course, it would all never happen if the universe ceased to exist as existence was still caught, and all time streams and dimensional streams would cease to exist as well. The Fate on Kul'mir had a flash of what was to be. Existence was still caught in the tide of erasure which dissipated all realities into nothingness. And nothing was safe anymore.

The vision for the Fate on Kul'mir was startling and disturbing, yet not particularly powerful. Everyone knew what lay ahead if the enemy was not stopped. The fact that she did not drop to her knees in a stigmatic ecstasy reminded her of how much of the war Fate always carried with her. Though it did cast gloom once again over her.

'What do you see?' the Hunter calmly asked.

'I see a place that does not yet exist but one that is still approaching ceasing to exist. The path ahead is uncertain,' Fate said with an almost disgusted regret.

She was the future, yet she could barely see her own reflection in it. Ominously, she was fast becoming blind to what was to come. All she felt she could do was watch as they lost everything to doom-fall. Fate continued to torture her fragmented soul. She conveyed her grim outlook to the Hunter who tried not to think of such things. Though the Fate confided in him with a resolute tone,

'The enemy has been given its form throughout their battles with existence by interpreting and transforming itself into an amalgam of all our collective fears and evils. We have been fighting generations of darkness at the end of their evolution. The Death of Death, on the other hand, is constructing itself from my battles with its dark spirit in my nightmares.'

'I know, 'Imiszi. Why else would you take it upon yourself to battle the Death of Death alone so that it may choose a corporeal form, and so that we can at last slay the Death of Death. A bold strategy to choose if all that will remain for you is to have the Death of Death in your nightmares.'

'Ever since our battlefield mind-link on L'Ja. The three that we are and will grow to become, have evolved our psyogenetic incorporation to become interchangeable and segments of one another, 'Iato. The three of us automatically search for more efficient psyogenetic sub-materials to interchange from each other to evolve us beyond that which we once could only dream of. Three have are now closer to one. For example, many of my enhanced reflexes are now H'Raka in origin just as you and 'Lus have enhanced At'Lann senses as part of your psyogenetic structures.'

She continued with, 'Our psionic mental functions has made it possible for the enemy to take on a more vulnerable form. My ethics may be forlorn to do what must be done but whatever I have become but I would never have been able to survive without some of your instincts and warrior's ways. Years ago, I was a pacifist and now I have become the blood-stained salvation of my people. What will come, I no longer see. The path ahead is uncertain.'

The Hunter was just as perplexed by what was already known amongst the Trinity to be true as he was by the uncertainty of the impasse ahead. Fate's words came not as revelation but that of the sacred truth of their path.

He could feel her temperance becoming a part of him along with the polish of the Aristocrat which became endowed in both the Fate and the Hunter. He wondered if a part of her simply did not want to tell him the path ahead was covered in darkness. The wildcard of their evolution was that they could now access the abilities of their temporal chromosomes, and existence would become a symphony of experiential multi-streams. Things had indeed changed.

The Hunter left behind sonnet and stanza for sword and shield, and in following the path of war had let so much of himself die and be consumed by battle that little of once was his art seemed lost in the flow of the Imperium Interface. He had lost his inspiration, his muse, from an enemy blitz in the years he was away from H'Raka, and had become consumed by his orgasmic rush that comes with battle joy. And though any joy in war is a scarce but necessary commodity, this war had began to cost him dearly. 'What have I become?' he wondered. He was H'Raka's blade and after L'Ja, he needed to once again hone his own.

Both he and the Fate wondered how many had they killed, and how many of their soldiers they sent out only to become fallen and dying like those left on the wrong shore of the Dnieper. They lived in times where even Atlas would have fallen under his burden and would lay crushed. The two walked on with their thoughts intertwined. They had to prevail in order to fulfil the promise of all their sacrifices.

The Hunter then threw a psionic harpoon into the jade waters just beyond the tranquilly harsh shores before the shore of his macro-villa. As the multi-tethered heads of the of the harpoon shot out in a fan like pattern in a mere blink, the scores of hooked tips surrounded and morphed to envelop a tan and steel serpentine shark of the N'mrada order, roughly the size of a mature redwood. Seems the Hunter had a change of heart about cloning and modifying the ancient Qus'na shark of the H'Raka of old. A psionic sphere of subtly crackling crimson energy trapped the stunning pursuer that levitated by and above the pair as the sun began to sink lazily over the mountainous and ocean horizon of this H'Raka world.

Fate looked up at the sphere cage that was thrice her arms length away from her right side. She gazed upon the great beast suspended in water and marvelled at its horned fins and seamless skin. Fate turned her gaze to the Hunter.

''Iato, what do you feel?' asked the Fate to an introspective Hunter who psionically held the beast above them with great ease. His words were also of revelation but a revelation far more cryptic in its scope.

'I feel that I am one with the path I have chosen and that I cannot escape my fate. But let your pain free you, 'Imiszi. Three are one and one are three. Let the Death of Death come to us. Why else would we be asleep? I sometimes see as you see and I will say the Two Ring beast will cast a shadow upon us until he reaches the universal core of the At'Lann system. We have time to prepare, and we have time to be ready.'

The Hunter with an Augustine confidence sailed the psionic sphere past the surf and back to being above the sea. He released the newly created beast with a splashy thud.

'But what of the shadow that which remains over us now?' countered the Fate.

The Hunter was reluctant but he did answer with what seemed a riddle for them both to ponder.

'We live as we should while time allows, and we should always strive to be what we are and what we shall become. If one is poisoned long enough in a den of vipers, one can live to another day', said the Hunter.

'Can they?', Fate countered.

'Only if their path is true'

The pair looked out to the glorious red sun and baked on the coral rock vista that they had made their way to. The Fate clasped his forearms then shook his hand and pressed his to hers as if to hold a pane of existence that bonds them together vertically from the ground. With a kiss on the cheek, she bade him farewell as she flash-folded herself back to the Lis'talla to leave for M'Goa. It was all so different after their time of battle on L'Ja, and now it was time to remember again what freedom is while there was still time.

Φ

Fate sat back on the centre-seat of the main bridge of the Lis'talla in what became the briefest of appearances since she returned to her ship to head to M'Goa. The sight of dwindled stars, and the once over-abundantly sparkling tranquillity the Lis'talla travelled through were hardly the graces to see that they once were to the Fate. She felt displaced and lost, and Fate felt emptier than she ever had before in her own flawed perfection. At least, 'Ivia's attempts to bring cheer to one so close to her left her in a somewhat mollified mood than she felt since the Trinity left L'Ja.

Still, the Fate smiled at 'Ivia as she produced two gene-storage slide amassed in their advanced Malthusian campaigns. She asked Fate which hand holds the entire species and chain of life of the Di'lora galaxy.

Fate chided her, ''Ivia, really. Your left has it and in your right holds the life components of the B'lka galaxy'.

Fate sardonically joked for her not to use them as coasters as she brought up on the holo-interface the extent of the Imperium gene-storage data-bank. 'Ivia tried to make her feel gratified that the length they had to go to probably saved the lives of all the life-forms threatened by erasure. But Fate needed time to be alone, and though happy for 'Ivia's company, told her what she desired until they would reach M'Goa.

'Ivia took her hand and kissed it piously before the Fate gently stroked her light pink rose cheeks before releasing her back to her duties. The Fate, from what she saw of 'Ivia, smiled as she left. She could see that she was only a few steps ahead on the path than the one from 'Xo. Fate did not enjoy her power as she understood the force that infuses everything with equality. She would hardly express this to her but she would watch as the daughter of 'Xo would grow and, perhaps, take a path like Fate's in a way all her own, and become what she could be.

'Ivia had become was a rarity amongst paths from the long ago days of decorum. Fate wondered if she could ever be something more or would become almost hollowed of what makes a soul so precious as that which she has pledged her life to defend. Fate made herself a 'Mura cream fizz cocktail, and used the gene-storage slides as coasters as she had faith in her technology.

Fate later cast out her mind to the main bridge and in astral and psionic form took 'Ivia's hand while psionically massaging her mind as Fate displayed her approval of the new At'Lann Imperium Fleet Admiral and now Ethnarch of the 'Xo. Their thoughts conversed again.

'Care to join me for another late night on M'Goa, Ethnarch?' the Fate asked.

'My pleasure is yours, Imperiatrix. Sy'dosa has arranged for an immaculate platform constructed in a venue he knew you would love for your joy for any time you wish to use it.

'Sweet,' said the Fate telepathically with a hopeful astral smile.

Fate later flash-folded to her sanctum and left the trust of her ship in 'Ivia's steady hands. She found a separate piece in solitude before she would bring herself to the wildness of M'Goa that would bring her soul rapture once again. And for the first time in a long time, Fate had something to look forward to.

Φ

Thick burning flares of multiple colours lit the sky of M'Goa as a welcoming to the intergalactic gathering which continued blissfully unabated. The fires could be seen from orbit as this was the first sight to greet Fate after the Lis'talla arrived. She could feel the world was filled to capacity with revellers. Fate could almost smell the flare smoke of luminescent hazard red, of bright malachite green, and subdued black light, which stomped along to the progressive beats of M'Goa and lit the surface more so than the gathering.

The thick haze, set aglow, was pierced almost magically by linear prism spectral charges. The Fate could already see in her mind her latest private platform, and one kept amongst those of gene-nobles, aristocrats, sovereigns, and notaries along with esoteric cliques would be her companions for her relaxing time that would escort and mix with the royal guests. Only this set was allowed to be in the company of the Fate but Fate was one to let whatever came her way enter her circle. Everyone always had initial equality, and after facing so much evil on the path of war, she found a talent in herself for weeding it out. She was as disgusted as she was saddened by the lack of diversity and variety for obvious reasons. Security concerns after the shattering of the First Ring inversely dictated a more intensive approach.

The Interface informed the Fate that enemy incursions were once again on the rise across what remained of the universe following the battle inside L'Ja. In this war, the strongest souls were the elevated targets in the sights of the Death of Death. Fate would figure out a way to get around the confinement of her free movement. Through it all, Fate still saw M'Goa as a refuge. A world that lay in the protected eye of the most destructive of storms. But even the paradise of sound had to thicken with internal and external protection.

Fate may have been denied the full flavour of M'Goa but knew that if only for a vacation, she would free her tortured mind. Fate resigned herself to doing so alongside the cream of the Imperium's noble houses. She flash-folded straight from her sanctum on board the Lis'talla to step out onto the platform with 'Ivia as the globally heard music of M'Goa entered their senses like a summer rain of steam dripping *novocaine* as she donned her M'Goa tribal necklace once again and moved to its drums. It came time for the house to become hard. The old school days were left to the past but glimmers of innocence and beauty remained to be embraced.

With the Imperium aggregate culture taking what was spun-cast to a higher state, it was an indescribable joyous return for the Fate. Blue and ultra-violet thumb confetti of tinsel light fell slowly to the floor as the music tranced into and from its house into something more. The vibe was set in motion as it was set off and everything started going off.

The venue selected by Sy'dosa was the aquamarine ovular coliseum Ni'lov', or translated from M'Goa, 'colossus court'. Fate's platform could accommodate thirty at any given time with ample space to move. Alpha genetic sequences were the only ones accepted and all at this party were gene-scanned before entering or exiting the spacious transparent platform that had the same seating area as Sy'dosa's had but much larger. It sadly cut down on the diversity but for those who remained strongest with the proper vibe, the songs of peace and love in their hearts still flowed into one and all.

From a dimensional pouch, Fate pulled out handfuls of solidifying glow-mist of variating colour, 'Mura'Lann Qal'atu nectar derivative dermal dispenser combos for those she would relax around, and even some temporary gender reconfiguring chemicals, as throughout parts of M'Goa, to add even more spice to the variety before Fate. When the Fate and 'Ivia hit the dance floor, she let slip a honey-melon hued glow wands with her hands raised in the air and bent her palms to face a star lit sky as she was curious.

Her body was like all those on M'Goa, 'Ivia moved to become united with the flow of the music. Every so often, glimpses of perfect clarity would overtake the masses, and in moments like these, everything came together. The sound of one like Wilson set the tone for the return to the M'Goa path. Like Canadians identifying themselves with what Americans could have been, the revellers dutifully picked up the neon, vanilla favours Fate left at her table, and continued in their fun feeling even more apart of the gathering celebrations. Who knew how many similar favours ended up in low gravity streams but the result was beautiful.

The M'Goa had successfully negotiated their way into the Tr'Lann system, and had acquired through their integration into the Imperium, the latest At'Lann technologies for their path of transual leisure. Fate thumb pressed a M'Goa dispenser given to her by 'Ivia. Fate decided against the precaution of an inhibitor though her Ethnarch of 'Xo did as she would have to eventually return to her duties. She always thought of them even on the hovering platform that had a freesia mist floating through what felt on the skin like running naked through silk.

After all the Fate had been through, M'Goa was better than ever before and M'Goa pulsed with a people mass of a gigantic size previously unknown for the continuing gathering. Sadly though, the war had changed the revellers of the M'Goa nightscape, and had worn itself into the portrait of what was now M'Goa.

Fate looked to all the platforms surrounding hers before setting her eyes upon Sy'dosa who gave her the At'Lann military salute to show his government fully endorses the efforts of the Imperium and all they fight against. Fate thanked him politely for being so formal and gave herself a little more solace knowing she, perhaps, had made a difference.

The Imperium women, on other platforms, danced like Valkyrie interwoven into the tribe of sonic faerie folk and the ecstatic princesses of tender moments of heaven alongside the more hardcore. It was wonderful to begin her vacation from the war for the Fate to see happiness on the many faces of her many peoples.

Minutes dancing grew into hours, and hours deep into the night of sonic electronic majesty. Sub-thermal fractures formed in the night atmosphere of the aether of M'Goa that grew from having their living energy thrive within it to a near psionic degree. The spectrum crossing life-force seemed to thrust itself like feral soaring cherry blossoms into her from the hot pockets in the sky.

It was like awakening from a journey of the dead into their self-actualised heaven. The heat was intoxicating and euphoric. Though an elevated being was above such things, the Fate had grown to hate the cold. But at least this beautiful place was still warm.

With so many star-fires extinguished, existence seemed far too bone-chilling at times for the Fate as she danced on with glowing, strobing psionic tracers surrounding her moves. Hope seemed to thaw in the heat of loving unity that came out of frozen cuts inflicted upon existence.

Fate appreciated the kinetic heat, and her body seemed filled warmth. The soul of the Fate was tired from her path of war, and she never felt so good to return to the throbbing sauna that was a path of hers as well. The glorious rainbow lights swirled about Fate like the serenity of dancing in the eye of a hurricane. M'Goa became more of a dream than reality with every movement. The nights would shine. Sy'dosa and the infamous Lt. L'krk from the Lis'talla, greeted Fate with revelling reverence. All that was the war for them was left aboard the Lis'talla, with her S'yana, with the 'Sonann'Nor, and with what was eating away at the cosmos. This was the other side of things.

Far too grandiloquent aristocrats and genetic kinsmen paid their various respects. Even those who chose paths of apathy gave home to Fate returned from the front, and somehow she was just as glad to see some of them. For the Fate though, the best nights came when things became egalitarian and individual souls intermix at levels those on any path can enjoy. Fate felt the sense of calm that M'Goa offered return to her with the fiery chorus of the goddesses of M'Goa breaking through the beats as the path of the music shifted into something more. Fate was glad to be back.

Lon'tus Imperium distillers, M'tak and M'taka, the always good lads who supplied the At'Lann cocktails and 'Qal'latu as well as other nectars of all sorts, made their appearance before Fate. The Fate was impressed by the variety offered to her and by the presence of two who made their residence on 'Mura. Their small pub, in the Lon'tus style, as was their heritage, on the east-side of 'Mura's shore had been a favourite of 'Lîna and Nul'lus in the days of their youth. A time when 'Lîna drank At'Lann blueberry vodka and Nul'lus always had a Lon'tus colonial rum when at the pub.

M'tak and M'taka were a pair of pleasant thinkers and the greatest of listeners who had always served their former princess by meeting her needs without her asking, and without telepathy as they would do for any. Their professionalism brought about their status as atmosphere makers. 'Lîna, who had always been one with the people, had always made herself a valued patron throughout all of At'Lann and 'Mura in her urban days of exploration. She was gracious to them as they had come to remind her, the people of 'Mura had not forgotten her, and they would do what they could to enhance an already great party.

M'tak poured a glass of At'Lann blueberry vodka, or 'Ia for Fate, one for his brother, and one for himself so that the three could toast the Imperium victory that had the interface ablaze with activity. They had a little drink, remembering raising the roof with Nul'lus and 'Lîna's castle-mates, Sn'bak, Vkv't the interface sculptor, and J'Gendo who danced over to join the Lon'tus lads who they had brought along to enjoy M'Goa with tonight.

Sn'bak and J'Gendo must have had to drop a lot to be here, thought Fate. The two were bio-quantum research scientists for the Imperium military as they still wore their lab tunics on this world of peace. After catching up telepathically, Fate left them at the couches as she danced and drank for a few hours.

As always this set of mates, whether on M'Goa or not, did not speak of the war which was all the more refreshing for the Fate. Though for all her efforts, the war remained just not the way that detested her most. She wished them well as they left in only a few hours to return to a critical experiment. The path of science had to continue they insisted as they wished the Fate farewell. She more than understood their faith and devotion as she watched Vkv't find a Lon'tus maiden to enchant his relaxing time, and thanked them all through her thoughts, for coming out.

Later that night, while enjoying a At'Lann cigarette, Fate was pleasantly greeted out of the blue by none other than Kir'rus. She almost dropped her smoke as he made his way to her through the throng of the club set. He seemed as silent as a desert wind to where she sat. He sat with her and took up her invitation to smoke as well. The two surveyed the throbbing throng on the platform that were as deep into the vibe as their M'Goa hosts who also joined them to be deep in the passion of the vibe of ultimate frontiers of transual defiance. Everywhere it was just as wild.

There was something about this one that drew the Fate to be around him. Kir'rus was an enigma. Like a polar bear's hunger for a seal was Fate's curiosity about this man who could make his way onto any stage where the daughter of 'Mura was present. Yet he never spoke of where he came from other than what he had already said, saying and insisting he was simply a fellow traveller of humbly minor means. One that said almost nothing of himself in all their moments.

Though Fate could not even psionically probe the mind of the mysterious stranger, she was certain he was a spirit of goodness from wherever he came from. Whoever he was, Fate thought him a fine companion to the festivities and could see he equally appreciated what they were a part of. Fate was never rude and did not pry any further about his path, and simply came to enjoy dancing with him at her side.

During a cigarette aside, Kir'rus said something in passing that was curious and almost cathartic for them both. He said,

'You did what was your fate on L'Ja. Understand your nature and you shall be as impervious as it. You are the sacrifice and freedom of life. You are Fate, and the path is yours.'

Before Fate could ask him further about the veiled truth he had spoken, Kir'rus was gone. She did not have a chance to even break her earlier resolution. But something was wrong that had nothing to do with Kir'rus. The peace of M'Goa shattered away into a nightmare motion. She could feel it. The enemy was here.

Fate dream-walked on a psionic level to the other end of the platform. There would be none of this on M'Goa, thought Fate as she moved through the psionic nightmare. She came before a seated chalk hued young man with adders for hair. Fate reached out to the demon and pulled him by his hair that bit away at her as she did, to see his face. The chalk pale and blue tinged face had a vulture's smile and hollowed out eyes. Fate immediately put herself in a fighting stance in the slow crawl of time as she drew herself away. It was a dead astral skin over the demonic evil, a herald, a fist of the Death of Death.

Without warning, suctioning and hooked cyber-optical tethers shot out of the hollow skin. Fate was hit with the speed of a Hagi strike. She was bit into, grappled and tossed with a vicious violence never before known to her soul, she was flung to the platform above hers before being tossed down with such hate that Fate splintered through the floor of her platform like Scholes ransacking his way through a Tartan fortress.

Fate fell in a Bessonesque descent with a Shatnerian visage into a glass breaking impact into the foothill piles of sharp-edged dispensers discarded by those who had went beyond Bolzonic excess. The glass crystal continued to shatter as Fate fell deeper into the discards of delight. The sound of breaking glass continued even after the pile buried and shredded her.

Time became hushed into frigidity as the music fell silent. Fate could see her obscured S'yana guards rushing to her position, and some like 'Ivia who took aim with a flash-folded side arm at the assassin, and the 'Sonann'Nor seemed more than in the air. Looking below, this instrument of the Death of Death, found Fate with her skull cracked and her entire body embedded with glass. It happened so fast as the psionic and reality merged, that no one saw the dark agent's attack.

Blood tricked in gushing streams of violet and lavender down the head of the Fate in the shattered glass grave. For a very unnerving moment, all was silent. Then Fate struck back. The pile below Fate's platform disintegrated as she shot out a contained tri-atomic blast laden with a woman's fury. The dark assassin stood alone in Fate's psionic astral nightmare and in reality looking down with Lucifer's gaze only to be met by an utterly destructive intensity of a blast thrice the power of typical stellar core energy.

A rippling blast of violet blue that was solely directed for the creepy thing in a dead skin burst forth. As it was reduced to the same nothingness for which it fought, Fate felt the same as she flew back to her relatively unscathed platform as M'Goa heard silence for the first time in years as everything stopped. But Fate would have none of this. She shot her mind out across the gathering.

'The party is never over!' Fate proclaimed and exclaimed as she brought herself up to stand atop the shattered and violet blood drenched glass.

She snapped her fingers and the music of M'Goa returned to grace them once again. Fate had 'Ivia, who joined her at the party at the most dramatic time, return back to the Lis'talla to make sure another security breach would not happen again tonight and preferably never again.

'Ivia's diligent eye would make sure it would not and she folded back to the Lis'talla to personally see it would not happen again. Fate was kind of sad to see her go after just arriving to enjoy the gathering with her though it was not near half the dismay that Kir'rus probably had swam to another platform when he vanished, and had disappeared into the crowd. She even wondered if J'Gendo, at his psionic card game, noticed the disturbance and the fluctuation.

On 'Mura, Sn'bak was busying himself with the current state of 'Mura's bio-chemical levels after he had taken care of his experiment, when he fell out of his seat as the readings went erratically off the scale. He looked to the holo-display of his interface with shock. He contacted Fate, through a secure interface channel, to show her his findings an hour after she healed on the attempt on her life. Fate simply said, 'I am one with L'unn,' and he understood.

Fate returned to the dance of prayers in the M'Goa style as the gathering returned to go off once again. The usually conservative scientist took one last look at M'Goa through the holo-screen as Fate danced away, and closed the communications link with an almost enlightened face of reason. He could see and feel how much she gave as she relaxed, and wondered how far she would go for them.

Φ

Fate came to relax once again in the sweetness of the M'Goa night. Fate thought of 'Temisa and wondered where she might be tonight. She knew she would see her again for she captured her heart in ways some would never know. Earlier, J'Gendo occupied his time with chasing skirts on M'Goa before retiring once again to his psionic cards that played like baccarat. Fate did not think this a bad idea again but it was her path not to chase them. Fate liked the chase to come to her.

She almost dropped her latest cocktail as she had a hearty laugh in a surprisingly slight Lon'tus accent at the thought of what would come during her time here. Though in the Trinity, she had been alone on L'Ja for far too many years, and she wanted to join her path to many, and hoped finding one to love might come to pass in a better reality.

Fate had a noble philandering lust about her, even after all these years, that rivalled that of Zeus, and she could feel it would not be long before her sensuous hunger was assuaged. She had a carnal ravenous appetite sometimes for those who worshipped her as much as she worshipped them. Fate had become reckless as the war corrupted her soul more than she realised.

Fate would not deny herself, 'Temisa would not want her to, and it would be a long time, if ever, before she would meet the one, and the M'Goa, more than any, would do anything to return a smile to her face. She let go of self-doubt, of everything except that which was her essence. Everything was fun and bizarre.

She watched the M'Goa dance on in their covenant that became their battle to exist. It was a beautiful trade with such a people as their thoughts soothed her soul that has seen far too many horrors in return for what passion they could give her. Fate, like Sheen, had always had an eye for making selections, and in this roller-coaster night, Fate also made time to send she could see as the carnal desires of her castle-mates she saw tonight, and flash-folded what they sought to wherever was their location throughout the system. Fate had an eye for moving the right paths together, and even in the relaxed insanity of war, dutifully selected paths that would only make her host smile. She had their faith but she would never do anything to lose it either.

Fate also sent a telepathic message to Sy'dosa to meet the needs of young Duke T'pata of the Lon'tus colony 'Nakala who she had met aboard the 'Tainja, and to her childhood mates of Vn'ru, and 'Aranek, who she saw on her platform tonight, and knew they would more than appreciate her kind gesture. With Duke T'pata she drank a toast with his three brothers, who drank a toast to victory for the Imperium.

She also chanced upon a joyously exhausted Vkv't who she bade farewell to. He had set aside his data-flow research long enough to find a little release with a M'Goa lass with light azure hair named 'Xili; a very hard-core Lon'tus dancer of peace. Fate waved to him as he swam through the lower gravity with his companion leading him on back into the thick of sweet things. He nodded his much appreciated thanks, and Fate was glad to see something before her that was well deserved for such a tireless worker.

Fate, alone in the crowd of her platform once again, cast her mind out across M'Goa, to invite eighteen of her elite selections to a night with her. As they all sensuously accepted, Fate flash-folded them to her platform for a night to never forget. No one turned down the chance to walk the path of fantasy. Since Fate sometimes dallied with the path of solipsism but her solipsism included and was all of existence. She would more than give them herself.

The Fate found before her a cadre of nymphal designs, sweet canvasses of athletic satin, M'Goa women whose fashion style seemed configured strikingly like her. They were all she psionically asked for and she was all they wanted. The sweetest of passions seemed to arise. Their perfumes, the tightness of their bodies, the beauty of their souls' peace striving for innocence, the smoothness of their legs, the softest of hot tangerine coloured skins, the sensuous curls of their dark navy blue hair, and the most kissable of their bacchanal lips, and the goddess like perfection of their slender curves. Fate felt at home for the first time since L'Ja. Her heart was truly made joyous that M'Goa was now part of the At'Lann Imperium home system.

As the goddesses of the M'Goa dance floors assembled before her wondering who would be first, Fate thought, 'What a bounty!' They were the ripe with one of the purest paths of goodness that the enemy, and this whole bloody war, could not tear away. Fate found their path of peace one that she would much rather be on but knew they were here because it was Fate's path to protect them and all in existence. She licked her lips as if before being about to swallow an oyster. Fate told them they would all be first as it was not Fate's philosophy not to run down for a wee taste but to walk down her mountain and take in the all the delicious delights.

She and her private party folded away from the smaller gathering on her platform. Their sensuous festivities lasted day and night and night and day again in a joining under a summer sugar rain where buckets of candy waters splashed down upon them. And bringing along the temporary gender alteration technology made it even more interesting than Fate could have imagined but their thought merged into nail-digging delights that went beyond anything she could envision. This was a path of Fate that allowed all the travellers at any point on any path to feast upon joy and joined the unity that is the ecstasy of life. How she bathed in their thoughts of peace and cleansed herself of so much of the cursed dirt of war while finding a little more freedom in herself and others to deal with what remains.

Φ

When Fate returned to the platform, she was without rest as she had been made so relaxed that she found a new joy for living that again became the peace of her soul. Fate wondered if a little corruption was a good thing. In her new moment of peace, Fate was joyously reunited with the Aristocrat, and the Hunter who decided upon a short jaunt to M'Goa from Kul'mir, and especially with the other daughters of 'Mura who could no longer remain apart and could not wait any longer to see her. It was the wonderful start of a brand new day on the path of Fate after so much release. If people only knew, Fate thought as she laughed because she knew they did.

There they were, Za'szu and 'Zaya, after all these years, Fate's sisters looked more than regal in their casualness, and though youth was still theirs for both their bodies and souls, they had aged well into new paths of beauty. It left both a sweet and bittersweet taste to see each other once again. 'Zaya still fretted and had her misgivings about anytime Fate exerted her power as she would truly need time to heal her still experimental psyogenetic enhanced paradigm, and it was probably by that fact alone that her sisters understood why Fate chose to come to M'Goa first. She could see they were still a little agitated after the assassination attempt as they felt her pain in their souls.

Still, when Za'szu looked into the war-torn eyes of those like one who had seen a liberated *Warszawa* that had been reduced to ash, brick, and rubble, which Fate shyly tried to hide. She cast any worries away as she embraced her sister who was so glad Fate was still alive. 'You are worthy of it all, 'Imiszi. You have kept us safe from the darkest of winds,' Za'szu told her with her thoughts as 'Zaya joined in. They gave themselves for Fate to hold. There was no further misery as Fate found herself with the company of her comrades and clan, and felt truly at home in all their safer hands.

Za'szu could hardly contain her excitement to bring Fate home to show her a L'unn growing into a refinement never before known. Regent Za'szu had brought their technology and the spirituality of the people to an efficiency unparalleled in the years Fate had been away. And though the darkness still lingered over them, the people still lived as they should.

She also told Fate that a city-bunker had been built, that would enclose 'Mura'Lann, as the last of the Imperium protocols to be met. 'Just in case,' she said. Fate felt only pride in her sister's excellence, and wondered if she could push on with her detail orientated work ethic to build a continent-bunker while she was at it. She hoped she would not. Fate told her if she was ever to fall, Za'szu would have to stand in her place. She said she remembered but somehow felt it was never to be her path.

Fate then turned to 'Zaya and marvelled at how her once youngest sister had grown into the most refined of 'Mura women in her absence. She was truly a treasure to their crown. She could see in her mind that she had also grown stronger in her craft of psyogenic construction and study.

'Zaya more than delighted in telling Fate her efforts in treating her body that sleeps has finally begun to move toward optimum genetic integrity. She had turned it around. But she cautioned Fate in saying she could not make heads or tails of it as her psyogenetic matrices were expanding at a slow crawling exponential rate with many new and unknown configurations coming into being.

'Zaya stressed this may have volatile side effect later on as she confided in Fate that the new genetic configurations were impossible to test as they only could exist within her genetic make-up. Fate, only wanting to enjoy her homecoming, shushed her not to worry.

Seeing Fate had far too much on her plate at this point in the extravaganza, the Hunter and Aristocrat waved as they flash-folded to another platform to wait for a better time to party and converse together. Fate waved an 'I'll be along soon' to them as they were pleased to see Fate happy by reuniting with the other daughters of 'Mura. 'Zaya then heard Fate speak tenderly in her mind, and told also Za'szu that they would meet on 'Mura at the recently constructed monument to their parent's reign, and honour that which has been made their grave, shrine, and tomb made by 'Za'szu for them in the strictest of ancient At'Lann traditions.

They danced in celebration for a few hours before Fate tenderly embraced each of her sisters as they had to return to L'unn. 'Zaya had to return to her research and Za'szu to the affairs of state. They folded away smiling as Fate made her way gracefully to the platform where she reunited with the Aristocrat who was decked out in the jersey, of his team, of the Lon'tus champions, and the Hunter was still in his more casual military lines for his attire.

It had been only a short time that the Trinity had been apart but it somehow seemed longer than the entire war so far. The Three embraced each other as warriors like those who had been and were still in a Ragnarok parade. What a heavenly sight. Indeed, what a heavenly time.

The Aristocrat decided to be at her side using the excuse of being there just in case another assassin might escape the Imperium rat-traps. Fate thought it all unnecessary but was glad to see the Imperator of Lon'tus once again. The pair enjoyed each others company far too much as their paths always intersected. He also came with a progress report on the new look of the Imperium which the Trinity chose as its path. The Hunter looked on and knew the Fate would be excellently impressed as Fate, more than any, needed progress.

The orbital unification of Rimisz'tii and Lon'tus had taken place as the new configurations of planetary bodies ahead of E'de and L'unn in the Tr'Lann system while H'Raka Prime would take solar orbit astern of L'unn. It would all be finished tomorrow as part of the defensive protocols of the last gate strategy that would soon become their path. To be absolutely sure of their agreement, the Aristocrat asked,

'What do the At'Lann say of this?'

'I speak for the At'Lann and I say proceed with our arms open as the trinity of our worlds becomes our home. Long may we protect them,' Fate said. The Trinity then shot up a sonic dampening field around themselves with a NATO shell's velocity as the Hunter entered into their thoughts, and Fate looked into his sharper eyes as she could see his time on Kul'mir was going well. His words were coated in positivist caution.

'I remind you, 'Imiszi, that the last gate strategy may permanently bond the paths of our worlds. The H'Raka once shared a path with the At'Lann, and the At'Lann may find the path taken together will be the regret of the path not taken alone. It may be a long time before our paths part again.'

'I understand and accept this as we must keep our worlds safe until we can find victory. There is no longer a path alone.'

She added, 'I thought our worlds already were bonded. Our path of paths, though sometimes straying and diverted from one another, is still a path always shared. Do you forget I am Fate. And I will have no regrets, I will only keep the memories.'

After Fate's words of quiet and solemn sincerity, the Aristocrat said, 'Then tomorrow it is. Let us continue to enjoy ourselves'. The Aristocrat added to the shared wisdom of the Trinity in the venture of tomorrow.

Fate then grabbed four dispensers from a nearby bucket as the sonic dampening field dissipated and the celestial music of M'Goa returned to them. She handed two to each of her comrades. While they danced the shows of light in the anti-gravity platform streams were as entertaining as the glowing dispensers in their hands. After all, she reminded them, the natives might also appreciate a show of some kinetic photonic sculptures. They would try to outdo the other artistically as a friendly game to play when the sound of one like Sneak rushed over them. They liked their art, and that much was true.

The reunified Trinity made themselves into a portrait of dancing peace on M'Goa as if they were the new canvas to be painted by the hand of one like Hearle. The Three lit their cigarettes in unison, and they flexed their thumbs in unison. They danced in harmony with the night, and the Three found a moment of peace, a moment to heal that would save themselves from heading to a burnout where one would have to land on a mined field just to refuel. It was a shame the Hunter would soon have to have to return to his torturous rituals but at least he would have nights of festival like these that were just as much his even if his was a path apart, thought the Fate. The music of one like Pappa or one like Creamer filled the air, and the style of everything seemed best for one like Karembeau. She could see from those around her many more from H'Raka now continuously came to M'Goa, that truly was their sanctuary. But the Hunter, ever the traditionalist, would give this up before returning to his path on Kul'mir. For he was not one to be gawked at, and he was on another path of war.

Fate looked at herself and her comrades to see their frames were now only the muscles of warfare. Too much time in the trenches, she thought, too much time. On another psionic level, she realised how much their psyogenetic structures stood out. 'How we needed to relax' seemed to be the theme of the night as everyone did and did their best to let it all go.

She flash-folded a holo-reflection compact to look upon her face. Not all her cuts automatically healed from her fall through the floor though something told her by their configuration that they fit the pattern of more ancient M'Goa traditions, and she decided to leave them as they were, and a few that covered her body in a enigmatic pattern that could not be passed off as random.

Fate looked around as she danced to the other platforms and saw how much had changed after L'Ja, and how much of what once was still remained. For even on M'Goa, the creeping winds of Alcatraz's musty cells had grown to weigh upon them all more and more though the majority of the M'Goa kept the faith, and kept it real. Even the championship team from Lon'tus were having a blast as only the music and the night mattered. But for the Fate right now, a Fate who had endured so much, it was all good.

Φ

It was soon growing into tomorrow, and it became time for the Trinity to once again to take their separate paths. The Aristocrat returned to a shore like that of

Sopot, a Hanseatic shore of an innocence remembered, and the Hunter returned to a different bank along a Baltic like shore. And the Fate remained but would soon shimmer along to her own shore. She remained on the gathering world as her companions on the great path attended to the call of home.

Fate enjoyed the full flavour of being entertained by the pleasures of a Trinity court now all to herself. The call to return to L'unn became the song that became her anthem on M'Goa, and she was once more filled by the path of peace by the end of the week. And soon tomorrow became today for the paths of the Trinity of the wind, water, and moon. The elegant spectacle of M'Goa was left behind for the light of new days that were still warm from the gathering night and nights. Their hopes would soon rest on the enlightenment of another path.

Φ

'K'nde D'le Snd'ar,' said the Fate as she clicked the heals of her high gloss boots together and straightened her right fist ahead of her as if she was almost about to fire a psionic bolt.

Fate saluted in the traditional and ancient way of the At'Lann military and acknowledged the struggle for freedom that evolved from a great myth and a truth believed that her people were once slaves to the Origin species. With erasure inching ever closer, Fate somehow understood how they once could have once been perceived in such a limited fashion and why they should remember how far they have come.

She was dressed in her black dress state Imperium uniform that was panzer drawn and tri-platinum adorned. The times made everyone a little fiercer. As Fate stood there in her smart uniform and in her black leather like gloves, she was joined by 'Zaya in an equally appropriate dark teal uniform of the At'Lann Imperium Psyogenetic Ministry corps, and Za'szu dressed in a jade and black uniform, in the same tunic style as her sister who once again returned home from the path of war.

To Fate, there was no one more befitting than Za'szu to wear the uniform of the Regency, and that of High General of L'unn's defence force which was represented by jasmine and gold intertwined adornments. The three stood on 'Nula hill; a hill like that of any found near Glasgow.

Fate felt so cold. If not for her psyogenetic discipline, she would have shivered. Za'szu and 'Zaya, on the other hand, seemed not to be bothered in the morning 'Mura'Lann air that was both sleepy and peaceful like the winds through a forest of silver pines ripe for the light of dawn. The sisters stood at the edge of the Nai'jan crescent peninsula. A path of onyx and pomegranate hued smoke swirl marble led to a triangular memorial of the same stone.

On the hillside about them grew long grasses of dark green and forget-me-nots blue blades that rose to their knees and seemed to stand with just as much a ttention as the Trinity of the Daughters of 'Mura did before the massive legacy stone.

The At'Lann sun rose and spilled across the V'nsz bay like an amazing grace morning of autumn dew over the highlands. The rays of sunshine soared like orioles across the horizon as the three sisters had an anime glisten about them and especially about Fate's tiara where sparkles of amethyst seemed to jump about her symbol of power. Fate's mauve and lavender highlighted hair was tied back in a set of cat's claws of curls and braids of hair and almost just as many strands of tied silver threads from what seemed to be over a thousand tied ends of her elegantly cut wiry locks. And for every battle remembered, there were many more were only left to the past.

Her skin had become a pastel lavender hue, which was still a landscape of dewberry hued scars. Her lips were a sandy purple. And for their own shades of life, her sisters were every bit the equal beauties as their thought offerings became a triune to those before them who had transcended. Their paths joined by Fate became much more.

The Trinity of 'Mura'Lann stood before the last memorial of their slain parents that contained their psionic holo-statues of all those past of the house of At'Lann. The last memorial to their Mother and Father who Fate almost despised during her time on L'Ja for leaving the war to their children's path but knew, through it all, that she could never escape her fate.

The faces of S'bel of the modern ancient path, and 'Usta, once their King who had victories near the measure of his father before him, S'Lanu, over the 'Komu'naz. The photonic sculpture of their former forms seemed almost as large as the entire peninsula in their eyes of those on Fate's path as the morning light shone beautifully through them.

The three sisters of the At'Lann Imperium looked to their left, to the rough as brutalist dark garnet pyramid that was about the size of a victory house. Atop the pyramid, a flame burned like a Venetian style fountain of white sugar fire that cast itself another thirteen stories into the L'unn sky. The two names of their parents were engraved into the base of the small pyramid shrine in the same colour as the cherry blossoms set along the path that came to it.

They stood in silence, in their salute of remembrance before names that turned into two others as they synchronously pivoted with their left heal and brought up and down their right to face the pyramid. The names transfigured to that of their full names S'bel U'Ani the Searcher, and 'Usta Es'lon the Dream-builder.

Such a terrible fate had fallen to them, lamented the sisters in their thoughts. Struck down in the first deluge before they could save themselves or be saved. No one carried the guilt of what had happened more than the Fate who had come to be called upon as a reality builder. She felt she had failed them from the way her path of war was still unfolding. She thought herself a terrible human in her spirit as she buried her emotions and turned away, with a beautiful face of stone, lit a cigarette. She walked away with her sisters at her side.

'Was that not a little too traditional even for you 'Imiszi? The 'Lann rituals have not been performed for generations', asked Za'szu calmly. Fate remained in silence after honouring the dead of their clan for a moment before saying with an air of absolution,

'I wanted to bring it back. Until we win this war, they shall have no peace, and neither shall I. Over two thirds of what was once the universe has ceased to exist. And I know Mother and Father are just as displeased about this as I am. I honour them in death better than I did in life. It is not as if they were fond of the path of my youth that took me away from At'Lann.'

The Trinity of the Fate, the Healer, and the Logic walked past the trees of fluttering blossoms back to their cities as swirls of wind blew past them like those over Dhaka.

'Stop persecuting yourself. The enemy does enough of that to us all. It is you who has been tireless for the cause. Their honour is yours,' interjected 'Zaya to Fate.

'It seems for nought,' Fate replied.

''Zaya is right. When you suffer, we all do, and we all suffer enough with this war. Let us not also lose the happiness of our souls to the Death of Death. We each have to take a path like even those of M'Goa', said Za'szu to a mollified Fate.

She looked to her younger but not so young sister with eyes that once pleaded and were now soothed by her words, and a little bit of her glacial wall of hard emotions melted away. Fate turned to look back to the pyramid and first saw the glow of Lon'tus and Rimisz'tii in blue and H'Raka in red in the still sky, and E'de below. She thought many on those worlds looked to the new blue light of the two blue and green worlds. The worlds of the Imperium Trinity were now within the walking distance of Hermes to each other. So close, and yet so far as they became a part of the At'Lann and each remained almost a path alone.

Za'szu and 'Zaya also looked up to the sky to see their space and system filled with life and looked also to just make out in the stars, the orange light of M'Goa burning on in the distance. Their space once shared with the Hy'Bor was now shared with many others. M'Goa was close enough to the *bleu nuit* generations of At'Lann, and far enough away from the more conservative elements of At'Lann to cause them any concern. Fate and her sisters turned back on the path as she spread a long blowing violet cowl unto herself as a tear of joy rolled down her cheek.

'Kr'va l'sza j'mura 'yalu', said Fate in At'Lann in what seemed the loud whisper of a child which, roughly translated means, 'give us all hope in survival for our home.'

As if hearing for the first time the BT enhanced call of one as sonically breathtaking as Plenty of Mclachlan, and always the multiple offerings that came from Tisto, Fate psionically split the white memorial flame open into sparkling streams that first flowed with the coldness of the waters of Bering and into pure waters with the warmth of Victoria over her falls as the waters of energy fire flowed onto the pyramid turning red, white, and mauve. As the once winter streams flowed across its sides, the pyramid turned to the colour of flames of liberation.

'That's better,' said Za'szu as she took Fate's arm and Fate took 'Zaya's as the Three walked back to their cities. Along the path, Fate picked up a white trillium flower and let it blow from her open hand into the wind and into the sea, and thought of her world. Fate had returned home to where a new world order had come to be and where its success could only be measured if there ever was to be a next generation.

Their true victory would be if there was to be a second Imperium generation. Worse still, Fate knew the Death of Death had been dissolving temporal paths, meaning even if there was to be a second Imperium generation, it was quite possible that it had already been erased from existence. Yet, Fate found there was still cause for joy before the family memorial that gave her so much cause for reflection as well.

For the first time in years, new stars in the sky were twinkling with light, and the daughters of 'Mura continued to look up as they continued to head back. And for the first time in years, there was renewed hope that life had it within itself to prevail. These were uncertain times.

'Where do we go from here?' Fate wondered aloud.

Φ

Days turned into months as the Imperium truly began to integrate as a shared system and as an integrated culture like it never had before. H'Raka soldiers frequented the commercial districts of At'Lann and 'Mura, and conducted themselves with such a respectful manner in the open market squares that one could have seen they had learned many lessons from the Lon'tus and from their own new respect for a people they now considered their siblings.

It seemed such a waste that so much time and issues had to pass before the Imperium came together, thought Fate. It reminded her of her zealously feisty challenges and conflicts with Za'szu. In both cases, too many games of chicken had been played where Fate had gone too far, and when thinking of such things, Fate always had a fretful face.

As she sat back in the sun on the platform of her lilac pyramid with her sisters, Fate vowed that those days were past and they would continue to look out for one another above anything else, and anything that creates grievances between them would be cast aside so that they may stand together. Trust in its purest form should always be found with family.

Fate finally came home to her family, and now a extended cultural family as well.

And now that she had two, now there was another reason for greater joy. Fate strived to be a nurturer and since she had not yet met the one to be by her side, she gave herself to the care of the Imperium. Using her enhanced psyogenetic intellect, she designed ways to make the gene-storage technology more efficient and even more micro-compact. Life forms from entire systems could be stored in the Imperium database with but a transmission from an Imperium listening post. Life forms not essential to the war effort were placed in storage. Even Imperium citizens were no longer spared.

So far this was not required for citizens of the Tr'Lann system though a significant percentage had volunteered to be placed in storage until the war could be won in exchange for either the honour of doing so or increased status for their children. Though day to day life continued to be maintained, it was in all these efforts of taking care of her families, and continuing different paths of war that Fate began to crumble.

Fate was exhausting herself: by continually remaining linked to the Imperium Interface, battling the zombie guardians of the soul-void that is the Death of Death on transpsionic planes, going off into battle to stem incursions into their remaining and receding space, her own excesses, and keeping the soul and peace of a new emerging culture, her psyogenetic structure was becoming far too overloaded for what evolution could allow and what she could bear.

She looked to 'Zaya, who relaxed in the sun beside her, and decided it was not best to tell her as she would let fate deal with her. Her condition was now above the measure of 'Zaya'a medical scans. 'I am taking on too much too soon,' Fate thought to herself. Something soon will have to change', she told herself in her thoughts. The Aristocrat and the Hunter began to be weary as well, as tiredness trickled onto them and neared overcoming them even though far less of their active service in the war on the front was required. It was the war at home, putting together Imperium peace, drained the Trinity.

The Trinity of the wind, water, and moon still assembled to command the fleet to isolate and destroy enemy infestations in space, against the Death of Death in the psionic nether realms, or by deploying the genetic inventions of the Hunter that fought infestation with infestation, and taking part in missions so secret even they could not remember them.

They had become the bored skills of perfection on the path of war. Their minor missions, all too often gave the Trinity far too much time to think about how the war had taken so much from them. It was probably their other nights on M'Goa or the relaxing moment of lounging around on her little balcony above 'Mura that Fate found herself doing what kept them going on the path of boredom that had merged with the path of war as everyone waited for it all to happen. It was the shell-shock of returning to the daily world, the coming down to a normalcy amidst chaos that seemed to revolve itself almost into a timid sorrow that felt as if it draped itself everyday, and at times, over the entire Imperium. It was hard to keep going with death hanging over your head and the Trinity, like the Imperium, did its best to deal with it.

What lay most heavily upon the collective consciousness was that entire races and species, over a quadrillion of them had their fate placed or placed their fate in the Trinity by being encased in data-storage crystals as their systems and planets were erased and the Imperium became a closed and enclosed population. So many species left to gather under figurative dust and a hygienically confined silence. It was a conformity worse than some might have known before, frozen in time, and waiting for a better day.

As Fate looked down to the Lon'tus and 'Xo shopkeepers in the central market square, she asked herself what had they become. Though Fate consoled herself and found she was able to relax with her sisters, she knew the final steps on the path of war would soon be taken, and she savoured the few quiet days that remained before the storm of nothingness would come to their door.

Fate came to bid farewell to this existence she helped bring together. The Trinity said goodbye to one another once again. Fate also came to bid her sisters farewell, as she did with 'Ivia, 'Temisa who she had many more nights with at home and away from M'Goa, and many others that she had met on her path. The Aristocrat left Lon'tus city, and the Hunter, who went from Kul'mir and briefly back to 'Vanx before departing as well. Fate felt it also time to leave, and the logical place to go was to return to themselves held in station and orbit above their respective worlds.

The Trinity would return to their sleep of no rest in stasis. Fate would resume an all-out attack on the dark realm of the Death of Death. They would rest once again to ready themselves to face the final assault from the horde and its evil face for their best chance at decapitating the vile beast. The time came to prepare for the last chance to give all their souls the peace of rest.

Fate's soul seemed to totter, and the dark circles underneath her eyes had grown far too dark for her liking. Her work, her path, her mission, seemed to fill her with worry. Though her sisters insisted otherwise, Fate felt unworthy of what she was and felt denied that she was not so much more. And even after relaxing at home on both Mura'Lann and numerously on M'Goa, Fate was tired. She had become fragile and at times could barely keep her eyes open as she languished, like so many, in restlessness.

Fate looked out to her system one last time. She looked out to: their Sun, Usz'shna (protected by the secret prototypes of the Hunter's genetic creations) the gravity captured carcass of a Two Rings planet destroyer, to Lon'tus, to E'de, to H'Raka, to J'Namu, the planet construct for At'Lann and the Imperium's energy resources. Fate looked out to M'Goa, to 'Xo, that had earned placement by 'Ivia's service to the Imperium, to Nu'Ata, and even to M'Gata on the outskirts as well as to N'Bira from the galactic museum which now shared system orbit with Tr'Lann. She brought her sight back to Usz'shna only to sneer at the melted hull of the large enemy tank-sphere she left held forever as a reminder of the first wave. Fate was as at home as she was homeless.

Fate hugged her sisters farewell for what would be another stretch of time apart and returned once again to space to fly herself to the At'Lann portion of the massive phase generator and back once more to the slumber of J'Poko. She was so cold, so chilled to the bone as she slipped herself back into her form still asleep under psionic blankets that were the only ones to be had and the only blankets to be wanted.

She first looked down at her peaceful self, and looked to her other reflection on a triangular, tall diamond mirror on the wall of this white and bright vaporous snow-white enamel chamber. Her reflection in the mirror seemed more like death than the chance to wake again. The Fate smiled one last time and found herself wishing for the serenity of her midnight garden before the final stand would be taken against the Death of Death. The Fate drifted like mauve satin plasma fire into herself that lay asleep under plum and rose lighting. Reality truly became a gilded prison and nothing seemed heaven sent anymore.

'Lîna was whole once again but was not at peace. Now and forever she was Fate. Her daydreams became a saddening sky blue and gold wheat meadows to fly through that took her to her midnight garden before thrusting her into the hell-heart of the Death of Death which the Trinity fought continuously to a nightly standstill. Even in sleep, her soul, and those of H'Renn and Nul'lus, languished in restlessness. Something would soon have to give.

31
The Battle

Her lungs filled with air for the first time in years in an ethereally visceral flood of screaming awakening. Fate's eyes opened to a pastel mauve light that matched the pristine gems that are her eyes. She first let her eyes close once again. Then 'Lîna opened her eyes again in the new unison of her being, and absorbed a long and massive download and upgrade from the Imperium Interface. It was time to return to reality and end this.

Years of psionic combat had refined the Fate and evolved her into a warrior that could even have changed the outcome of a dreadful 1795 in Europe. She could feel the moment and the days ahead could be seized. Fate took in the purest of aether still tinged with the tighter shackles of erasure, and her body automatically adjusted to her specific and optimum psyogenetic output levels.

'Lîna and Fate were one. She almost felt like a complete being once again to see the world through living eyes for the first time in years, and Fate, who was all paths, felt more whole than she ever had before. She was a professional, and with every step, she evolved to another level to be ready. The Fate, returning to the living world, felt like Dhurya before the siege.

From the nights in stasis, Fate fought long and hard in the Tekken style of Michelle with the tenacity of one like McCallister. Her years away from the real world had been spent mind-zagging about the dark matter of the Death of Death; hyper-spin-kicking away at its psionic armour of tar hued jagged hell-shard and blade. In her Tekken-esque attacks, Fate's obsession became a flurry of kicks to dislodge the faceless face-plating of a Styx of secret and polluted waters. Indeed, this menace was a phantom. It truly was the life from the lifeless, and the Death of Death remained the nihilistic prophecy of the battle of last day.

'Lîna had evolved to become the maker of Fate, and now fate was her only path. She carried a little fear with her but she carried faith found in arriving at her own awakening, a faith she had to keep strong enough to keep eternity alive. This was the path of Fate, and these were the last few steps on the path where victory is life and pain is only what forges one. She walked towards destiny, and she was Fate.

She keyed a short data-sequence into a interface panel beside the stasis chamber, left open with *cere* laying scattered across the pillow framed module, as if discarded from an ethereal chrysalis.

Fate transformed her gentlest clothing into her black Imperium garb as the cere still lay there ruffling in the particle winds. A door panel opened by going into another phase and disappearing and Fate walked through to a small control chamber, the size of a loft, with a tall nave window and interwoven holo-screen below a white crab claw like arch that rose from the ground. The arch was covered in interface control tiles and activation controls for new data-streams.

She began the activation sequence with her mind fully linked with the Aristocrat and the Hunter, and the systems of the phase generators that began to come online. These were the final steps to be taken in this transfixed church of technology. The Trinity began to be once again whole, and Fate let her mind reach out across the Imperium. Fate then swam the deepest depths of the interface data-streams to activate Tr'Lann system wide At'Lann Imperium weapons platforms in the form of delphinium hued luminescent pyramidal spatial buoys that acted as both cannons and mines.

Za'szu was placed in command of the remaining Imperium fleet. The Regent of At'Lann had spent the years preparing by immersing herself in the most advanced forms of tactical training that she and the Imperium Interface could provide, and she too was ready for this day. She stood on the bridge of the Lis'talla and looked out to the view of the pressing emptiness of null space that they would wage war again with. The reunified remnants of the enemy fleet would emerge from a darker space. The First Ring returned to grace by the puppet master's hand of the Death of Death and would soon engage all that remained.

She was as impatient as Fate to end this war and all its misery but most of all she wanted Fate to truly return home. After all the hardships of coming together, the years away from 'Imiszi had been years missed and had been empty years. It was time for their sacrifices to end. She thought 'Imiszi had endured too much suffering to save their home. Za'szu put her feet down in anticipation on the path of war cleared by the Fate. She greeted her sister and this day of reckoning with a quiet dignity that had always been her path.

Za'szu inter-linked her mind with her revived sister's and swam in the thoughts of one that had chosen a path of thorns still dripping with her violet blood, and all the blood of life within reality. The battle plan became laid out for their minds. Fate was more than impressed by the efficient logical nature of Za'szu's tactical designs as she was always impressed by her. She vowed to Fate that no enemy ship would break through their lines to interfere with the launch. The sea lion would not find a beach to land upon. The enemy would be returned to the purity of nothingness and only the evil that tainted it would be the only thing erased. The sisters said a prayer to one another for a morning after, and returned their minds to the paths of this day.

'Ivia was on board the newly constructed 'Xo flagship, the T'Kala, an E'de class vessel built on 'Mura, and in its triangular and yet gothic configuration, it was approximately the same size as the Lis'talla, and was a gift to her peoples fleet. The Ethnarch of the 'Xo would co-ordinate the Imperium fighters with the exception of At'Lann squadron 303 and H'Raka squadron 189. The H'Raka elite black squad was commanded by Y'vis's nephew, H'khnn, who had become their greatest ace. These brave pilots flew a separate path, and from their gallantry throughout the war earned the distinction of autonomous command.

She could feel Fate inside her soul as their minds linked and blessed one another for what was to come. For all the Imperium had given their people, 'Ivia would not fail a people that had sheltered them so selflessly in their equality with them. The Ethnarch reassured Fate for whatever reason that she believed the path ahead would not end in a dead end.

'Ivia was ready for whatever lay ahead. As both could feel the end surrounding them, both became a little more afraid of the dark prospect that erasure offered, and after the plan was relayed, both returned to their vigilance of a horde that was soon to come. The last battleground of the Imperium was the merged M'Plura and Us'ka galactic systems in what was now the entirety of the universe. Fate moved on throughout the souls and minds of the Imperium, and her path was the hope of tomorrow.

Fate inter-linked her thoughts with Val'damus, who transferred to command the K'rana, a Lis'talla sister ship after having lost the Kam'manu in the years Fate slept waiting to be unleashed. The Kam'manu had been destroyed in an enemy incursion three years earlier which took place in the 'Vulura sector of space of all places. Fate chided him not to lose his ship today, and if he did, to not to go down with it. He said it would all be good, and that was enough for Fate. Everyone hoped for an opportunity to break out the garage.

He walked the path alongside Fate too many times not to be one of the best field officers to ever wear the uniform of the At'Lann Imperium, and Fate knew he would not fail what was now the last cause. His path had taken him to too many vessels that had fought in most battles throughout the war, and that was the simple reason Fate placed so much faith in him; he was both an optimistic survivor and one who had slain many dragons to get where he was this day.

Val'damus's heart had not been turned bitter by the sardonic gibberish that life became in war, yet he walked the path of war as the bravest of warriors. And he fought with only one goal in mind: to end this destructive conflict. Along this path of war he came to understand destruction all too well. He placed his faith in Fate to bring about peace, and Fate confident that he was ready, moved on in her thought streams.

After her brief inter-link, and with her thoughts merging with that of the great minds of the Imperium, Fate returned to the activation sequence. She could see Val'damus on his bridge giving her a salute for what lay ahead as his crew followed suit. Everyone knew that this was for it all. Her mind linked and reached out across the Imperium that gave her a strength in faith that she had never before known. Their strength was hers as she prepared herself for what lay ahead.

Fate's psyogenetically enhanced mind multi-tasked by diving deeply, and she worked her way across all data-streams of the Imperium Interface to make the necessary calculations to begin the convergence. Like jumping her way from glowing obelisk to glowing obelisk miles above the ground, as if she were one like a raider of tombs, Fate's mind made its way across the entire data-flow and fully integrated with the Interface.

Her soul drew form and infused all the souls of the Imperium with her might. The power of her mind became more united than it ever had in all her years of evolution. There was no time to ponder the choice of paths, there was only time before the horde arrived to make the decisions of the day. The universe was a small place now, and she could see everything. All she could see beyond that was the dark storm of the horde they would soon face again.

Fate could even see, Kir'rus, of all people, stroking his beads, watching it all unfold from a rooftop balcony on M'Goa where the dance of the gathering was at its hardest and fiercest yet. It was if he stared at her with trepidation that was in the hearts of many this day. As he danced united in the vibe, the peace of M'Goa left those who awaited the Death of Death totally unafraid, and probably would not even have time to see it coming. She took one last look at one whose secrets, even now, she could not unlock, and waved goodbye to the mysterious stranger of her life before moving her mind on also looking at a few of the great many Fate came across along her path.

She could feel within her thoughts, Sy'dosa who always went out of his way to make sure M'Goa was a beautiful journey, to sweet 'Temisa, her luscious courtesan, whose lips she could still feel pressed against hers. Fate embraced her thoughts to say goodbye to one who gave her the hot icing of M'Goa. Her thoughts continued to flow to so many such as Sn'bak, Vkv't, J'Gendo, L'krk, Mu'tolma, M'Tak, M'Taka, and so many more who she met along her path of exploration and the exploration of war. 'Zaya linked thoughts to and told Fate to give her all, and wished for existence the best of luck. Fate readied herself to tighten her link with the Hunter and the Aristocrat who went about similar regimes. She walked forward on a path of convergence that Fate hoped would lead to a restoration.

Fate breathed in a deep breath, she felt her heart was a little afraid as she did her best to be stoic in the sombre excitement of beginning the path that would lead to the final outcome of the war. Fate pressed the final interface key as she did when she opened and activated the last of the Imperium protocols, and as she pressed the key with her thoughts, she spread her arms out to form a living cross.

She closed her eyes to await the synchronous launch. The interface control panel surged with flickering light until it came to its most vital output, and the At'Lann phase generator hummed with a power resonant with Fate's own. The psionic phase generator seemed to burst with surging power that it could barely contain as its systems came on-line with bolts of every possible colour and description of energy shooting outward into space like a planet size chandelier exploding into millions of energy ribbons shooting out as two massive energy spikes ripped to the macro-phase generators of the Lon'tus and H'Raka as two came from each of theirs to hers. What was left of the universe and reality as set ablaze as what was dubbed J'Poko came to life.

A crescent wedge module of the J'Poko phase generation array separated from the main module to carry Fate to the transport point of her convergence where the Trinity would once again be unified. The convergence of phased and psionic power had begun just as the enemy ships of the horde murderously broke through the darkness cast by erasure and poured into the central and only remaining galaxy where the last stand would be made. A blood soaked circular rain seemed to drench itself upon the Imperium fleet. Fate had no time to look back as the Imperium fleet of brave hearts engaged the Army of Two Rings, the reassembled from the dead army of the Death of Death. The last steps were finally here.

Φ

The Fate of yesterday's future turned to the Hunter, deep in the currents of another temporal stream, with tears flowing down her ice steel veneer as she looked into the combat focused eyes and darkest of wolf blue eyes of the Hunter. Fate smiled slightly but even after all this time, her smile seemed barely there.

Her smile seemed laced with the lament of the loss of her innocence that was taken by the talons of the enemy, and the talons of the bloody war left long ago behind but always remaining on their paths. So much had been taken from them in a war that no one had wanted. Not even the Hunter was left damaged as she looked into his eyes. Fate bore the guilt of the universe upon her shoulders for one that had fallen so far away from everything she once held dear.

Even with her wisdom and youth working in tandem to keep her alive all these empty years, she could not contain the reflections made from the fullness of her memories. Their eyes seemed to shine with the same sheen of the energies that lay outside the temporal night train. Fate started to laugh sardonically,

'Do you remember this day now taking place, 'Iato?'

'I do, 'Imiszi.'

'It was all such a waste, was it not?'

'Was it?' the Hunter slyly smiled with a tinge of cruelty, despair and only a glimmer of hope.

Their souls were aged beyond most, and now carried themselves in the most calm and gravest of fashions. The scars over Fate's heart seemed to almost reopen as did the secret pain of the Hunter. Their path shared together became awkward for the first time since their early days spent together.

'I thought I failed you that day.'

'How could you have, 'Imiszi? You have done more than any could have asked. It was I who failed.'

'We have spent the last three trillion and three years wandering, trying to piece together our shattered souls. All those years you spent alone, trying to find warmth in J'Namu. I realised that no one failed us but we all defeated ourselves against the Death of Death. I simply did not have it within me to save our existence, and I have hated myself for it ever since.'

'You have isolated yourself too long around those who would never know what loss you had overseen, 'Imiszi. And you are right, we did defeat ourselves.'

After a pause, and just before the inter-temporal engine core of their ship would bring their ship back into existence, Fate responded to the Hunter's words that seemed to stitch together a few more pieces of her soul. Her words seemed to flow like those of Faust in the madness of one like Hamlet's life that could not accept itself.

'All this time I thought it was just me, 'Iato.'

'An oracle once told me that I would slay one more powerful than any of H'Raka had ever done before…I am still hoping that it will be the Death of Death.'

Though his words came with great confidence, the Hunter truly had been torn apart by his path so much so that he had no further words to say. Fate took his shoulders with her soft and slender hands as she leaned across to him.

'You still can. You have found balance in your soul once more, 'Iato…and you are worthy of it.'

The Hunter smiled for the first time on his path of redemption that was his path of being a slayer. The Aristocrat, by the command interface console, smiled as those on his path came together as he keyed in the final sequence into the temporal ship interface while he looked back with remembrance to the Fate and the Hunter. He could see how their wanderings through rusted relics had made their souls flow in the waters of the deepest thoughts, and the Aristocrat, also a soul of exploration, also took the pondering path.

After all that remained of the empty cities of splendour laid to rest in the coffin like confines of planet-bunkers and their own devastation, the Aristocrat had had enough of automated systems and remained on the controls of their ship that took them on temporal rails to their destiny. And it was a destiny that the Trinity had almost collectively forgotten but deep in their hearts never could. The sting of their paths, thus far, had returned them to their sole path.

And for the first time in a long time, their soul paths merged and began to emerge to break the solitude of anchorites and exiles so remorsefully contained. The balance of eternal wisdom was once again theirs for the taking, and the one who had taken the path to simply prove it could be done, the one with the exemplary manner of a neo-renaissance diplomat, steered them towards the end of their punishing quest.

The Aristocrat who also walked a path of an ennobled Cincinnatus from the tropical sands of Rimisz'tii that found themselves upon the 'Paradia province of Lon'tus. He had found equals of souls, and he had once again found his forever friends. The Aristocrat continued to key the sequence into the temporal ship interface technology that was the full evolution of L'Ja and Imperium technologies, and he listened on to what could be the last conversation of his comrades.

'I understand your soul, 'Iato. You do not have to say it. No one wanted things to turn out as they did but we, above all others, cannot escape our paths.'

'Who knew the path towards peace and freedom would come with such costs beyond those we were willing to give, 'Imiszi. Even you were blind to your own path. I want what we all want, and I want what you want. Though the path ahead might not exist, there can be no turning back. Are you ready for what you must face again?

'I am no longer afraid, 'Iato. We are the future that comes to pass.'

Fate took a moment and then added, 'Do you think we will ever learn to forgive ourselves?'

'Perhaps one day. Have you? How have you spent the last trillion years?'

'I spent most of it looking inward to see what I truly was and to those once upon my path… I know what you are, 'Iato, just as much as I know 'Lus. We should not drape ourselves in tragedy any longer. And speaking of 'Lus Su'han. Status.'

'We will meet the point of convergence in less than one hundred temporal distance units. May the Imperium prevail.'

'K'nde D'le Snd'ar'

Fate reached her hand out to the Aristocrat who joined her as she took the Hunter's. She took the hand of her eternal kinsman, and to the great warrior of their peoples, as the Trinity was about to take the last steps on their path. Their inter-temporal ship was about to shatter itself into a fiery ruby energy flowing nexus that was the end of the line for them. They held hands and waited for the end, the miserable nothingness they had escaped all their lives. Now, the Trinity would throw themselves like the Sati into the flames.

''Lus, we *are* going home', Fate said with a peace in her voice that only comes before death. The Aristocrat smiled and the Hunter smiled with the same peace as their ship began to rattle apart. The Aristocrat looking to the warning flashing interface display, and he only had time to shout,

'Brace for temporal impact.'

The shores of a blissful Pal'lana never seemed so far away as they did now.

Φ

'Enemy fighters coming in.'

Lt. Commander L'krk said it to Za'szu who sat back as if she were Rodin's Thinker that became the thoughts of mortal combat. Za'szu brought her mind to inter-link with that of the interface of the Lis'talla and the entire Imperium fleet. As one of the best minds of the Imperium, Za'szu swam through the tactical data-stream rapids with the grace of perfect calm to find the perfect target locks on and strategies to use against the locust siege, and like Fate, she knew what she had to bite. The Lis'talla lay ready for her gambit.

'Change heading to mark 6-0-6 mark 33. Maximum power to the shields. Attack pattern 'Mura 7-12.

'The Imperiatrix's manoeuvre,' L'krk thought at his station on the bridge.

It was the first course correction taken before the ship would go into a negatively-sloped spiralling dive into the maelstrom that surrounded the Imperium fleet that was spread across what was left of the universe. The Lis'talla flew through their fleet pocket, zig-zagging the greatest armada the Imperium could assemble before diving into the wall of locusts as it came out the underbelly of the pocket of ships with all guns blazing.

To buy the Trinity as much time as possible, Za'szu brought the Lis'talla directly into the den of vipers. During her stasis, Fate in holo-interface form, once commanded the 'Mazopolo, an Imperium super-dreadnought of integrated At'Lann and H'Raka crews and systems, when her bridge crew were incapacitated from the bombardments from the enemy advance, and used the same manoeuvre to wipe out the incursion.

Though on this day, Imperium once again outnumbered, and as the Lis'talla began to climb slicing its way through the wall of death, this two wave attack pattern became the most efficient suicide run against the void-walkers of the Death of Death. Whatever the cost, Za'szu vowed, the convergence would take place.

As enemy weapons fire tore into the Lis'talla as they edged ever higher, Za'szu looked and became every part the thinker of logic that was at war with the greatest chaos ever to come to their path. Her path became Fate's and everything upon it that was worth pursuing. Using the interface, she incorporated her warrior's ways into her own. As Lu'va was knocked away from her post by an exploding and falling bulkhead, L'krk, took over the helm as Za'szu shouted out to him, 'Steady as she goes. Fate must prevail.'

Their fighters flew about them engaging the enemy with the diligence of Bishop's passions and the essence of the Kosciuszko squadron that seemed to flow with the same force in the At'Lann 303. If only there were more like Zico to come to play. The dogs of war were let slip into a mauling rampage. The shrinking border of the universe became the smoke, fire and blood falling over the cliffs of Dover. Fate was right, Za'szu thought, there was no turning back. The die was cast, and judgement day was upon them.

The Lis'talla, surviving the energy barrage, flew once again in a downward trajectory deep into the loose conjoined ship wall of the First Ring as the Second Ring of Erasure moved so quickly that the plague of necrotic locusts collided with the At'Lann fleet pocket. The Lis'talla's white hot guns shot out Black Widow like web blasts in what was fast becoming a vain effort to contain the tsunami of death.

Several dozen enemy warships exploded about the ship as Za'szu held the course. Time was running out as Za'szu made the second pass. The flagship of the At'Lann Imperium continued the second pass as the ship descended into the valley of death like a raven of purity to blow away another round of the enemy that seemed sure to overtake them at any second.

Za'szu channelled her mind deeper into the interface, and she established a communication with L'unn. Her mind linked with 'Zaya in the At'Lann Imperium central command headquarters, who also swam into the data stream. 'Zaya activated the 'Mura'Lann city bunker, as both she and her sisters could see that the Army of Two Rings had rendered their phase inversion defensive technologies all but useless. The enemy had adapted as it pressed on. The horde had broken through their lines and had begun to carpet bomb L'unn. There was no escape.

The cities were as safe as they could be as 'Zaya folded over to the Lis'talla to fight the remainder of the battle at her sister's side. The youngest daughter of 'Mura found herself on the smoke-filled main bridge as the Lis'talla pulled away from the dark locust storm, and was taking heavy fire from the ever flowing onslaught. 'Zaya inter-linked completely with Za'szu and the interface.

She took her sister's hand before taking over vessel engineering as Za'szu continued to make instantaneous course corrections and fleet strategy changes directly into the interface. They could feel they were knocking on Death's door as two heavy inter-spatial charges hit the Lis'talla with such force that the ship barely held together as half its systems were knocked out. The Death of Death seemed to surround them as the dark force of evil moved in for the kill.

'If we do not succeed, I am glad to face the end with you, 'Zaya.'

'Keep your faith, sister. I still have faith in tomorrow. 'Imiszi will come through,' said 'Zaya with hopeful expectations as interface consoles crackled into static and exploded about them.

The rest of the bridge crew lay dead about them as the sisters left their hopes and prayers with the ultimate product of their genetic inter-trade. It was up to the Trinity to bring about the convergence. Their fate rested precariously above the rotting jaws of the Death of Death who had begun to consume their home as the battle began to burn away the heavenly space of their peoples.

Blasts of black light from the 'Xo ships, white from the 'Raanu, blue from the Lon'tus, red from the H'Raka, mauve from the At'Lann, and bile yellow from the enemy began to shred space apart as the battle progressed to the point where Imperium force were pushed back to Tr'Lann.

The daughters of 'Mura pushed on through their path of war. This was for it all. This was for existence. This was for At'Lann. And this was for the Imperium. The guns of the Lis'talla kept firing on at targets everywhere. Space became a flood of screams.

Φ

Val'damus was in a fire-fight above M'Gata. The enemy was constantly adapting to Imperium attack techniques, and it only seemed a matter of time before the end would come. The horde, demonically reinforced extra-dimensionally, continued to grow and grow as the dwindling Imperium fleet was either shot into erasure or blown out of space by the barrage of the First Ring in an ante that was all too excessive and expensive.

Val'damus left his bridge as his ship's propulsion systems were knocked off-line from continual enemy ramming attacks. He now manned the main weapons platform, symbiotically becoming a part of the gyroscopic interface controls of the main guns. Ship after enemy ship in his path was blasted out of the way as the universe faced its final moments before its very death. He could see the erasure and the very end coming as he continued to fire away and hoping the Trinity would save him. He seemed utterly unafraid as the end came closer and closer.

He kept on firing as his ship was once more surrounded by enemy fighters. He found no end to the continuous targets. His vessel was grazed and gashed wide open on its starboard side that took on and repulsed most of the enemy fire and kamikaze runs. 'Valis Val'damus, yet another son of the clerisy of At'Lann, and one in the middle of the storm of the path of war. He felt no pity or second thoughts as death crept closer as he fully rotated the interface gun-pilot to fire upon another wave that was about to claw its way like vultures across his ship.

He smiled with a sigh of relief as the siege against his ship abated momentarily as Imperium fighters flew through the exploding enemy wreckage that had moved in to kill him, and once more into the maelstrom to take on the dark storm. Val'damus could make out H'khn's fighter zooming past like a blood-lusting shark, and leaving a little less for him to shoot at. He also looked out to near home where At'Lann's elite squadron taking care of business. He continued to fire as the systems of his ship were overloading to critical levels. He was so sickened by this war as the enemy continued to pour in. Erasure was only a few light years away. So this is doom, he thought, so this is doom.

Φ

'Ivia sat back in the captain's seat aboard the T'kala amidst the frosty haze of her, also smoke-filled to choking thickness, bridge. She felt as if, at any moment, an enemy torpedo would pierce the hull and blow her ship to bits. The Imperium fleet was losing too much ground too quickly. The dark horde was trampling its way into the very heart of the Imperium. What was once paradise became the battle-ground of apocalypse. The enemy was shredding away everything they held dear. Judgement did not appear to be in their favour this day.

'Ivia was growing more nervous by the second. The T'kala was being pummelled by blast after destructive energy blast. And though she kept firing, she felt she was in the centre of one like Zeus's kindling and like one left in the shooting gallery of Ragnarok. Her dread became reinforced as erasure edged its blade closer to the throat of the Imperium. Impending doom was everywhere. 'End this. End this,' 'Ivia prayed as her thoughts became the most dreadful of pleadings as the T'kala fell into the no longer escapable pull of erasure.

Warning lights and sounds filled the bridge of the T'kala and its holo-screen. The warning siren became the only sound heard as the dead lay scattered and eviscerated about her. The Ethnarch of 'Xo set the auto-destruction of her warship as enemy fighters swarmed in and on her position. Erasure was only a light year away. 'Ivia watched in silence as the countdown began that armed the ship to blow apart like a shattered subspace singularity.

She looked to the dead 'Xo who had followed her and for their faith lay charred, smouldering in what their existence had been reduced to. She stared out to the holo-screen filled with self-destruct countdown warning flashes and the bloodshed of battle everywhere. The T'kala's engines began to overload as 'Ivia went into prayer for salvation. The horror awaits, she thought in the full suffocating grip of fear, the horror awaits.

Φ

Aboard the N'Lurr, Mu'tolma chanced upon the predicament of the T'kala, and had 'Ivia and the rest of the survivors folded aboard just before the 'Xo flagship exploded in a blaze of sad glory that hindered the enemy for only a moment. An'sze was at the executive officer's interface station verbally feeding Mu'tolma course corrections with their H'Raka third officer, J'bura, firing on every conceivable enemy threat for their K'mja festival of death for the enemy fighters that hurled themselves at the N'Lurr.

The T'kala exploded in dual symmetric aquamarine hued mushroom clouds like those once over Nagasaki and Hiroshima atop one another before the explosion itself was swallowed whole by erasure leaving behind only a trail of grey and pink smoke that only added to the grim *danse macabre* of the battlefield of shredding space.

The crew of the N'Lurr raised their fists and cheered as the forced scuttling of the T'kala took four hundred and seven enemy warships and fighters along with it in the sector of space where it exploded. Fate seemed to still smile upon 'Ivia this day as she had bought a little more time for the Trinity and the Imperium.

She fourth-walled her way to the bridge to join Mu'tolma and An'sze to continue the attack. Za'szu had ordered the fleet to begin a firing withdrawal to the orbit of J'Namu at the border of the At'Lann central system where the last stand of this battle would be made on home space. The N'Lurr, like the rest of the Imperium ships remaining, fired the last of their current rounds, and by way of subspace hyper-corridors, made their way to the heart of the Imperium. Would love shine through?

As the darkness of the locust horde moved ever closer and the Imperium were pushed further back, 'Ivia went to another interface sciences station and the command controls of the automatically piloted Lon'tus ship K'manu (not Captain Val'damus's former ship) and inter-linked with its interface. The K'manu had sustained heavy damage, Captain 'Damaris 'Galnovu and all her hands were dead. The ship had repaired itself, and 'Ivia, as if by the hand of Fate, found an opportunity to return to the front.

However, she chose to hurtle the ship into a large enemy fleet pocket of over six hundred ships as the hyper-particle grid sprang forth from At'Lann weapons array that were one of their few remaining lines of defence that sub-atomically grated thousands more. She detonated the ship in the centre of the pocket with the same effect that the T'Kala had previously upon the encroaching army of the Death of Death.

Across the ever shrinking existence, thousands of enemy ships were skewered like pins through crickets but with the universe being so small their rate of extra-dimensional rate of replacement was that of only a few seconds short of instantaneous. The shock-wave from the explosion of the K'manu even could be felt on the N'Lurr as it collided with the ship with a thudding bump.

Enemy fighters still pecked away, and the Army of Two Rings still forced every step of the Imperium fleet withdrawal. The enemy seemed only seconds away from closing in on them. And that was the least of their worries. Then suddenly, out of the blue, Mu'tolma came to the front as he came through more so than he already had and elevated his soul to the path of one like Galahad.

Times became such that even he chose to return to the path of war, and finally took a stand against the peril of a forever laid silent. And just as much as Fate would be, 'Ivia was more than pleased to see that he decided to change the direction of his path even if it meant taking the new path of boldness directly into an armada of pursuing enemy ships.

Mu'tolma reconfigured the N'Lurr's heavy cannons to form multiple quantum singularity streams vertical in axis to the armoured hull of the N'Lurr and had An'sze change course to turn about, and take out as many of the enemy ships before colliding with the fast approaching wall of erasure. Perhaps 'Imiszi knew, 'Ivia wondered. Their pride in his boldness and bravery was not even noticed by him.

The Ethnarch, as did those aboard the N'Lurr, understood what was to be done and met the moment with the peace of the sounds of Transeau heard over M'Goa. The energy surged into tremendous spatial disruptions that ripped through huge sections of the enemy infestation before their final moment came.

'Ivia, Mu'tolma, and An'sze, facing one another, gave each other the Imperium salute in their last moment as many of those aboard hit the emptiness with more faith than they had ever known. Theirs now became the inevitable silence that follows the end of a party thrown by ones in the vein like Reubel.

Φ

The erasure oozed ever closer as the Imperium fleet raced home to the central core system. Even their minefields no longer deterred the onslaught of the hungry vermin. Captain 'Valis Val'damus's face was in shock, for he believed that Fate would have found victory long before this.

It had finally come to be, he thought. He watched from the K'rana bridge as the K'manu, or son of J'Namu, exploded as he watched the drive-field tracers stream and trail away from his ship. He watched as the erasure itself began to overtake his ship, and at that moment all he was left with was the hope that the Trinity would prevail. He continued to transmit as much tactical data as he could through the interface of his warship to the rest of the fleet for as long as he could.

He turned away from the nothingness swooping in towards him displayed in all its vulgar glory upon the holo-screen of his bridge. There was no time to react.

There was no time to blow the ship. And then he turned to look straight into the motionless, silent end.

Φ

Za'szu, the Regent of At'Lann, sat mashing her fist into an interface console at the side of her centre throne on the bridge of the Lis'talla as their losses continued to mount and erasure continued to advance. She hoped her sister knew what she was doing. They were outgunned and surrounded. But her time on the path was still not over. Fate had to liberate them from evil.

She continued to swim in the data-stream of the interface re-targeting their main guns to near instantaneous realignments. The holo-screen of the main bridge displayed two enemy vessels shattering apart from the trionic plasma blast cannons of the Lis'talla. Everyone was playing for keeps.

The Death of Death had forced Za'szu to follow Fate on the path of war, and now the Imperium path of war seemed to be coming to a literal end as she sat in her smoke and fire ridden bridge. Nu'Ata, M'Gata, N'Bira, and 'Xo were already lost to erasure. Just like that, half of their system had been torn away. Things became even worse as an enemy fighter managed to break though the Lis'talla's defences and broke through the hull two decks below.

Za'szu almost overloaded her mind from her link with the interface as the casualty reports from the lower decks flooded in. 'Zaya, who had folded her way to the Lis'talla, to stand the last stand with her sister, pointed to the holo-screen as she entered the bridge and soothingly took Za'szu's hand as it now displayed the erasure that awaited. It was all up to Fate now as the end drew near like a burning tundra below an ashen sky assassinating what had once been the most beautiful of winters.

Za'szu clutched 'Zaya's hand tightly. 'She is Fate, is she not? 'Zaya asked serenely amidst all the chaos. Za'szu did not have time to answer as the erasure tore into the Lis'talla finally overtaking them in the most stalking of pursuits. Their path came to its omega.

Φ

Fate was the human cross in lilac and *lazulum* hued fires of swirling psionic energies as she was about to take her path into the deepest extent of the sinister nothingness as the full power of J'Poko flowed into her trillions of various gene structures. Her very being was slipstreaming into the very heart of the Death of Death, the great puppeteer who desired only an end to everything. Reality splintered away in a glass like shattering of crystal exploding plumage that grew into a brilliant psionic fire that seemed to be the only speck left in the vast infinity of nothingness.

The Libra's balance had been knocked fully askew by the ancient evil left behind as the pollution of those who purified their souls and transcended beyond reality and non-reality along the way to the purest of paths of enlightenment.

The Death of Death was the frozen bitter steel plate armoured warrior sarcophagus that contained the pus ridden tar residue of all that had been left behind, and flowed ever stronger with every death it encountered and had taken. The void that encircled the last speckle of reality was moving in to deliver the very last killing blow. But now the Fate was here, and she walked into the new reality of her soul's path, and walked into a path where *Doshin So* would steady his sword.

The living nightmare, from all her travels through the psionic realms of existence, had an eerie familiarity to it. This arena of death was like facing, for the first time, the greatest of bosses of the greatest and deadliest of games. The battleground chosen was the rocky bone-yard of a world like Lit'vaa, and a horizon of Volhynia. Nothing remained but the Death of Death standing atop a dark red gibbous, powdered tombstone ground.

'How heinous, how vapid, how I shall kill you,' thought the Fate as she steadied her thoughts as violet psionic energies crackled about her. From her once tender hand, she fired a mauve hued psionic blast at the standing horror that was the Death of Death. The strength of the blast increased successively, as the Fate became so psyogenetically advanced that her modifications to herself made her more powerful than she had ever been. A march of Bikini test blasts psionically shot into the armoured chest of the darkest of beasts.

The Hunter and the Aristocrat, also at peak enhancement psyogenetic equilibrium, fired from rocky ledges nearby as they opened their own gates and came into the venomous heart of a place beyond Tartarus. Fate could see them and feel them now in her mind as the Trinity reunited on the path of war and triangulated their attack on the Death of Death.

The Trinity continued to fire away at the Death of Death with the purest force of sharpest of thought projectiles that could be fired from the most evolved psyogenetic structures in all the Imperium. The Three were hell bent on turning the tables and consuming the dark beast, ending the misery that had plagued life for the last ten years once and for all. The Trinity continued to try and quench their thirst for its blood as their shots became even more destructive.

Much to the greatest of their dismays, the Death of Death stood through it all unscathed as if he were Foley taking a thousand chair shots, and a Flair walking into a collapse.

It was time to be as direct as George II. The Trinity flash-folded and descended even further into the dark heart of what could be their final nightmare to where the Death of Death stood ready to do battle with them. The Trinity of the wind, water, and moon, found themselves in the dark dungeon of the mansion of what war had spawned. They were now residents within evil. Fate slid a bolo of At'Lann maces out of a sub-psionic pouch that served as her arsenal, and tossed it to strangle to darkest of beasts with such force that she could have cut a black hole in half. As time began to grind silently into the thinnest moving pace, the Aristocrat and the Hunter reached into theirs.

The Hunter gripped a sword that one like Takamatsu would even covet. The Aristocrat pulled forth a Lon'tus claymore style sword called a 'Kamasai, and a gauntlet of morpho-psionic alloys that grew across the knuckles of his other hand. The Fate chose to unsheathe her At'Lann straight blade as the moved in for their long awaited true showdown with the Death of Death.

The Hunter passionately yelled an Imperium battle cry, 'H'Rak K'mja 'Ki'. He screamed his way into the ever more violent battle as the Trinity moved in. The Hunter leapt into the Death of Death with a front kick before a barrage of side kicks while arcing his blade to open particle fissures everywhere it sliced. But for all his effort, the Death of Death parried his attack. His blade could not scratch its way through an armour that easily became composed of nothingness.

He was repulsed away with an armour of stalactites glued together into the fist of the beast which struck the icon, the warrior of H'Raka. The Hunter flew into a nearby rock face amazed that he was not able to damage the shard-scale plating that covered the great beast. The Hunter had managed to strike every Achilles point his mind and soul could see, yet his multiple fists, feet, and blade of fury were easily warded off by the Death of Death. Time seemed to fall into rotating, flashing snapshots of itself, as the Death of Death shot out at the Hunter a blast of chalky glint grey psionic hell spikes. Unfazed by what came at him, the Hunter routed the blast with his blade with a *Jodo* like block.

The Aristocrat flash-folded a plethora of roundhouses at the Death of Death in the combination strike of the Lon'tus style of fighting that had the panache of spicy Rimisz'tii thrown into the mix. It was almost grandiloquent but it was an immensely powerful attack just the same.

But the Death of Death was always able to out-fold the Aristocrat and his ethereal mountain shattering blows. The scent of Digweed's heaven seemed barely there. The Aristocrat countered by hyper-warping himself over the sharpest edged ablative armoured shoulders of the Death of Death to reverse German suplex the armoured spectre into a cliff wall. The Trinity continued to adapt as their minds became more and more psionically linked in order to pierce the shell of a still-born soul.

Fate lunged at the darkest of beasts and struck its chinless faceplate with a flash-fold twist into an uppercut. The Death of Death flew three stories into the air before the darkest warrior fell back to the ground and toppled to its side as the Aristocrat managed to somehow shove two short Lon'tus claymores into one of its spiky forearms.

He continued in a psionic zag-stream before throwing two At'Lann *sais* like

Exorcets at the Death of Death which was bringing itself, as if undeterred, to its feet. With the quickness of a piranha in its first bite of food in a day, the Death of Death swatted off the latest salvo from the Aristocrat. The Fate rolled out of the way as the empty anger that was the most demonic of puppeteers lunged his spiked fist at her like a strike of the most vampiric of fangs. The Death of Death came close to ending the path of Fate as it was able to shear, with one of its sharp stalactite like appendages, a lock of her ivory and mauve hair that had become combat tangled and with every lock knotted in platinum wire braids.

Inter-temporal mult-angular sidekicks. Blocked. Psionic scissors quick and ballistic psyogentically enhanced punches. Blocked. Desperate lunges of all sorts. Blocked. The Trinity's attacks with their swords were parried as well. The Hunter jumped even more into the fray as he attempted to slice through the empty ghoul on a near infinite number of psionic planes. His warrior spirit had awakened from what had been far too long a slumber, and as the drums of Death thumped on, he could feel this was for it all.

Fate steadied her sword and tossed another bola of maces that seemed made by the hands of Hephaestus himself, at the throat of the Death of Death once more. Her blade only clanged against the armour of the dark beast as she finished her faster than spatial-folding slash. Fate then converted her weapon into a At'Lann staff of swords made from high density 'Mura ore that moulded itself perfectly in the psionic nightmare reality.

She crouched and side-kicked at her final foe as the Death of Death lunged a punch at her, and she pushed her foot into the handles of the imbedded blades in its forearms. But it was all to no effect as she could not push them deeper into the dark flesh as she slashed the other fist of the beast away with a slash of one end of her staff of swords. She tried not to watch in horror as the blade shattered apart against the dark armour. Fate withdrew and flash-folded a few steps away as she watched the brittle bits fall like silent snow to the dusty ground.

The Hunter folded in from the dark beast's side with a H'Raka machete and attempted to wedge the blade under the plating seam that grew into the chinless and chiselled chin of the mask of the Death of Death. He seemed to ache for something like a chain-saw and brought such an instrument into reality to use against their greatest foe. And though the Hunter was precise in his latest killing strike, as if he were the essence of a Stuka attack, the shards of his last called upon weapon fell to the ground as the Death of Death shoved him away with a blast of tainted psionic energy.

The Death of Death could be seen as a dark opaque cloud within its formidable armour that seemed to move as if to spit with a sneering scoff, laughing at their attempts to win this final battle. The Aristocrat thrust his newest *sais* of Lon'tus diamond-steel as if in a Sten bullet strife across what his psionic sight told him was the weakest points of the Death of Death's armour. And though the Fate's last blow to the dark beast was full of the power of her faith, she only dented the tile and spiked dark exoskeleton. The Aristocrat could not pierce the dark armour as well. Things seemed to slow to the whisper that follows the final kiss of life.

Fate stared down at the pieces of their shattered blades as the Hunter and the Aristocrat tag-teamed to grapple with the Death of Death. Fate picked up a shard of 'Mura ore, and stroked it with her index finger until it bled. Drops of her violet and rose blood fell into the now dust consuming ground as if dirt was just thrown upon their graves.

Fate could feel her very faith had been shattered as much as the once indestructible piece of crumpled metal in her bleeding hands. The Death of Death is winning the day, and with its every ominous step, Fate lost her confidence. She was not invincible and she felt that she was not mighty.

She was once an observer, a listener, and an explorer. She had become a warrior who suffered by not being all things, and Fate made herself suffer even more as something told her it was not within her to win this day. Fate had not stopped the coming of the war, and Fate could not win it now. Fate crushed herself in the guilt of one like the Wandering Jew. She had to stop herself from destroying herself. The Death of Death was attempting to infest her. Fate had to return herself to the path of one like Moses and get what she had wanted all along.

She re-forged her psionic spirit and refused to submit to the suffering of the Death of Death that kept trying to eat away at her already eaten away at soul. The tide of his essence of faecal despair attempted to flood into her and grew ever closer. Fate gripped the shard tighter as a little more blood gushed out from her hands before she let what was left of the shard fall to the ground. She looked down to her blood drenched hands and seemed to find oracles of truth by the sight of her caking and drying dark violet blood.

She saw Za'szu and 'Zaya, and watched their strong souls perish in the onslaught of erasure. The last of the Tr'Lann system, the At'Lann and Imperium home system, was being swallowed up before her. In one sickening instant, everything that was life fell to the twisted zealousness that had pulled the strings over all of nothingness. The Death of Death was overtaking and adapting to the Trinity as its mind now worked to decrypt their psyogenetic structures so it could become the worst of monopolies. Their universe was swallowed up, Za'szu and 'Zaya were dead, and the Imperium was no more.

In a rage summoned from the life fires of sword lilies and the furnace that lit the fires of the deepest parts of her soul, Fate tossed aside her At'Lann *bo* and her Lon'tus *kamas,* and vented all the rage of her loss by flash-folding a front-kick that jammed another Lon'tus *kama* into the most wretched beast's throat. The *kama* was the last one that the Aristocrat had lodged in the thorn covered exterior neck bone of the darkest of beasts. Fate shattered it into the dark armour and outward into high velocity splinters.

Unfazed, the Death of Death twisted free of the once tight grasp of the Hunter and the Aristocrat, and struck the Fate with a power punch that struck her at its full force and threw her in the highest of psionic velocities to another rocky outcrop. The Death of Death easily tossed the Aristocrat aside leaving only the Hunter to face the beast who had consumed almost everything. The Hunter summoned his strength once again into his blade and readied himself for the next salvo.

The Fate had been hit hard and her skull had shattered and was crackled like a broken ice floe. Her eyes seemed nearly welded shut by the force of the blow. She felt her thick blood ooze from her scalp that almost hid the latest sets of damage inflicted upon her. Fate felt very faint and longed to fall into the bliss of eternal sleep. Everything seemed sure to be over.

The Aristocrat had been thrown a great distance away and could not yet force himself to rise from the charred and gnarled dust ridden ground as the Death of Death seemed to walk in a predatory slowness towards him as if across a dead crystal lake of sorrows. The dark beast of all ghouls grabbed the Fate's neck and lifted her dejected form triumphantly over his head. An equally bloody and broken Hunter continued to concentrate his might into his H'Raka broad sword that he held out before him. He readied his mind to move in for the kill.

The darkness of eviscerating and blood-clotting evil grew even more cohesive with every step. Its dark armour was already beginning to heal itself as it held Fate's unmoving form aloft. The Trinity had to move quickly. The minds of the Three moved towards a greater and greater inter-link. The time to move was now. The Trinity was all that remained, and all that was left for the path of the Death of Death.

As the Death of Death held Fate aloft, leering at her all but defeated form, the dark beast, before readying itself, to discard her by tossing her still form to the hard dirt below. The Hunter, now shone in crimson H'Raka fire, and with all his might, shoved his blade out. The Death of Death, in a disgustingly neat shattering flash of time, lifted Fate outwards by crunching into her its spikes and held her form hostage in front of him as the blade designed for the great enemy impaled her, and all of reality as if it were Rome ceasing to exist.

The long blade violently tore through the heart of Fate and sank far off its target into the side of the armour of the Death of Death. It finally happened. Doom finally happened. Death came to strangle the soul of Fate in a gurgling and drowning of her own blood that overflowed out her mouth and pierced chest. Dark lilac blood splattered across the ground and onto her tiara as the soul of Cronos seemed to explode viciously apart.

The Hunter stood in the madness of a warrior's orgasmic climax screaming from the reality that had become his prison. The Death of Death had adapted to every weakness of the Trinity, and had countered their power to not harm one another. Everything became terribly wrong. The corpse that reality became had ravished them and all that now remained was the dead womb and its necrotic semen stained walls beneath the crackling sores of labial lasagne rotting ever quicker away. The Hunter was buried in the madness of the horror. Death had become all innocence lost.

Fate could see her blood covered fingers as she fell further into the abyss of erasure. The Aristocrat lunged forward in psyo-adrenalised shock. As reality slipped away, all Fate could do was look at the blood on her hands. Her existence seemed to drift toward liminal revelations as everything grew dark.

Her life was literally before her eyes. For one shining moment, all of existence and reality became clear. For a glint of time, Fate understood it all. And as quickly as it came, all was lost to her. What was once the perfect logic and chaos, became knocked totally askew. Pain became the Trinity, and all at once, pain froze their souls as what was to be the convergence shattered them.

They fell away from the path, in broken little pieces, falling to the defeat of nothingness. The falling shards the Trinity's souls fell quietly into the darkness that was the last breath of a dying eternity which had strived to keep life alive. The erasure flowed over them like stale dirt onto the coffin of a universe. Complacency was destroyed. The darkness and the horror became all consuming. The phase-generators exploded into nothingness. Was this surrender?

32
Exiles In The Wastelands of Splintered Souls

Fate fell into and became the nothingness as if the erasure had swept across everything. Fate became the totality that she had tried to prevent. Yet, Fate was not dead. A dream remained, or a nightmare of Golgothic misery depending on the perspective. Yet a mere dream did not yield to the nothingness. And Fate was that dream.

Fate lay dead in an aftermath of evil attaining victory before defeating itself. The sword of H'Raka which had pierced her heart was gone but blood still flowed freely from the gaping hole in Fate's chest. She could not understand what went wrong, and why the sword was able to pierce her heart.

Her transpsionic body was beginning to regenerate. Her battle garb was caked with her drying violet and lilac blood. She drifted out from her union with not existing. And now Fate was but a ghost who was left to wander somewhere else. Her eyes shot open, and she was not sure if she was alive, and Fate was no longer sure what was real.

Fate lay in an illuminated circle before a pointillist like etched council of graiae over-souls who had the power to decide if this truly was her journey's end. Souls of those who had built the technology of worlds like L'Ja sat in pious shadows over Fate's still form. Fate was now in the hands of those who were the path of the Origin Species. They sat in stoic apathy etched as much with silent driving faces as they were etched into the shadows that seemed to assemble for the petty matter of a dead girl before them.

They sat over one who had fought all the evil they had cast off when they had transcended with the result being that she was as dead as her people and her existence. But she was Fate, and she just had enough strength to bring herself to her feet to look around to souls far beyond her path and to see she was cast grey under a dim spotlight. Fate struggled with her words as her throat was still choked with her blood.

'… I did not find… the victory of peace.'

Her strength left her as she fell to the cold and sterile ground. She collapsed as she was left without the strength of what she was. As she descended into the silent cold light of burial, and as Fate hit the frozen Darwinian ground, she thought she saw Y'vis as one of the assembled before her.

The room began to spin in spasms of vertigo, and Fate could swear she was watched by the ancient rulers of the Imperium, her family, and even all those she knew in the *genro* before her. Nothing made sense anymore as she fell deeper into the madness of Death. A soul that had many of her paths flow into existence by her empathy wilted under the cold light where all feelings were constrained. There were only walls of haunting silence surrounding her. Fate hit the floor that became thick with her still pouring blood.

Reality seemed an illusion. Everything was wrong. Fate fell further into the darkness where no one remained alive to reach her. As reality became darker, Fate thought she saw her parents sitting removed from it all. So close, and yet, so far away to be sure. The music from one like Trevor seemed forever gone. Her mind and soul were shattering apart. Her path was no more. And then everything faded to black.

Φ

Fate awoke in the debris field of ships from the first wave, the second wave of the Two Ring horde, and the wreckage of their destroyed phase generators. The first thing she felt was the knowledge that the Death of Death might not have been able to destroy existence but had been able to destroy almost everything that had mattered to her. The Death of Death had eradicated the peoples of the Imperium. All her psionic links to them had been cut and her thoughts found no else that had remained. It was as if awakening as the last one standing, and as one that had not fallen to the Black Death.

Time churned in a ill fashion to move on once again. The once heavily melted hulls that had made for a noose shaped graveyard were as cold as her once powerful psygenetically created flesh. Fate was still lifeless and far from the sun that somehow still burned on. Lying in the midst of the debris field of wreckage, Fate could only feel that she was walking through death and felt left to be exiled to the emptiest of spaces.

Fate felt more like a ghost than the ghosts of ships that lay floating around her in their stagnant orbit of hollow mausoleums. Fate finally awoke to a silence that could no longer be enjoyed. The life of her universe seemed forever gone. Fate was as parched as if with the dry mouth of one like Bacchus after a binge with absinthe and ambrosia, finding himself in the morning after.

She was the drought that remained behind after extinction left to thirsts to be quenched in the fermented rains of sorrow over her shattered soul. Fate awoke to the empty new day and a universe spawned by all they had lost. Her thirst needed more than a few drops to numb her pain.

Fate awoke to what felt like a caged tomb emptier than Spandau, and yet for all Fate suffered, she only wished it worse upon herself for all the faith she had failed to live up to. Fate could only believe that she had failed existence itself. The explorer Fate became her own worst gallows. She was the shattered ice, the path frozen, and the path left to a death of exile, left to a death of one like Scott. Yet, for all her path had taken her to, Fate was not dead, and Fate was still there. This was the tomorrow she had always feared. And now Fate was left to walk the wastelands of the splintered soul. The Three had been lain to waste. The Trinity was shattered.

Fate shivered slowly to life. She was so cold. The darkness of space was almost uninviting for her. She opened her eyes in time to watch the expansion of the new universe and reality move out as if it had climbed out by itself from the dead womb of the last. Besides what wreckage remained behind as the tombstone of the Imperium, a few pieces of the macro-phase generators, this reality cut its own umbilical cord and grew itself out into eternity.

Such moments were once times for wondrous joy for the Fate but after so much sacrifice, so many ethics tossed aside for the sake of the path of war, joy had been lost to the abyss of misery for all. Liberation had not come to be for those she vowed to protect. In this moment, she did not see her quiet path as anything more than the beginning of an imprisonment for those guilty of failure and for the suffering that could never convey all that had been ripped away from her.

Fate had once tortured herself to continue on the path of war, and in this empty place she once called home, she seemed bent on continuing her sad penchant. With what little strength she had, Fate pushed her spirit to move, and the Fate slowly flew home to a desolate L'unn, to a desolate 'Mura'Lann. Fate knew that even though existence had survived, it had become a fenced path.

As she flew home, the Fate tried to grasp the enormity of an entire universe erased and figured that all but three percent of all genetic sequences had survived degenification. Fate's path had brought with her all its defeat, and what was left behind in the aftermath.

A few days later, Fate made her way to L'unn, and in her homecoming, she was greeted by a world that had been ravaged into ice-ash and bomb craters. The lush forests of Kem'ja Khonn, the once tranquil atmosphere, the river K'urszt, the exhilarating oceans of 'Mura'Lann, all life, gone. Utterly gone. All that Fate once held dear had vanished into erasure. In space, Fate turned to look upon E'de. The world had become a become a swirling ball of dust over a wide array of decomposing carcasses of once great beasts and base sequences that were once the greatest achievements of the At'Lann and the Hy'Bor. Namistai could no longer be heard. Fate turned her gaze to Lon'tus, to H'Raka, only to see worlds as scorched as her own. The music for one like Fleming that once was the pulse of existence, no longer played, and in her world, there was no more love from Russia.

This brave new universe held the splintered seeds of the genetic remnants that the Second Ring of the Death of Death did not have the chance to eat away at. Fate tried to find solace even with the deep wound from the Hunter's sword that the Death of Death used to kill her. The only thing that kept Fate going was that at least some of what was, even if it was only three percent, was spared. Though the Tr'Lann system survived as tombstones around the sun, the universe had become another Mount Pleasant.

The Fate kept flying on until she reached the entry point of what had become their continent bunker. Even after her death, Za'szu still continued to impress Fate in how hard and how far she went. She had spared no expense. Perhaps her love for her clan and her sunny memories kept Fate going as she stood on the barren, ravaged, and defeated world that was her home. Before a charred interface console that dimly glowed in the silver sheen of L'unn, Fate keyed in the decryption sequence and psionically changed the phase variance inside the city-bunker, and she opened the great door to the cemetery that was her home.

Fate had returned and Fate's sight could only see such emptiness, such silence that was sadly so welcome to her, as this was more than a city-bunker. Fate found the oceans of At'Lann a frozen slab, without any wakes or waves, and without any temporal movement but she did find her oceans.

Fate re-routed power from their heavily drained and damaged Imperium Interface to re-ignite the thermal core of L'unn. The waters of L'unn instantaneously began to warm up in what she knew could only be the 'Mura'Lann defence bunker. The islands and a large proportion of the land remained. And though the environmental controls were brought back on-line to what Fate had remembered them to be. Fate was still left wounded and shivering.

She walked the winter beach that melted like frying butter on a pan, and as the interface did its best to bring things back to Fate's optimum comfort level, the Fate tried not to think of all the emptiness of life that was all around her. Fate focused her path on returning to her home amongst the lilacs.

When she finally made her way to her pyramid, Fate found that her lilacs were left brittle, freeze-dried skeletons of themselves. Her home, once beautifully restored by the hand of the sister she was so proud of, had never before been left so tattered and torn. Her home and hearth had become a dusty tomb. All her people were gone. And not a trace of any life of the Imperium, which once so fruitfully thrived, remained. She could even see that the gene-storage crystal depository had been erased of their priceless data. All but the dejected Fate remained, and no one else had survived.

Fate fourth-walled through the quiet structure to her sitting room and increased the temperature by five levels. To her astonishment, her quarters were nearly immaculately intact. She made her way to her bed that she rarely used and rolled taxingly into the sheets. She no longer seemed desire her eyes forged by the path of war, to look out to this hollow world for awhile. Her eyes, surrounded by thick black circles from all the pain she came to exist in, were such tired eyes. So with an almost primordial desire, Fate, with all her guilt, fell asleep amidst the tombstones of what was once her existence.

Φ

Fate awoke from her narcoleptic binge in a shiver and a shivering that brought her from the realm of sleep to arise to reality once again. There was a light coat of dust, as a pinching of time had passed over everything in the 'Mura'Lann bunker. Fate brushed the thick pinch of dust off herself, and walked outside to stand on her terrace, to see the empty streets, the great buildings, the silent docked ships in the deserted space port at outside edge of the city.

Fate psionically brushed off the last bits of dust off her dry blood caked body, and without almost knowing it, ran out to her silent and still sitting room. She returned back to her bedroom contemplating returning to slumber, and saw the sheets were layered in the tawny dust that had passively overcome her silent home. Fate brushed off her night stand interface display that was less dim than the bunker light whose artificial rays shined in just outside her bedroom door. Fate brought 'Mura'Lann's self-cleaning systems back on-line with a few slides of her tender and still scratched fingers. At least the interface was more functional than it was when I first arrived, Fate thought as she tried to think optimistically.

Fate had slept for a long time. The interface brought up scans of the other worlds of her home system. M'Goa had especially suffered and its new rings forged in tragedy seemed to strangle the still and lifeless world below so many of the small worlds of various species of the Imperium that had been reduced to orbital rubble while others were left barren. Sister Bliss was no longer heard and even the echo from long ago days was no longer there. Thanks to the pull of the once again expanding sun, both that of what remained of J'Poko and M'Goa managed to keep their other planets in the system which seemed just as scarred as Fate's home and centre system. None of her home worlds had escaped being ransacked by the Army of Two Rings, or the cruellest hand of the Death of Death.

She shut off the cylindrical and rotating holo-display that had arisen from her night-stand, with little motivation to see more at the moment. As her home began to clean itself as the dust was trans-atomically cleansed away, Fate teleported herself to the beach before waters that barely became waves in the stillness of it all. Fate continued to walk in her warrior's garb as she removed her boots to walk in the sands. Wanting only to see warmth upon her soul, Fate made the molecules of L'unn transparent in the rock walls above her.

Though time no longer mattered, as Fate had slept through quite a few eras, she still wanted the warmth of the sun to shine contemplative rays down on At'Lann for the first time in years. Fate walked into the oceans and boiled them into the heat of the hottest of hot-springs. Her bloody garb disintegrated as Fate lay floating alone in her oceans. She looked into the light of what seemed an almost different sun. Fate then telekinetically activated an interface to change the orbital position of L'unn for better rays to melt the sad ice of her shattered soul. She lay floating in what seemed the aether waters of a place that was once as glorious as Olympus.

Fate floated on without movement and thought of the Hunter and the Aristocrat. Gone from existence. Gone from her soul. Perhaps they were on other paths she could not see, she hoped and tried to believe. But they were gone. She hated the thought of the Hunter's final moment being the fulfilment of finding victory in what could be only thought of as a lost campaign. If he came to exist like Fate, she thought it would be hard for him to continue to exist even if he survived. Their so-called victory was indeed far more bitter than defeat. So much of what once was had been exterminated and erased from existence, wiped away in the sheer totality of the last stand.

Fate longed for the side of the Aristocrat, and wished that on some path he had returned to the lush tranquillity of satin quilt caressing oceans. She found it far too tragic that one who had fought so hard simply for the honour of doing so, could not have returned to his favourite beach side plantation estate. His world should have been spared the hand of the Death of Death, leaving Fate's shattered heart full of the greatest burden of the silence about her. Fate wished she could forget it all.

The Trinity had integrated itself into so much of Fate that its defeat and its loss to her soul left her without that which made her what she once was. Her memories were fraught with the same stale tinge that had marred and destroyed their struggle. Fate hated what she now was. She looked to her wet and tanning mauve and lavender skin of her body. On her chest, remained the largest of all her scars as if the broken stones of the walls of Jericho had been the shrapnel that had torn its way through her heart.

''Iato, how you must suffer with yourself. And how we all suffer now if you walk the barren path as I do. The Trinity is no more, and the enemy greater than the Death of Death is ourselves. The Death of Death had an easy time with us. And now my soul seems lost from too much war. How much did the darkness poison our hearts?'

Her thoughts seemed to pour away in the heat she so craved. Fate kept L'unn's orbital position stable to what little joy she could find basking in the light that her pale body seemed so remote from. The last daughter of 'Mura floated herself into distraction and away from her loss of faith that had wavered into a last day of sale decline. The ocean waters boiled around her to the point where it would consume flesh but even they could not melt away her frozen soul. At least the empty beach still looked beautiful, she thought as she floated back to the silent shore as her restored garb grew back onto her form cleansed of blood and had a little more of her colour return to her.

Fate returned to the lilac pyramid where her lilacs began to bloom once again amidst the stillness of 'Mura'Lann. At times, its quietly screaming walls were far too deafening for Fate as she tried to block it all out by climbing back into her bed and a state of rest. Fate fell back asleep in the tomb of her heart.

Φ

After a restless sleep of only a few years. The Fate came full circle on her barren path in the wastelands of her soul. Fate became obsessive to remember the memories of what was. For weeks at a time in her sitting room, she would put herself into holo-interface programs of holo-film taken from Imperium warships. She would interact with the holographic versions of her comrades, acting out past battles, or battles like that on L'Ja. Her favourites became the gambit in the M'Kema system, in which she took the Lis'talla to the core of a enemy hive ship to detonate it from within, and the siege against the 'Xo home world before they joined the Imperium home system which Fate modified the holo-program to win the battle.

Fate sank into the memories of what was on her barren path alone. In the days that followed, she even came to enjoy walks in the virtual country sides with Za'szu still challenging her as she always did, and with 'Zaya who would explain to Fate her latest psyogenomic theories. Fate tried to find herself again around her artificial sisters that held a small remnant of their virtuousness and the great wisdom of their souls.

Fate did everything she could to battle the silence. Battle re-enactments, strolls in the woods with those she cared for who shared her path, M'Goa parties, confession, and even reconfiguring the interface to bring all its scans of the new existence into her sitting room that became her holo-room as that which became her days. She tried to separate herself from her fantasy world by studying data from the various probes the interface had launched for her, though she did so with a holographic 'Zaya at her side to confer with.

After a while, the empty days spent with photonic company seemed all too fleeting and far too punishing for the Fate. She made it worse on herself by spending far too many days at a time in the confining corridors of L'Ja lamenting all she had lost. Ancient combat scenarios of all she had endured no longer was enough to keep her going. It all made Fate far too uneasy with herself. On her last day in the virtual world, holo-Za'szu and holo-'Zaya, as usual, wanted to know of every nuance of the enemy technologies, and Fate, much to her surprise, remembered them all too well.

Fate hugged her interface derived sisters goodbye as she quieted them to end their friendly debates and conversations, and Fate shut down the holo-room to return it to being the silence of her sitting room. Everything returned to its stillness and the stale silence which now ruled L'unn.

Fate did her best to repair the interface and return the cities in the bunker to the beauty that they once were before the dark invasion. Fate changed the phase variance of the 'Mura'Lann bunker and placed it in temporal stasis to keep her home as she left it. Fate sealed the bunker as she departed its confines and left At'Lann once again, and separated herself from her empty home drenched in the breakdown that follows information overload.

Φ

Fate had had enough of reliving what was, and she flew away from what she could never escape. The nightmare of what was seared into her mind branded her like a slave with her own dreadful misery, and the nightmare that always stung at her wounded heart. Fate did what she could, and thought leaving home was the best way to live with it.

The new path alone had evolved to where there were things worth seeing once again in the reality that imprisons her. The Human species on E'de, created from the genetic remnants of the Imperium, had both expanded their evolutionary path as much as they were constrained by the innate path to seek out what they might have been. They still were a young offspring born from the loss of what was but Fate thought life beginning anew was one miracle that the Death of Death could not take away.

The children of E'de still resigned themselves to intra-species civil economic war but those times seemed drawing to an end and a divergence of market flows when their wealth became overabundant. Their primitive capitalism and economic systems had begun to evolve like never before when it became financially feasible for private industries to pursue space exploration, mining, after geological surveys were carried out, as well as colonisation.

All of which led to corporate and governmental convergence as individuals in the economy of socio-economic contrasts bought their way out of financial obligation through purchasing large blocs of stock in ultra-corporations, and which coincided with Human colonies becoming reality on what they called Luna and Mars. And moral human individuals released many of their own kind from wage and financial slavery until all humans had more freedom than their constrained species had ever known.

As wealth became overabundant, social capital increased to the point where the only differences in equality arose from paths of individual choice, and what one had done to better themselves. As the Human race expanded outwards from their home system, they did what Fate could not, and let themselves go from the war against themselves. The Human species, though aggressive, arrogant and adversarial, had grown into explorers of knowledge, and that gave Fate's scarred heart a small measure of peace.

Human data, intercepted by the interface, detailed how ores from Mars could be molecularly combined with what the Humans called Earth minerals to produce hulls for space faring ships at a fraction of what was the previous competitive cost that multiplied the effect of their economic expansion in one of their most historic drives of market innovation.

When the Human race became a space-faring people, their economic markets were transformed as their markets had grown to be dominated by multi-planetary corporations. When their interplanetary economic systems came into existence, the face of this new humanity was changed for the better. It seem more than ironic that the very financial wealth that enslaved them was the same wealth that liberated the path of their species. Yet Fate was still hardly aroused by it all.

Fate had another reason to leave as her neighbours were now the living embodiment of all she had lost. She vowed to still tend to them and perhaps have her path join theirs when the need arose. For the moment, Fate chose to remain alone on her path. There was now a large enough universe to see. She would have the interface contact her if there was need to return home. And then Fate flew out into space to find herself once again.

Resting in the silent tomb, like all markets, became governed by the law of diminishing returns. As Fate flew out, she thought of the Human markets that were saved by first contact with a similar species, and Fate hoped to find one like her to set the balance right. She thought of how she should change the dynamic of her existence just as the path of Humanity changed.

After the first official first contact, the Humans developed an elaborate barter system where goods such as genetic sequences or technology were traded for other technologies, mathematical theorem for mathematical theorem, literary and artistic databases for literary and artistic data bases, and so on and so forth.

The Humans had advanced their existence enough to have crude molecular replication technology become publicly available. Consumerist paths of wealth accumulation largely went to the grave, and the occupation of advancing themselves in life became the reward for training and study. Compensation in life came from the benefits of the path chosen aside from neutral worlds where previous market structures continued. Fate wondered what benefits she would offer to one like her.

Fate left the grave of the Tr'Lann system, she left with a new faith that her home was watched by those worthy of a path to At'Lann in, perhaps, times to come. The Humans had evolved enough to unify their governments into a interplanetary system of governance and a society where, once every genetically incorporated citizen, and now either a citizen of the neutral path of capitalism continued or of the interplanetary government, was driven to expand new markets with the allocation of most of their resources towards innovation, efficiency, creativity, education, exploration, and career. Fate wanted to free herself just as the Humans had with their technology that still paled in comparison to the At'Lann.

At least Fate knew what remained the universal currency should she desire to encounter anyone along the way. She tried to find the same liberation as the day when a single percentage no longer controlled the wealth of an entire economy. She centred her natural greed on the same path that was that of humanity by returning to exploration, and by seeking both technology and new artistic concepts to give her some release.

And as the Humans unified away from their formerly brutal ways to one where every citizen was a stakeholder in the Human path to compete against the universe, Fate would once again competed for hers. She thought it all about time, for the Fate had rested too long. She flew away from her home and that of a thriving post-consumerist culture, and she flew on with a little caress of happiness that her home system was fully populated. And like Humanity, Fate left as something more.

Fate made her way to the Imperium debris fields that her probes the interface sent out had either cloaked or melted down into exterior core elements, leaving the enemy and Imperium property safely hidden, and counter-intrusion technologies took care of the rest. She psionically scanned what remained of the technology before moving on to take her path into the wilderness once more. What she found seemed to release her soul a little as she flew fast through space once again as Fate, in the prison of her own defeat, returned to her solitary path.

Φ

Fate returned to At'Lann years later with her soul having healed somewhat, and in seeking what she sought for herself, returned with a treasure-trove of trans-temporal technology originating from a wide variety of sources. She also plundered from the Trinity's macro-phase generators components for all she sought to do. Her soul had brought her onto a new path. Fate now had it within her to construct a means to once again breathe in the life of sweetness that was the love of her soul, and revive the murdered body of the Cronos of another path. After so much pain grew into her after all her losses, Fate craved an end to this alien and, at times, isolating moksha.

Fate dutifully assembled her creations in the shadows, and in the dark. For a time, to complete her new task, Fate like an anchorite, fled into the wilderness of darkness and away from the sanctuary of day. Fate no longer felt the need to make transparent the mantle of L'unn. The aged shards of her shattered soul had learned to live with the torment of pain that gnawed away at her every moment. Fate was at a cross-roads, yet strived to the high voltage voyage sounds of one like Graham to fully return to her.

As Fate finished the latest phase of her new technological endeavour, during the latest perigee of her new existence, Fate realised how far she had to go. After all the time Fate had spent encountering billions of error paths to reconfigure the interface to run her new creations, her mind was reaching burnout from data-overload once again. The years spent away from the icy grave of her civilisation had been rough ones in terms of they brought the way of Fate's path. And sometimes she could not stop her thoughts from her soul crying out, 'Someone on this path save me. Save me from this. This suffering I cannot take anymore of it!'

In spite of how far her soul had walked through the bitter wastelands, Fate remained constantly imprisoned, and not an end appeared in sight for one that seemed eternally damned. Her old cigarettes seemed stale but she smoked on anyway in the underground, in the tomb that was the constant reminder of everything that was, and the one that became her own personal and private prison. After she had finished all she could now, the Fate forced herself to leave for the sake of her own sanity.

Fate flew back into the skies of space until she came to the skies of E'de, and fell without regard to the world below. Fate let herself fall away as all her sorrows followed her everywhere she went. She crashed through the arctic ice like a faster than light meteorite into the firmament below, and through frozen waters left brittle and broken by her. Fate had fallen so fast and so hard that she came out of temporal sync, and found herself in some other time. The cold winds that swept across her face blew across all of her as she embraced the chill of Death.

In the centre of the ice-shard crater the size of Anfield, Fate started to laugh as tears rolled down her bleached mezereon cheeks, amidst the sardonic misery of where her path had brought her. The cold air of this place was beyond that of Ulan Bator but as the cold numbed her, her body of bones snapped and crackled, for she was a soul that had fallen onto the path of apathy.

Her psyogenetic structure popped her bones and musculature back into their optimal placements. Her dark violet blood plumed and froze in a lotus blossom of the damned amidst the shattered ice, in a stark and agonising sad vividness of her colour. Fate laughed as she could only think of how, in too many ways, she remained immortal.

The Fate, in all her sad glory, once a bloody broken mess, lay nearly restored by her auto-regenerative transpsyogenic healing factors. Fate's body slid down a valley of melted ice until she slid to a clearing where she chanced upon a hunter of unknown species origin trying to shoot down a polar bear, a variant of the At'Lann Utupuku from what had been their U'linn bears that had more the look of elongated jaguars.

Fate rose from the wind-worn ice and now frozen waters. She could not let the creature die as it had been far too long since she last saw anything similar to the beautiful ursine gaze, so strikingly similar to those of her favourite of a home that was lain to an ashen rest long ago. It disgusted her that such a poseur of a hunter was so obsessed with killing such a creature. The sound of the ice shattering from Fate's descent into E'de was left ignored, and only death would bring satisfaction to this poacher. The obsessive nature of it reminded Fate too much of what she hated most about her way.

This little one seemed far more unique than any of its species which she could see beyond the horizon. This one was smarter than your average bear. The polar bear moved fast enough to dodge the harpoon like projectile shells that hurled silently past it. Fate could see the evolving genetic mutation beneath its form that had produced a shining intellect. She could see the bear had within it the ability to walk and talk.

Fate saw before her a living embodiment of an evolving gene-link to something more was being preyed upon for what could only be the dirtiest of profits. She saw before her such a creature of balance, living in a perfect harmony with nature and existence. The thought that someone would harm such a creature reviled her spirit. Fate had to intervene.

As the bear fell in the snow, tranquillised from a shot from the vile poacher, Fate chose to stand on a path that she had not in so many years. She would not have harm come to any of the noble divine creatures under Ursa, as she rushed towards where the bear put its paws over its eyes expecting the dark thunder of the impending doom from a scavenger, and expected death one that seemed nothing more than a poverty strewn Loki. As the poacher in tarnished garb and skin of soot and grey stood ready to take away the innocence of its life, Fate steadied her own thoughts. The traitor to capitalism moved in for the kill shot, Fate incinerated the poacher in a highly vicious psycho-kinetic plasma and particle violet flame storm.

Fate stumbled toward the sovereign creature of this hinterland. She fainted into unconsciousness as the last thing Fate saw was the polar bear, which Fate would come to call her Utupuku, investigating by sniffing Fate's bosom in snout pokes of curiosity as everything went dark.

Φ

Fate awoke to the smell of freshly bitten seals and the smell of snow. She had been carried by her Utupuku into its den of ice. The natural grandeur of snow light silently filled the air. The tpk had neatly stacked three freshly killed seals with one above the other at the opening end of the ice cave. Though the bear was only an animal, Fate was impressed and curious about its cognitive abilities.

The nine-year-old polar bear bit them one by one and tossed them by the scruff of their bulbous necks, flinging and batting them further to Fate with her strong and powerful paws into a similar looking stack that flew and slid until they were in front of where the daughter of 'Mura lay.

Utupuku was a sovereign creature both as humble and confident as the ice, water, and sky. Fate could see in the bear's thoughts that it was a true gift to existence. Fate was more than obliged by the hospitality of her host who had also taken the path alone. As Utupuku began to eat her single seal lain aside for herself, Fate could see this noble animal had both the civility and intentions of a proper host, and she watched as Utupuku used her pretty eyes watch her food, to her nice little teeth chew away on the most favourite of its treats. After all the creatures she had seen on her travels, few seemed as unique.

Fate watched as Utupuku sunk respectfully and hungrily into what were her dreams. For her, this was the blessed bounty from a creature willing to share an innocent dream. To be a proper guest for the evolved polar bear, Fate took a bite of the meat that steamed in her mouth. The daughter of 'Mura found the texture curious and could tell by the taste that its seemed in balance with the selfless fruition of one like her. As Fate swallowed, for whatever reason, it reminded her of what the ancient H'Raka used to eat.

Fate appreciated the kindness of one like her who found a home in a land under the sun and moon, a home always in search of the dream that brings tomorrow. For the bear who shared her den with her, this was her castle in the sky amidst the ice. As Fate sat up, no longer bloody or broken, the young eyes she saw contained a suffering Fate knew from her own reflection, and she could see the same pain drowned in clarity. The path did not seem lost. Fate converted the other seals that her host thought her slender form seemed well in need of, into a sparkling, floating raspberry, carrot hued glitter of psionic energy and fed some to Utupuku as she delightfully ate the food she was offered.

A storm of wind and snow continued to blow by outside as the two souls began to spend many a night before strolls during the day together in the way that enlightened Fate to see a different path of ursine tranquillity other than that of the Lit'vaa. Fate let Utupuku be her guide of this path of existence before she came to leave. But before she did, Fate ensured that her little friend who led a life alone and had not ever had any cubs, would have the gift she so craved. Fate saw another at her side who walked with peace in a beautiful bond with nature and the land, and she decided to reward it to one, who in many ways, was on different paths ahead of hers.

Fate imbued Utupuku with one of her psyogenetic components of her enhanced genetic matrix and sub-matrices. In return for her kindness, Fate made Utupuku an enhanced being. Fate flash-folded a small arsenal of Imperium weapons from 'Mura's armoury. Hyper-pulse rifles, sub-spatial mines, swords, trionic cannons, she spared no expense for another one who now would find superiority in their humanity and what they exist as. She also left her some data-crystal recordings of essential mixes from M'Goa which she handed into her new friend's paws, and told her friend in her thoughts . . .

'Let only those who are one with the ways of existence of your species hunt your kind, solely if they are in a worthy hunger. Your kind should be rarely feasted upon. You now have strength on top of strength. I cannot free you from the path of the survival of the strongest but for all you have done for me by letting me into your thoughts and exploring the ice expanse, I leave you its guardian.

If you are disrespected, I have prepared you for what must be done. We now share a covenant to watch over one another, a covenant I have not shared with anyone for a great many years. Farewell, my friend. May you always remain on your path, and find all you seek that brings you joy.'

Utupuku, who in many ways, had a way about her like Za'szu's benevolent toughness and nurturing, brought a little solace back to Fate's soul. Her whole experience on this path reminding her of the way her sister used to be; always rushing to the aid of any pain felt by others. Always rushing to hearts of goodness, Fate lamented. Though she loved her sisters equally, the loss of Za'szu to Fate was much harder for her to take than any. The flow of the path changed. She had to push on as the Fate did what she could to leave her new friend in safer hands, she let her new friend walk the path of humanity if she chose.

Sad to see her leave, Utupuku asked why the daughter of L'unn had to go. 'Lîna, as she let Utupuku call her, told her further augmented and ennobled friend who shared her path that the misery of her future's end could no longer keep her here. Fate promised she would return if she ever became whole or if in need of her. Utupuku embraced Fate in such a lovely hug that her hollow fur to keep her warm was filled with as much love that grew in her heart. They both shared paths to balance freedom, and Utupuku knew Fate had a long way to go on her path. Fate did not want the kindness of who was once a stranger fall to feeling as imprisoned as Fate felt about her existence. Fate flash-folded herself back into space, and tpk bade Fate farewell with a still wave from her immaculately carved paw that grew into a slender, almost light silver hued, hand of a woman with perfectly manicured moonstone coloured nails.

Φ

For a time Fate languished in a restless sleep in what remained of her soul, as she walked on as a ghost in the wastelands that seemed stretch on forever. Fate could not find peace. Part of Fate could not forget, could not let go. Fate flew into the core of her system's sun, and even there she could not find rest. Fate found no rest in the storms of J'Namu, in the 'Vanx catacombs, submerged Lon'tus, anywhere on her path in this existence. Even the sun was not enough for her. Fate still remained cold. Fate once more set out on a path of exploration, and left the Imperium system, which remained extinct to her. She seemed to walk into a wonderfully divine light that cast itself once again over her and had the taste of the ecstatic nights on M'Goa.

Fate returned to the path as the explorer as if she were a frozen Scott wandering home. But Fate brought her path only to the ruins of what was, and that was also symbiotically a part of what was new. The only thing that kept her going after she returned to At'Lann, only to find that the gene-storage data-crystals had been wiped of their memory, was that she tried to leave each dead world a little less despondent than before. The Fate began taking her path to dead worlds that thrived as something else as well as new ones she had never encountered before.

Fate passed herself off as a citizen in some and less than what she was in others, and on the deadest of worlds she stood alone. She even joined the crews of ships lost in space until they made their way home or lived on space stations in far away frontiers. As Fate ventured deeper into the her essence of exploration, learning all that can be learned, seeking paths that join and cross your own, Fate seemed to become something more than she ever was. She was not sure if she was healing but she felt more whole than she had in some ages. Fate seemed to once again be on the path of what was to come.

Fate began to walk with a greater clarity as she continued on her path towards the secret truth. Fate had found the path, the Trinity, the way home. She somehow kept on because she knew eventually she would be there. But something else remained.

33
The Path Home

As the flash of the spatial fold ceased, Fate stood alone on the transport pad, in the middle of the path, that should have taken her away along with the Hunter and the Aristocrat back to L'unn and back to At'Lann. She had not left with the Trinity but she had reunited with the path of souls to complete the ultimate convergence.

The Fate had simultaneously stepped onto the ice of L'unn and stepped back onto the path. For a moment, the silence was almost deafening as Fate stepped off the Imperium technology transport platform. In the distance ahead was a ballet of mauve and delphinium violet light. Like the speed of Whitfield after a sprint in the deep funkyness of one like Onionz.

The sonic gushing buckets then became a new expedition. Fate fell to the ground by its sheer trance symphony of beauty that went all the way into her mind. Her faith wavered with uncertainty. The curiosity of it all was enough to keep her conscious as defeat grew to overtake her inside herself, for she had not felt beauty of the path in some time.

Then a miraculous sight gave her the strength to remain alive. A soft gentle hand of one who shared the path of her existence before reaching down for hers to grasp. Everything seemed in a purple haze, and Fate could not make out the form that made its way to her from the distance ahead, and had taken her hand to raise her from the ground. Fate took the hand that seemed to save her battered and war ravaged soul. She knew who it was the moment she felt the touch of one for an angel. Perhaps she had wanted this more than she thought, or else this was the path that answered her cry for help. Reality seemed to fill with the tranquil air of destiny. Fate's eyes met Kir'rus's once again.

As they stood before one another the wind swept across them in the heavenly glory of transual summer mornings gazing out from a wondrous place like Plâge de Préybré. The psionic vision of such a view became the reality. The two were everywhere and nowhere in the universe amidst the stacks of universes where every existence was a mere molecule to the next with a path of paths running through each one. Few ended in nowhere but all were in limbo towards somewhere and Fate's path came to overlook the frozen fountains of time.

Fate clasped Kir'rus's hand before turning to see a sleek modern gothic intertwined building, an evolved Romanesque structure with a high tower and steeple that also had a manor's cut set in a photonic glow of lilac and dewberry. They walked in sand by cedars with the wind at their backs with a gaze at one another that worked to let each of them in on the other's thoughts. The two walked briskly and soon made their way into a great hall. And this became the moment that so much became clear to the Fate.

The high-order transpsionic hall became the world around the grey and tan silk marble that grew into the mauve and moonstone walls with a high ceiling amidst photonic marble statues of those who had seemed to have come before. The ceiling was a fresco of constellations and galaxies that mapped paths across entire universal bodies. Everything above them was cut in a way that seemed almost classically obsolete, and yet every moment became ever more contemporary.

As Fate continued to hold Kir'rus's hand, she became more than able to look through what was corporeal and further into the shimmering streams of that below the genomic and of the soul sphere of spheres. It all became clear. Enlightenment filled this holiest of grounds on the path. Fate confirmed what she had always known and that had kept her on the path ahead. She always knew he was not the one but he was the continued promise of the forever path.

Fate smiled proudly at Kir'rus as she finally made her way into his thoughts as if to the beat of some Northern Exposure playing inside and out of reality.

'You know I never asked you for your full name, one of M'Goa who seemed more At'Lann than M'Goa. You too share a path that is walked forever. Tell me your name.'

Fate asked what she always wanted to know, and knew the answer as soon as she finished speaking. The question was a part of the path that had driven her here. The temporal and existential alignment rotated through the streams of universes they could see, and was another small movement toward what was to come. Kir'rus spoke the words she said aloud in her heart.

''Imio Kir'rus N'P'Goa 'Mura'Lann K'hana 'Maq…I am Fate, 'Mura'Lann generation thirty seven.'

'A temporal tourist and nothing more?' Fate asked with her thoughts to the future kinsman that she could now see had been just as scarred by wars as much as 'Lîna had been.

'Lîna, who always had walked the path of Fate, was now so far away from the torture and pain of her soul as another Fate came before her. He was truly the continuance of her species amidst a heritage of genetic inter-trades of generations to result in the man who stood before her. She felt bathed in the light one sees in their eye when they close them. Kir'rus was At'Lann Lon'tus as his path with touches of H'Raka, Hy'bor, M'Goa, along with future races the At'Lann would later encounter in his reality such as the N'Pol, K'Rua, and the K'hyn 'Ro. His hair became a raven shatter of feathers with tips and whisps of light and dark mauve. 'Lîna looked closer to see he had the eyes like those of Za'szu's, and those like 'Nuli, a pre-At'Lann Matriarch. The two Fates were now together on the cross-roads before all paths. He bore a faith that would have pleased her father's eye, and he too was chosen to walk the path of Fate.

There were others in the great hall of ecclesiastical trappings of the soul where reality meets no reality. A younger woman, who seemed by her soul only ten years older than 'Lîna, and told her she was Fate, generation five. Her genetic structure appeared H'Raka dominant, and had been enhanced using a psyogenetic variant. The room was filled with Fates of every path. Kir'rus became the friendly swash-buckling of what was to come.

An aged woman and man in slit At'Lann soutane told her they were of Fate, generation twenty six as they followed a Gemini path. They were inter-temporal war aces in the finest tradition that were also 'Mura, generation thirteen. A man that would be and was a psionic sailor, told 'Lîna he was generation twenty-eight, and like her was a sovereign along a path like Cincinnatus's who told her she would refine the P'rynn into the 'Nla 'xen genetic path of the At'Lann, which would culminate in the advancement of their evolution by At'Lann generation thirty-three of another path of the path. So many realities, 'Lîna thought.

'Lîna, Fate, 'Mura'Lann, generation one, was in the dizzying swirl of every temporal path of what was, what is, and what could be. She looked to Kir'rus and realised . . .

'I have no place here, my path has ended…yet it always begins again.'

Her path of Fate had been preordained. As the Fate, 'Lîna realised she walked a path of chance and what Fate seeks towards fulfilment. Fate's soul began to enter the convergence in the temple of her soul. As the Fate, she stepped across existence, jumping playfully from one to the next, hopping above and jumping past pillars and platforms of reality. She saw the truth of Kir'rus's path.

His path crossed hers while returning home after finding victory in a war between what became and remained of the Imperium and a species called the Q'cyn'qulov. A rather brutal war he told her without elaborating. The Q'cyn'qulov were vanquished in one cross-temporal day that was for Kir'rus many years. For him, it was a day thrice as long as the daughter of 'Mura's had been after her Trinity had fallen and shattered. Though he told her it was an uneventful day for Fate, generation thirty seven. Another Fate, three-one-nine, an ethereal figure of temporal fissure streams, watched on. This Fate spoke to 'Lîna.

'Welcome home, 'Mura'Lann generation one. Soon you shall forget what this is, or you might not, until you desire to return.

Kir'rus turned to her and said, 'I came to M'Goa to rest after walking the path of war as you once did but it was Fate that let our paths cross and during our crossing. Links were joined on the path of timelessness that exists on M'Goa. Though you may not yet understand, you are Fate generation one, and one that quenches the thirst for what is to come.'

Another voice of Fate said, 'We are Fate. We are all Fate. We do not violate what will be the way of the path, for a path is always there. We do what we can to see it come to pass. But this… this is your path. Destiny collides and Destiny grows inside Eternity.'

The somewhat enlightened daughter of 'Mura responded in the bliss of peace that was her temple of the cross-roads, 'I understand what is to be, I see now that all of it is within me, and all who walk on the path of the Trinity. The evolving temporal seed will break through the soil once again.'

The Fate seemed to become all that remained in the temporal intertwine. A glow of amethyst, emerald, and sky-water blue filled the transpsionic aether as Fate, 'Mura'Lann, generation one, watched as the perpetually evolving, cosmically existential fresco grew around her. A voice reached out to her,

'It was always within you. There is nothing left to reveal except that which has already been seen, heard, and felt. You have seen what you always will see and what will always be seen by you.'

Kir'rus's voice echoed psionincally across her. It was a voice that ethereally bonded to the clarity of her soul. Fate looked around and saw what was to come as a plethora of paths shot out and shattered the stiff silence.

'I understand what will be and I vow to cross onto the path of legacy once again. In the path of the Trinities, I will continue to walk and flow into paths that can never be shattered. I will liberate myself. Prosper and evolve, my kinsman. May all be infinite in eternity', Fate said with a restored passion for existence. Fate released her youthful hands that still held the path of Kir'rus and maintained her veteran's gaze.

'K'nde D'le Snd'ar, 'Imiszi of 'Mura'Lann. May your path always be there. Prosper and evolve, may we always find infinity in eternity. Farewell, mother of many paths. Farewell Fate.'

On the path of the temple of the cross-roads, the convergence became the only path. The Fate could see Kir'rus fading away from the psionic realm as he took his path home, and faded into the inter-temporal expanse and walked into infinity. Though Fate found more than one path to return to, this was her path. The nothingness could no longer constrain existence.

Φ

Fate stood impaled from the blade intended for the Death of Death. Her eyes shot open as if with the energy of a thousand screams. Fate's path had taken her and left her to wander the silent dunes of extinction. Everything became so precious and so clear. 'Iato nodded his mistake as if nothing had happened. No member of the Trinity could harm another. But he knew. He knew. Fate could see it in his eyes. He knew it all, and so did she. Nothing was lost.

His eyes, like those of Nul'lus's knew the burden of over three trillion years of walking barren paths. 'Lîna could see in the Hunter's grey wolf eyes that he acknowledged that he had been a professional whose path had been left to the chaos of complete randomness. He, more than any other, was pleased she had survived the descent.

Before the Death of Death could react, Fate attacked with a flash-fold backhand fist, to elbow, to fist, until the swarthy beast released its grip. Fate liberated herself from its clutches but before she could move away from the great beast, the Death of Death impaled her once more with its fist spikes into the same spot the sword of H'Raka cut through her heart. It grew and jammed its way deeper and made the whole in her chest wider. There are no words for what is beyond pain. Another stalactite pierced though her right leg below her hip. Another through her stomach. Another flew through her so fast it cut off her lower three left fingers.

Fate felt her soul shatter once more as she was caught, and was stabbed through the back. And then she started laughing as if after walking through the deserts of Tartarus only to have the rains of heaven shower down upon one at the last step of a journey. Fate rotated her shoulder to the point where she nearly dislocated it, and in a mauve and violet chorus of lightning flash-folds, shattered the instrument meant for her execution in one quick elbow. Fate ripped the repugnant spikes from out of the wound and tossed them to the ground as if she had freed herself from the shackles over her soul. The poisonous spikes in her stomach and leg crackled into dust. All of its evil was cast out of her as she psyogenetically regenerated. Her form was left unblemished. The scars of war were gone but Fate would always see them, and the scars of war would always be there. Fate flash-folded to a further distance away from the centre of the battlefield.

The Aristocrat, who had slept soundly through all nights of long knives, yet found no rest on his path. He looked to the others of his path in silence. One flew back into the fight without regard for all that had occurred, yet the sword of H'Raka was still embedded in her chest. The Death of Death trans-psionically pulled back and tossed Fate to the ground before grabbing her by the throat as if before readying to behead her with all its rage and hate.

And the Aristocrat turned to look at another, who still held the very sword as the one in the heart of one on their path. He could see the path of the Hunter had attained a new perspective on existence after all their years of burden and exile which came in one quick twisting of the blade. It was a perspective that only the Trinity could share. The convergence was upon them. The Aristocrat fired another transpsionic bolt at the Death of Death as he strangled the Fate with all its efforts as it realised she held the key to it all. Its grip seemed to all but crush her throat. Her violet blood dripped down to the cursed earth of this final battle.

For the Fate, there seemed no escape. There was nowhere to run. Yet Fate did not want to run anymore and did not have to. She looked down to see the broadsword of H'Raka in her chest. No matter what she did she could not escape the Death of Death who now knew all her secrets. Fate had to stay strong. The Trinity had to remain alive.

Time seemed to drag itself out like the end-storms before what once was. The Aristocrat watched as everything seemed to become the wind-ravaged world of Ra'laris, a Lon'tus moon where the Aristocrat sought the fires of one like Sarasvati amidst the ruins of the throne world of the Lon'tus Imperium. A ruin of a world that was a sad sight for one that set a better example for his people away from their grandiloquent flows of thought.

That was the paradox of the Aristocrat, he could be one to drive a decades old Jaguar puffing away on a European tobacco cigarette but only after what must be attended to is taken care of. But he was something more. He was not an aristocrat after all but everything any aristocrat aspired to be. The path of the hyper-clerisy of the At'Lann, or the warrior's path of H'Raka became his path, and became the path of Fate, and with hers, joined the path of the Hunter. The convergence was finally here.

Reality seemed to shatter and reform with every passing moment. The soul interlace had begun as the Trinity of souls reunified. The cherished tortures of where their paths linked again waged war against the nothingness surrounding them. Like one of the most fondly remembered sunrises over Tonga and Kirabati, the moment their souls had waited for was beginning to come to pass. The moment when all became clear for the Trinity, who had over-killed themselves with suffering, waiting for their victory that remained unattained.

Existence began to spiral in a transpsionic multi-spectral glitter that began to grind itself once again to a halt. The Hunter threw his harpoon at the head of the Death of Death cracking off the mask in a lightning shatter from its dark armour to reveal a perfectly empty shell. Nothing there. But he could feel the thickness of evil in this realm. He could smell its almost overpowering stench. He watched as it reformed instantly as the Death of Death.

Fate pulled the sword viciously from her chest with all her strength as the Death of Death began to strangle her with its crushing grip. The Death of Death pulled her around and was about to go for the killing blow when Fate, in three swift movements turned the blade around, and jammed the sword that was once through her heart, through the dark armour of wretched emptiness. The blade passed without obstruction to where a heart should rest, in the now rusting armour of the Death of Death. The blade pierced through her and out of her, and remained wedged in the empty heart of darkness.

Fate freed herself to make her final stand to end this and flash-folded to a rock face that shot up from the ground in a tidal wave of dust as if it were a coffin that rejected itself from the soil. The Trinity surrounded the howling dark beast. The daughter of 'Mura watched as her eyes came to look upon the dark armour of the shrieking and screaming dark beast amidst what seemed the fireworks of a world commercial. The Hunter and the Aristocrat continued their attack for a moment kicking and attacking the darkness and wedging the blade ever deeper into its evil flesh. The Hunter took the blade of H'Raka that remained in his hands and plunged it into the beast to converge with the one that had pierced the heart of Fate.

They triangulated their position ever closer around the Death of Death. Fate looked over to see the Aristocrat stare into her eyes as he rose to his feet once again and watched as their life-forces flew into one another as his noble fists still smoked and swirled with fused transpsionic energy. It was as if his fists were sculpted like those of Rāma before his moment of battle came with Rāvāna. Fate looked to the Hunter who had walked the path of redemption and balance to restore his path as the time was at hand to release the final barrage.

The Trinity would at last put an end to this entangling snare over all they held dear. The ancient data-stream filled them with more power than they had ever known. Fate released her clarity to the Trinity as she dropped what weapons remained with her and sealed in her arsenal pouch, and steadied her mind by moving herself into her most intimidating posture for the Death of Death and watched as the Hunter and the Aristocrat did the same.

The enlightenment of a new moksha swept across the Trinity as they stood surrounding the Death of Death. The storm of souls fell into an end-sleep of quiet and serenity. Each of the Trinity looked within themselves to unleash the new path to stretch into the living future. As they cast away violence, and gave in to pure thought, each soul began to lift away to what would be.

Fate dove into the temporal data-stream of her mind to find the genetic flaws that were all that were left to open the gate to move beyond what was the final assault on erasure. Fate found an adaptive component in the 'Xo genetic structure that had served their species well during their battles against the Army of Two Rings, and also found a genetic variant that impeded their genetic integration. The enlightened Fate easily fixed the flaw and the Fate integrated the desired adaptive component after modifying the 'Xo genetic matrices to have the choice to fully follow the path of the At'Lann. Fate then realigned every infinite psyogenetic combination for infinite diversity. Everything began anew. The Death of Death was a virus that Fate twisted into and its heavy dirty locks over existence and began to fling them away from everything that it had infected.

The Hunter cast the chains off his soul as he made his way out of the ethereal labyrinth. He looked to Fate with a new spirit of peace in his soul as he realised his misery had come to an end as no weapon of the Trinity would harm one of their own. He knew how far she had gone. And now all of existence held its breath for peace. The Hunter marched his way though the unholy darkness using his every step to bring misery to an end.

The Aristocrat fed the triangular psionic flow and fires as his thoughts became the balance of perfection. He had returned undaunted to complete the journey that had cost them all so much. It was as if he had prevailed over the storms that had swayed Eiffel's tower in which no wind of death could knock him down. The winds smoothed as the Hunter became the wind as the Aristocrat became the water lit by the Fate.

The drops of the oceans of the thoughts of the Aristocrat became the new waters of refined souls which grew into new streams to run. The dark winds of the Death of Death became the merest of zephyrs as the Aristocrat's path joined the Fate's and the Hunter's as their souls converged.

Fate did not yield her light to the darkness of the Death of Death. Her soul looked outward. L'unn would never again leave its place in the eternal sky. Existence would be maintained. But Fate began to drown in such cathartic waters even though she was willing to give it everything. Her body seemed to pore away in a stabbing baptism of violet blood. Yet Fate would not yield. Fate unleashed the secret truth against the Death of Death.

All that was, is, and would be was psyogenetically data stored and compiled in sub-matrix three of Fate's being, as it was in the entire Trinity, and only they had the power to once again unlock reality. As their souls were inter-sliced into one another, so too were the inter-slices of all genetic existence of their universe.

And more than what was living but their entire universe itself. Everything would be set free. Fate spread herself out to even find herself inside and far away from her generational temple of the cross-roads. In the fiery ecstasy in more than a thousand nights in the burning bliss of it all, and their everything became their here and now. The past had become the future and the future became the present.

The Trinity had always had the power to defeat the Death of Death and the Two Rings all along though even they did not know it as it was a secret truth from themselves. And now they had found it after taking the most torturous paths to have searched for it. The Trinity imagineered reality as everything became the purest unity, and the purity of the Trinity was now unleashed as every soul and every life flooded through the Death of Death breaking its dark dominion. It was as if the dams of the Ruhr had been flung apart by the fist of a disappointed Odin, and he watched without remorse as everything fell into the waters of the soul.

The convergence was fast becoming complete as all the stream-dropping power of existence flooded out of the Trinity. All became nothing but the pure non-existence that lay beyond the good and evil flows of reality. Time became the sleeping awakening into the here and far away. Then far away at first, the psyotemporal spindles of Cronos reborn danced away like Shiva into what felt like the close stillness of what felt like celebrating the last day of civil economic warfare on M'Goa.

Like Gates conceding most of his fortune to the path towards the future on a path that Fate had once watched below her, the path towards balance, towards peace came to be theirs once again. The K'mja returned to the Hunter and to the Trinity. Its strength entrapped the dark beast as the serenity of the Fate, and the passion of the Aristocrat, enslaved that which had enslaved them all.

The Death of Death was stripped of its shell of slag tar, the dirt of resinous darkness. Nothing and everything cosmically danced under an ambient sonic terrace like Shiva finding new energy with one like Plush, like Raissa, like Copeland, and one like Warren in the dawn breaking over reality once again as the path of life took another step forward in a transual thump of hymnal bells from one who walks the path of progressive nations. The souls of the Trinity had been rendered shells and now the Three were once again re-forged stronger than ever before and left with everything from the journey of their path.

The once dark spectre of the Death of Death fell to the dusty ethereal ground below. The Death of Death fell away into an eternal scream of silence. Its armies, its dark force that were once held a murderous grip over reality, the walking dead, all that the Trinity faced was wiped away as the Three inverted erasure. The songs of M'Goa seemed to pierce louder into the blossoming of reality with their ethereally pulsing beats and rhythms beyond any before known.

Nothing became everything as the path of infinity remained unbroken. The Death of Death lay slain as the forests grew once more over L'unn, and the oceans of 'Mura'Lann danced under the sun to wash happily on her shores. The 'Mura'Lann citizens were restored as much as their troposphere returned to existence. The 'Mura'Lann bunker returned the sky to her returned people and was deactivated. Existence returned from the last genetic sanction of the Imperium protocols, and protocols which were never revealed to the Three by the Interface. The data-stream flowed fully into them now. Restoration of reality held and shared by the Trinity became the only victory of life. All that was existence returned through the transpsionic vessel states of the Trinity which vanished in and out of existence.

Planets, stars, nebulas, Ram'szas, galaxies, the universal alignment of life, populace, species, gods, god-flows, and the path to the next state poured fourth to fill the emptiness. The glorious existence flashed into bloom and spread out into that which became a great eternal expanse as if awoken to the sound of one like Kleinenberg. Their lost tribe had been found. Life's pastures spread out over reality once again. The convergence of the Trinity from three into one became the now, and it transformed the souls of the Trinity. As Cronos reset himself, three trillion and thirteen years on the path of war for the Trinity came to an end. Their souls had survived the reformation of their universe.

After so many great costs, after all that had been sacrificed, after going so far and yet having gone nowhere, victory had finally come. And victory, freedom, came almost as quietly as just another day made long ago into a day of global celebrity. For those who toiled below on E'de, it was the first day and first steps into freedom away from so many things that were once their path. Souls, life, energy, flashed back into existence. Almost everything flashed back into existence.

The path of the future became the path of possibilities once again. Ideas, thought, emotion; everything that was held sacred, made their way back into reality. The macro-phase-generators had served the Trinity by helping take them full circle for their paths to path of salvation. This was a day, the first day that reality tasted freedom and yet remained just another day. The empty torn open armour which once held so much darkness faded away into the grip of erasure.

The phase-generators of the Trinity exploded and their debris floated in a ring where the advance of the Death of Death was halted; the hammered bracelet which lay past H'Raka. And in the debris lay floating an awakening Fate. The emotions and the spirit of life flowed back into as her soul became hers once again. She was the sentinel of empathy on the path of Fate. All was returned to its rightful place to what is and what is not reality. The Imperium was restored. Existence grew to expand beyond the womb of the soul of souls.

The convergence became one and everything with existence. Fate swam in the folds of reality to hold the hands of Za'szu and 'Zaya on the bridge of the Lis'talla. On another path of reality, she took the hands of the Hunter and the Aristocrat at the same time. The path of trinities was restored. Living worlds thrived back into their glory.

The permanence of the Imperium, held in the salvation of the Trinity, was restored as Fate looked out to space to watch the universe expand outwards with much more exhilaration for the event than she had the last time she had witnessed such an event. She could hear the music of M'Goa once again filling space and every cosmos as every awe-inspiring balance of existence was brought back.

The living dream became existence as reality was brought into a perfect moment of peace. The Fate awoke from the torture of the path of war, which would always remain with her, to the beautiful sounds of living worlds and a living universe. And everything was upgraded. The P'rynn were brought into genetic harmony with the Imperium taking their new steps as the recomposed, 'Nla, or new breed.

The Lit'vaa once again happily roamed the grasslands of their world in the delight of their existence once again. Utupuku's kingdom was restored to the prosperity of the land of snow, ice and sun. Fate touched the soul of one of her favourite warriors, 'Ivia, and freed her from the pain of war that had gnawed its way deep into her as well. She gave another path to Mu'tolma to find what he tried to hide from himself and to finally find what he always sought.

Fate watched as the Aristocrat found paradise in his soul once again. She watched as the Hunter chose his path and yet left it wide open. As if freed from the shackles of genetic and consumer corporatisation that once held E'de prisoner, and like that plague, the greatest plague to face the Imperium was eradicated. The plague that inspired the creation of a new existence for their reality was gone but its memories would remain embedded forever on the Trinity as all paths flowed outward once more. At great costs, the Trinity had found their option of choice. Their journey's end came amidst the silence and amidst the almost disbelief that everything worked according to plan. Reality was saved.

On the Inter-temporal cross-roads, the Imperium came to exist away into an infinite number of paths. For the Trinity, all became one and the many simultaneously. The vibe was back. After walking the path, for what now seemed as if it were the blink of an eye, the souls of the Imperium Trinity made it home. Their paths and their souls, united forever into one, and also theirs became their own once again. Almost as quickly as it all had ended, the three souls found themselves on their own worlds once again, the reality of all they had done set in, and their lives became their own to live once more.

After walking and continuing to walk the path of Fate, 'Lîna returned not to At'Lann but to what was now officially the 'Mura'Lann Imperium to find a hyper-luminescent ticker-tape laden celebration as she returned home with her sisters to 'Lunn. The 'Mura'Lann Imperiatrix almost felt ashamed by the attention of the cheering crowds and the girandole trionic displays brought out only for her. Yet, sparkles were the only way to go.

A gravity-flux platform, like those on M'Goa, except one with all the trappings fit for one who had swashbuckled her way through history. If only 'Lîna could have told them of how barren her path had been. But she remained happy, and as bitter-sweet as it was, the Fate found victory, and 'Lîna found everything she had wanted when she found peace once again. Fate had restored the Imperium, and all those that they had lost in the war, for the most part, had been liberated back into reality.

She could see it in her sisters that they knew it all and said nothing and thought nothing other than extending the love of their bond to her and all their sister had been through. In many ways, Fate was beyond them, and in too many ways she was not. But not even the Death of Death could shatter the bond of the first generation of the 'Mura'Lann to come since their earlier time.

Though Za'szu probably thought maintaining the Imperium had been a wrong move and was still hesitant about it now, she still left her fate to the will of her sister who had saved them all. The Trinity had endured, and 'Zaya felt even more at peace as her constant interface scanning revealed the current levels of their psyogenetic enhancement had stabilised into a perfect psyogenetic interlock.

The platform carried the daughters of 'Mura above the main boulevard as the three waved to the crowds of their equals below. The crowds were vast but also sparse as the memories of the war had been too painful for some to celebrate its end. 'Lîna let fly the doves of her thoughts of peace, love, and freedom for all those who united against the onslaught of the once great horde. She let those, who had suffered in far too many ways protecting existence know that they had not been forgotten, and that it was time to forge ahead on the new path. An ultra-violet heaven found itself way out west once more.

Everyone and everything had fought the Death of Death in the end, and no one had been spared the unmasking of the true face of evil, that which was behind the mask, and for far too many in the war found too much of what they had fought in themselves. Though everyone did find the release as the erasure became, literally, no more. Nothing became nothing and everything did its best to carry on. The daughters of 'Mura were reunited, and like the Fate's, everyone fell into the happiness felt for the beginning of a hard fought day. The prohibition of reality was no more and the denial of existence finally ended. And everyone could see forever.

It may have been that the Fate and the Trinity had not saved everything as approximately three percent of what was once existence remained lost to erasure. But this time now was their well earned time to have fun, and as 'Zaya and 'Za'szu held aloft 'Lîna's humble arms, this sister knew their would be plenty of time to find all which remained lost and left to decrypt. The prison of reality crumbled and became the long awaited shore.

'Lîna eventually got into the spirit of things and came to find the festivities the succulent icing to the sweetness of returning home to a world full of life, and to her family that she had gone without for so long. Peace swept deliciously over the sea set in the sweetest of lavenders for all the souls of the Imperium to gaze upon. After sacrificing so much and evolving so far, her path of liberation finally became hers. Her tender, cathartic laughter delighted in the beauty of existence and reality restored.

'Mura'Lann threw a gathering of celebration that night as if their world were M'Goa. Fate found the bliss of peace as the celebrations of the 'Mura'Lann victory gathering stretched on for the once quite staid 'Mura'Lann for far longer than a day. The path ahead could wait as her people could finally relax as the path of war became no more. Paradise was everywhere as the sounds mixed by one like Fontaine started going off in the pristine world that so many gave so much for.

The Aristocrat returned to the neighbouring Lon'tus home world, and from his throne and castle, he looked to the sky to see the other worlds of Lon'tus found in other parts of the system with the majority of them now in orbit of M'Goa. He could not think of a better new home for them. Nul'lus also looked to the towers of his home city which were ablaze with the spinning fantails of enhanced pyrotechnics and hyper-pulsating, growing photonic spheres.

He waved to the crowds and the Lon'tus warships that flew by overhead grazing the atmosphere before changing the colour of the sunrise to Lon'tus blue above 'Mura'Lann mauve that flowed into H'Raka rose red. He looked out past the city to the beach filled with people dancing and letting loose the way only the Lon'tus knew how. And though some Lon'tus probably would never remember that he once returned home to victory, the Aristocrat knew he had earned this moment, and for this day he was only glad that it had come to pass. For his people, today he was the man of the match as what sounded like Deep Dish found its way to the rising sun.

The Hunter returned to H'Raka free to step out in glory as the moment where K'mja became everything was finally grasped and the savannah of the universe was their to once again walk. 'Iato, after the barren path war had brought his way, was not surprised when he returned to find how much peace had imbued itself into the soul of the people of H'Raka. It was as if Maas were on the decks. Perhaps, they were homing in on our destiny or else it is a destiny we need for a time, he thought.

For now, the time of war was over. H'Raka had to rest after such a torturous feast. The Hunter was uncertain but he felt free. He had placed his faith in the Imperium once and saw that it might not be so bad if the Imperium remained. He let loose a loud roar to the assembled thousands of H'Raka warriors around him that had waited far too long for this day. He laughed with the glorious joy for a victory he at last savoured though redemption remained a continuing path. The sounds of Potente made their way into the sky once more with a little less worry than before.

He looked around and saw that Y'vis had not returned. 'Iato somehow knew his father was pleased. The Hunter survived the greatest of hunts and the Fate seeing all that he was and would always be. He was almost unnerved that one of the greatest victories of peace found at the end of this path of war was the solace in knowing that 'Lîna had forgiven him for all that had once come between them. The hunters of H'Raka fired their weapons into the air in thumping tribal pulses to fire up the crowd as the Hunter blew off his own cannon, and laughed in victory as the blood red sky of the sunrise on H'Raka was set on fire with the most golden of flames. The Hunter barely had time to glance a lone H'Raka warship being sent straight into the sun of the Imperium home system in a move of disarmament that would rid the Imperium space of his surplus genetic creations aside from those which guard the technology of Usz'shna and that left behind in the now slightly larger Third Ring. He did not have time to notice that the ship did not burn in the sun but strayed off its trajectory and was lost in space though that is entirely another horrendous story.

The war that had cost the Trinity so much had come to its final end. The calm waters of Fate's joys returned as 'Mura'Lann became her home. The path continued but it was a new age for this first generation that had moved beyond the powers of psyogenetic enhancement. Their faith was never broken, only lost for a time. More would follow on the path of Fate. And as for this Fate, she found she had much further to go, and no where to go at all. For there always would be paths and possibilities. And the Trinity would always be a part of her. Her soul could finally rest in the celebration of peace amongst Lon'tus and H'Raka who continued to share the rays of the sun with her people.

On M'Goa and on the cross-roads, Kir'rus watched on in the living future made by those of the great Imperium worlds, and one who was once a young princess of At'Lann who left home to explore existence. Fate had continued the path, and the M'Goa around him revelled in every moment of their after-party. What more could be said by one who was once a mysterious stranger who seemed to have the sounds of Hotel Costes imbued into him. It was all good.

He saw 'Temisa dancing on another platform as if she were soaring into the contentment of being a sparrow. He wondered how soon the daughter of 'Mura would make it this world once again. Kir'rus flash-folded out of time and continued his path home with a Heh! Heh! laugh knowing that it would probably be sooner than he could imagine. Just as history records and as all became revealed with time, he thought.

Somewhere else entirely, Y'vis laughed in a lion-wolf's roar. The glory was theirs. Now all that was left to do was to wait for 'Iato to join him on the next path of battle for those on the path of the H'Raka. If they only knew what was in store for them, Y'vis thought. He laughed as he continued on his path, for it was a new day.

As S'bel and 'Usta walked the path into eternity. S'bel chided her eternal companion for not thinking that one of their next generation had it in her. Fate had continued the path in ways they could not in another dimension of infinity. As they moved and looked back to see her tell her sisters that those who became before had become something more, and that they would join them at another time as their path would always be intertwined. They walked with peace in their souls as freedom came home, and found the burden of the path of war for all life ended. The long awaited dawn reached every world and every path as the three souls found home.

Φ

In a outdoor patio café, by a tropical beach above a vast stretch of the abandoned ruins of the Hy'Bor who seemed to have went the way of some colonists of Roanoke, the Trinity reunited on E'de along one of De Gama's paths to hear new songs for ones who are game-masters. The war had ended months ago, and though their memories remained, they could not help but bask in the natural tranquillity of the afternoon sun which relaxed those around them to another day to play dominoes amidst the clear azure sky and the music of one like Sa Trincha.

And even more so was their joy of having their paths converge once again. Only this time, their shared path was under the happier circumstances that was never theirs when their paths came together but was found when they had the time to leave the war at the door. They looked out to this place to see that this world had progressed to a more evolved path.

'Lîna turned from her chair and lowered her bright lilac hued sunglasses to read the latest news headlines for this world that flashed out from a simple holographic note pad display left on another table. It read, 'Poland wins thirteenth World Cup over defending Scottish champions. Canada, a six time world champion, narrowly defeated England for third thanks in part to a spicy English player that was sent off.' Surprisingly, Fate read that there were no riots even though there had not been any in years as the English were gracious to lose to what they considered one of their grown national children, and after being banned from six world cups, after a winning a record six straight, they had finally learned their latest lessons on the path of football. The Fate found it pleasing that the only shred of nationalism left only remained was in sport, as every former nation of E'de now had colonies throughout the third quadrant of their galaxy. All the while, unaware that an Imperium existed over most of the universe.

'Lîna caught up on the latest colonial reports broadcast live from the Intersystem government news bureau on what those of E'de called Pluto and which those of the Imperium knew as Nu'Ata. She returned to sipping away on her tea and enjoying the few cigarettes she now occasionally smoked as she shared the round table alongside the Nul'lus and 'Iato. The three laughed together as they raised glasses of the island's domestic rum to one another, and also their tea which was left to simmer.

And though taste and texture were an occasional dalliance, their true joyful feast was that of the rays of tropical sunshine on all those who survived. As they drank, she could see the faces of all she came across on her journey in the victory crowds that first greeted her, and it returned another joy to her as she had done it all for them. And she thought of the day she told Za'szu, a few weeks later, that she would leave 'Mura'Lann to explore once again, and that she would now become Imperiatrix as was the way they had always agreed to lead.

'Lîna told her she had earned it but Fate's path was to go another way. Za'szu told her sister she would protect their home so that it would always be theirs to return to. After a ceremony that was a happy one, 'Lîna left 'Mura'Lann, in the trust of the strong and tender hands of her younger sister. For the moment, 'Zaya declined the Regency even with 'Lîna's blessing. And like Fate, who takes herself completely away on the path of exploration, 'Zaya could not yet take herself away from the path of science.

'Lîna's comrades on the path of war and on the path of life wondered what she would do now. 'Nothing too surprising,' she told them as they looked out to the yachts and their tall fluttering sails in a bay shaped like the tiara 'Lîna still wore. And she thought of her cousins 'Xona, 'Mura'Lann minister of the data-flow, 'Trvi, the couturier of the Imperium elite when not assigned to the fleet, 'Ellyra, the 'Mura'Lann minister of sport, who she thanked for sending 'Lîna the supplies and data she had needed to survive L'Ja. And she thought of their mother, Ulana, and felt at peace with herself that she did not let anyone down from the house of T'Koris.

For the first time since she had forgotten, 'Lîna felt so warm in the luxuriously hot tropical air. And as the Three chatted away psionically, they all felt as if they sat beside Hephaestus's furnace. Someone inside the café put on some classical trance of many years before that sounded like Atlantis, and the three clinked their glasses together and had another round only this time with some Qal'latu nectar they flash-folded in from M'Goa.

'Lîna turned the tables and asked her mates and companions on the great path where their paths would now take them. Nul'lus retired to his summer manor on Lon'tus 4 which orbits M'Goa after transferring most of his powers to his Lon'tus Imperium Prime Minister and would return to Rimisz'tii later that year and would attend the release of the M'Gata populace from genetic storage. While 'Lîna had left them in data-stasis, she made a few changes as she did for those of E'de. She could tell Nul'lus longed to once again swim in the waters of his home world and relax knowing he had earned it all.

The Hunter's path also changed as well as he would have to return to leading the H'Raka to a new era in their Imperium. He also wrote a collection of poems that he used to inspire other H'Raka hunters to share their culture of honour with the rest of the Imperia, and to once again choose honour before the path of war and before the path of the hunt.

And after only seven days of universal peace, the H'Raka were brought in to settle a dispute between two feuding worlds as life returned to normal. The Hunter dryly laughed that some things would never change. And whether as peace-maker or warrior, the Hunter walked a bold new ground with every step. Even 'Lîna could not tell him where things would go. He told his comrades, that these were interesting times.

The music shifted to play the sounds of those like the Thrillseekers as if it was mixed by some Sirens, some Chicks With Decks by the beach. 'The wonders of what their 'internet' spawned,' Nul'lus laughed. 'Bless those humans,' 'Lîna said as she took a drag of 'Mura'Lann lilac vitamin enriched tobacco in a short violet leaf roll. The three, relaxed as they never had under the sun. Their conversation lasted well into the moonlit night. 'If they only knew,' they all thought.

Days to relax the mind and soul and enhance their paths for knowledge down less strenuous paths were theirs once again. Everything was the Ibiza, the Muskoka, and Ayia Napa of something more as reality seemed totally anew. They once again walked the shores of complete meaning and as they sat back before it all. Weeks later, taking their paths would be in different direction once more, they felt the beauty of everything that was wondrous about existence.

And before the Trinity would take to their path, they took the time to indulge in the vacation that was a long time in coming, and enjoyed what was like a Copeland closer. They once again existed in existence, and through it all, had survived to make it to what seemed an optimistic eternity of infinite choices and the responsibility of freedom.

On their last morning before returning to their paths, the Three assembled once more at the same small café beside the ocean, as 'Lîna poured a fourth cup, and set aside another chair though it would probably not be used. All just in case a stranger with a good soul might come to share their path. After flash-folding onto the beach, Fate's companion, joined the three by their table as 'Lîna slyly took her last sip of Earl Grey, and told her comrades it was time for her to go. With her hand on her hip and the stance and the beauty that was always hers, 'Lîna's companion awaited leaving on the path out into space.

'Temisa's tangerine skin never seemed so radiant. Her body was soft yet tightly sculpted from dancing so hard in faith to many, many songs that made her rise up to, as she stood their patiently and succulently waiting to depart. 'See you on the path,' 'Lîna said as she flash-folded away with 'Temisa. 'Iato turned to Nul'lus and said, 'Fate really does like to have her cake and eat it too.'

'That she does,' Nul'lus said with a laugh. 'That she does.' The pair raised a glass of rum to her, and to all the veterans of any war. For without those who fought for freedom, one would never know it. At long last, the universe once again became home.

Epilogue

The winds of time could never tear away at the path of the three souls on their journey home, and when the three finally found home, they returned to worlds that were brave and new with the songs of their day and all those to come. Their suffering had transcended into what seemed the blissful peace of what lay ahead. But the three would always be on guard. The winds of time did, however, move them along on their various paths. And together, it was a path, even at its most distant, was a path always shared.

The great path of life is the living promise toward the continued search for better ways of existence. Music always was and would eternally remain their sweet house. What seemed lost would always be there. Conscience and passion once again became the cores of their souls that forever walked the infinite paths. They were now refined beings and complete as they could be for their current paths. The war would haunt them always, but for the three souls, there was no going back on what had made them what they were.

Home for their souls became what their souls surveyed on their travels through life, and the infinite bounty of all paths of creation; with creation being another diamond of the soul. The trinity of the past, present, and future, became their playground of life. Triumph came with the price of the memories to get there, and what it is to be Human. Curiosity once again became a worthy pursuit and the noblest drive of their immortality. Their true power came from the powers of the mind fully unlocked for a moment of time that gave them eternity once more. They had survived both an exhilarating and horrendous path, and as the path of war seemed only a shadow in the distance, the three souls who found home had finally moved on to happier pursuits.

The way of the Trinity became ideals both sacrificed and refined into eternity through the three being left to only judge themselves. Life once again became an adventure, a path to greater knowledge and to greater paths of evolution. Though sometimes finding that knowledge is entirely what one does not expect, and sometimes too much information leads down paths of darkness of the greatest abysses, their way was to explore all that existence offered. But the path of legacy could always be found as another path towards the freedom of home, and the three souls who found home were now the legacy.

The great path was forever immortal as a path, once one of sadness, led to one of the most joyous of the fulfilment's of life. The trinities of souls and time, now walked a path on both the corporeal and not corporeal, and beyond what words cannot convey. They soon may journey out there once again in the pursuit of betterment for all who come to walk on brave new paths, and those who come after them to find the hidden weaponry of peace waiting for them to use to defend reality. For everything and everyone walks the paths of what was once thought of as God and gods. Interconnection is existence. One does not have to bow to have faith but one must find peace in themselves before one finds peace in existence. Though what ones soul becomes depends on how far one is willing to go.

The End and what is The Beginning.

Fate will return in
Fate: The Path Of Her Dominion.

Glossary

Agent 27: an At'Lann medical technology.

An'sze: First officer of the N'Lurr.

Aristocrat: A wealthy and enlightened soul called away from his home. Ambassador Nul'lus becomes the Aristocrat in the future. Part of the Trinity of Fate, Hunter and Aristocrat.

Armn'dallos: located in the H'Nua galaxy and location for Imperium war supplies.

Army of Two Rings: the dark forces controlled by the Death of Death.

At'Lann: Name for the people who populate L'unn. The term also means oceans and island jungles as well as origin and existence.

B'Dak: Royal tutor who taught in 'Mura.

'Ea'tel'som: World capital of M'Gata.

E'de: Planet also known as Earth and location of the Hy'Bor colonies.

Ersz'ta: extinct reptile of E'de.

Fate: An explorer of the universe. 'Lîna 'Mura becomes the Fate. Part of the Trinity of Fate, Hunter and Aristocrat.

G'arja: At'Lann warship captained by General 'Ivia of the 'Xo.

Gatan: At'lann term for an evil force which brings about unintended positive change.

G'jara: rare Lon'tus spirit not made for centuries.

Gn'rys P'rynn: World Systems Operator for the P'rynn of M'Gata. Chief operator of P'rynn financial markets.

H'Bdkas: An alien species encountered by the Imperium and lost to erasure.

H'Raka: World of the Hunter and also known as the name for a legendary race of hunter warriors.

Hunter: A great warrior and combatant against darkness. I'ato H'renn becomes the Hunter. Part of the Trinity of Fate, Hunter and Aristocrat.

Hy'Bor: Colony of former At'Lann citizens; diplomatic relations no longer existed with the At'Lann Imperium.

'Hyn: high gods of the H'Raka.

'Ia: At'lann blueberry vodka.

I'ato H'renn: Great H'raka hunter and warrior. Represented by Hunter in the Trinity. Son of Y'vis.

Imperiatrix: Title of 'Lîna 'Mura.

Imperium Protocols: Classified noble technology unlocked to alter evolutionary processes and enhance them in response to war.

Imperium Trinity: Empires of the At'Lann, Lon'tus, and H'Raka.

Imperator: title for either 'Iato or Nul'lus

'Irilis: a world visited by Fate.

'Ivia: A general from 'Xo serving with the At'Lann. Captained the At'Lann warship Gar'ja.

J'bura: H'Raka officer serving aboard the N'Lurr.

J'Gendo: At'Lann scientist of known repute.

J'Namu: Planet construct for At'Lann and the Imperium's energy resources.

J'Poko: At'Lann classified defense technology.

'kamasai: a claymore like Lon'tus sword.

K'Nang Soong: Imperium supply vessel.

Kem'ja Khonn: forests of L'unn.

Ki'Bur: At'Lann supply escort.

K'mja: H'raka name for the ancient spirit of combat and battle.

K'or: Title of a leader of H'Raka.

Kul'mir: H'Raka noble estate world.

K'urszt: famed river of L'unn.

L'krk: At'Lann officer serving aboard the Lis'talla.

Lis'talla: At'Lann flagship.

Lon'tus: People of the planet of the same name.

Lon'tus Commonwealth: Cultural and military ally of At'Lann which became the Lon'tus Imperium.

'Lîna 'Mura: Eldest sister of Za'szu 'Mura and 'Zaya 'Mura. Represented by Fate in the Trinity.

Lis'talla: Flagship of 'Lîna 'Mura's fleet.

L'Ja: Ancient desert wasteland planet.

L'unn: Planet also known as Earth's Moon. Capital is the city-state of 'At'Lann with second capital of 'Mura. Orbits the planet of E'de.

Lu'va: Lon'tus officer assigned to the Lis'talla.

M'Gata: World of the P'rynn.

M'Goa: A peaceful and continually-evolving world where art is the primary life function.

M'on: a Lon'tus fleet admiral

M'Plura: Home galaxy of the Imperium.

M'skoto: cousin to 'Lîna and Mu'tolma.

'Mura: Capital of the planet of At'Lann.

'Mura'Lann: A name chosen by Fate and also the name of an Imperium Protocol file.

Mu'tolma: Cousin to 'Lîna 'Mura. A first officer of the Lis'talla.

'Nakala: a Lon'tus colony.

N'Bira: Planet that orbits the Tr'Lann system.

N'Lurr: An At'Lann destroyer.

'Nuli: pre-At'Lann matriarch of 'Lunn

Nu'Ata: Planet also known as Pluto on other inter-connective paths.

Nul'lus: Ambassador to the At'Lann from the Lon'tus Commonwealth. Close friend of 'Lîna 'Mura. Evolved to become the element of the Aristocrat in the Trinity.

Pal'lana: an ocean of L'unn.

'Paradia: province of the Lon'tus home world

P'rynn: Race of financially-motivated commodities traders.

Qus'na: breed of H'Raka shark

Qal'ha: rare H'Raka liquer not to be confused with Qal'latu

Qal'latu: M'Goa beverage popular amongst the At'Lann.

Ra'laris: a moon of Lon'tus.

Ram'sza: beasts indigenous to swimming in nebula gases and prized by the H'Raka.

'Raanu: member of the At'Lann Imperium.

'Ri'Muria'Lann: ancient Mura'Lann

Risz'tii: Nul'lus's home world in the Lon'tus Imperium.

Rz'hro: a species integrated into the H'Raka Imperium.

S'bel: a Queen of At'Lann and mother to the daughters of 'Mura.

S'Lanu: a king of At'Lann and grandfather to the daughters of 'Mura.

S'linn K'jak: Imperial palace of the H'Raka, located in the capital city of 'Vanx.

SL'ona: global capital of Armn'dallos.

Sol'linko: Classified Lon'tus defense technology.

'Sonann 'Nor: H'Raka elite guards, the north blade.

Sy'dosa: World ambassador of 'Goa.

Ta'al: At'Lann noble house for those of the line of T'Koris.

'Temisa: a member of the Imperium court from M'Goa.

T'Kala: name of the 'Xo flagship.

'Tainja: At'Lann warship.

Tazi'ma: At'Lann Imperium member.

Ti'mat: H'Raka giant squid.

T'Koris: 'Lîna 'Mura's legendary uncle.

Trinity: The combination of the souls of Fate, Hunter and Aristocrat.

Tr'Lann: Home system of the At'Lann.

U'kra: a galaxy in the Imperium.

U'linn: ursine forest creatures native to 'Lunn

Usz'shn: At'Lann term for prisoner.

Usz'shna: Planet closest to the Tr'Lann sun.

Val'damus: 'Lîna's mesomorph science officer.

'Vanx: Capital city of H'Raka.

'Verga: At'Lann supply escort.

Vkv't: 'Mura'Lann scientist.

Vu'latta: planetary system within Imperium space.

'Xo: Race allied to the Imperium, as well as a planet of the same name.

Y'vis: Father of 'Iato. Imperial leader of H'Raka.

'Zaya 'Mura: Younger sister of 'Lîna 'Mura. Also the creator of a beverage called 'Zaya's Ocean as well as being known for in being at the forefront of At'Lann genetic research.

Za'szu 'Mura: Younger sister of 'Lîna 'Mura. Sometime ruler of the At'Lann Imperium.

Zun'oon: Imperium supply vessel.

Utupuku: Bear rescued by 'Lîna 'Mura.